MILADY
SalonOvations'

COSMETOLOGY DICTIONARY

Edited by Linda Athey Gately

Milady Publishing Company
(a division of Delmar Publishers)
3 Columbia Circle, Box 12519
Albany, New York 12212-2519

Cover Design: Brian Yacur

Milady Staff
Publisher: Catherine Frangie
Acquisitions Editor: Joseph Miranda
Project Editor: Annette Downs Danaher
Production Manager: Brian Yacur

COPYRIGHT © 1996
Milady Publishing Company
(a division of Delmar Publishers)

Printed in the United States of America
Printed and distributed simultaneously in Canada

For more information, contact:
SalonOvations
Milady Publishing Company
3 Columbia Circle , Box 12519
Albany, New York   12212-2519

6 7 8 9 10   XXX   01 00

Library of Congress Cataloging-in-Publication Data

SalonOvations' cosmetology dictionary.
    p.   cm.
ISBN: 1-56253-214-6
    1. Beauty culture–Dictionaries.   I. SalonOvations (Firm)
TT951.S25 1995   94-23230
646.7'2'03–dc   CIP

❧ Contents

PREFACE   v

PREFIXES   1

SUFFIXES   5

COMMON WORD ROOTS OR STEMS   7

COSMETOLOGY DICTIONARY: A-Z   9

❧ Preface

As new techniques and methods are developed in the cosmetology arts and sciences, new words are created that become a part of cosmetology terminology. Although many words used in relation to the practice of cosmetology and its related fields can be found in a standard or conventional dictionary, words with more than one meaning can be confusing. For this reason, the *SalonOvations' Cosmetology Dictionary* is comprised of words and phrases that are used in connection with cosmetology and are defined in their sense of relationship to anatomy, cosmetic chemistry, electricity, dermatology, esthetics, hair structure and chemistry, nutrition, color, massage therapy, and professional skills.

This dictionary has been prepared to keep abreast of the times in cosmetology language usage and to provide clear definitions as they relate to cosmetology and associated fields. It has been designed to provide cosmetologists with a practical reference that is comprehensive and professionally correct, yet not so technical that it fails to serve the needs of today's students, teachers, managers, salon owners and practitioners. It can also serve as an ideal instrument for classroom instruction for use in preparing for state licensing examinations.

For the convenience of teachers and students, many of the main ingredients used in cosmetic preparations have been listed in this dictionary.

The terminology used in cosmetology reflects the mind and spirit of an industry. When a profession or vocation is developing new techniques, its language will be expanding and moving forward. Every new thought and every new fact becomes fixed in words and language that reflect the spirit and progress of the industry itself. This dictionary is intended to capture that reflection of spirit and progress and make it available to the entire industry.

We wish to express our sincere appreciation to the many cosmetology educators who have contributed their much valued advice during the preparation of this dictionary. This edition contains updated terminology prepared and submitted in part by the International Haircolor Exchange, for the purpose of providing a standard vocabulary of hair coloring for our industry. We wish to also thank Pivot Point International, Inc., for their courtesy in granting permission to include a number of widely used Pivot Point terms in the *SalonOvations' Cosmetology Dictionary*.

MILADY PUBLISHING COMPANY

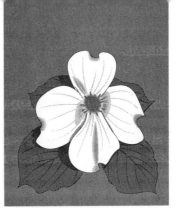

Prefixes

Following is a list of prefixes, suffixes, and stem words along with their meanings. A prefix is one or more syllables added in front of the stem to further its meaning. A suffix, likewise, is added to the end of the word. Suffixes often denote a diagnosis, symptom, or surgical procedure, or identify a word as a noun or adjective. By breaking the terms into their parts, the logical meaning can be derived.

PREFIXES

A careful study of the following prefixes will enable you to grasp the meaning of many anatomical, medical, and electrical terms or words.

Word Part	Definition	Example
a-	absent, without, away from	**a**bacterial
ab-	away from	**ab**duction
ad-	to, toward	**ad**duction
ambi-	both	**ambi**dextrous
a-; an-	without	**a**typical
ant-	against	**ant**ibody, **ant**idote
ante-	before	**ante**rior

1

Word Part	Definition	Example
bi-	two	**bi**ceps
bio-	life	**bio**logy
carcin-	cancer	**carcin**ogenic
circum-	around	**carcum**vent
co-	with, together	**co**operate
contra-	against, counter to	**contra**indicate
de-	down, from	**de**scend
di-	two	**di**ssect
dis-	apart, away from	**dis**locate
dors-	back	**dors**al
dys-	abnormal, impaired	**dys**function
e-	out, from	**e**metic
ect-	outside, without	**ect**oplasm
end-(o)	inside, within	**end**oderm
epi-	upon, over, in addition	**epi**mysium
ex-	out of	**ex**it, excrete
extra-	beyond, outside of, in addition	**extra**cellular
flex-	bent	**flex**ion
front-	front, forehead	**front**alis
hemi-	half	**hemi**plegic
hetero-	the other	**hetero**sexual
hom-	common, same	**hom**ogenous
hydro-	denoting water	**hydro**therapy
hyper-	above, extreme	**hyper**tensive
hypo-	under, below	**hypo**dermic
in-	within, into, not, negative	**in**ternal, inept
infra-	beneath	**infra**spinatus

Word Part	Definition	Example
intra-	inside	**intra**venous
leuk-(o)	white	**leul**ocyte
macr-	large, long	**macr**ophage
mal-	abnormal, bad	**mal**practice
medi-	middle, midline	**medi**al
mega-	large, extreme	**mega**dose
micr-(o)	small	**micr**oscope
mon-(o)	one, single	**mon**olith
multi-	many, multiple	**multi**ply
narc-	stupor, numbness	**narc**otic
ne-(o)	new	**ne**ophyte, neonatal
nutri-	nourish	**nutri**tion
para-	next to, resembling, beside	**para**lysis, paraplegic
path-	pertaining to disease	**path**ology
per-	through	**per**forate
peri-	around	**peri**osteum
poly-	many, much	**poly**unsaturated
post-	after, later in time	**post**humous
pre-, pro-	before in time	**pre**vious
pseud-(o)	false	**pseud**onym
quad-	four	**quad**riplegic
re-	back, again	**re**peat, review
retro-	backward	**retro**fit
sub-	under, below	**sub**scapularis
super-	above, in addition	**super**ior
supra-	over, above, upper	**supra**spinatus

Word Part	Definition	Example
syn-	together, along with	**syn**ergist
tri-	three	**tri**ceps
uni-	single, one	**uni**lateral

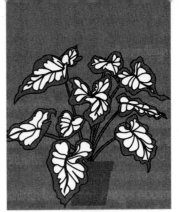

Suffixes

SUFFIXES

Many medical and anatomical words are of Latin origin. The following endings will enable you to tell at a glance whether they are singular, plural, or possessive.

Endings or Regular Latin Nouns

Singular:	Plural:	Possessive Singula:
...us —Nasus	...i —Nasi	...i —Nasi
...a —Ala	...ae—Alae	...ae—Alae
...um —Labium	...a —Labia	...i —Labii

Word Part	Definition	Example
-al; -ar	pertaining to an area	femor**al**, clavicul**ar**
-ase	denoting an enzyme	lact**ase**
-algia	painful condition	neur**algia**
-desis	a binding	teno**desis**
-ectomy	surgical removal of body part	tonsill**ectomy**
-gram	a record	sono**gram**

Word Part	Definition	Example
-graph	write, draw, record	electrocardio**graph**
-ia	a noun ending of a condition	leukem**ia**
-ic	a noun/adjective ending	pelv**ic**, hypodermi**c**
-ide	names of compounds	bacteric**ide**, germic**ide**
-ist	one who does	art**ist**, antagon**ist**
-itis	inflammation	arth**ritis**
-ize	transitive verbs	steri**lize**
-oid	resembling	styli**od**, lip**iod**
-ology	study of, science of	bi**ology**
-oma	tumor	carcin**oma**
-ostomy	forming an opening	col**ostomy**
-otomy	excision, cutting into	lob**otomy**
-pathic	diseased	psycho**pathic**
-phobia	morbid fear of	claustro**phobia**
-sis	inflammation	pityria**sis**
-tomy	surgical procedure	colos**tomy**

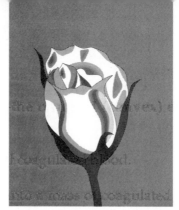

Common Word Roots or Stems

Word Part	Definition	Example
aur	ear	auricular
arth(ro)	joint	arthritis
brachi	arm	brachialis
cardi	heart	cardiac
cephal	head	brachiocephalic
cerebr(o)	brain	cerebrospinalis
cervic	neck	cervix, cervical
chondr(o)	cartilage	osteochondritis
cost	rib	intercostal
crani	skull	cranial
cyt	cell	leukocyte
dent	teeth	dentine, dental
derm	skin	subdermal
fibr	fiber	fibrositis
gastr(o)	stomach	gastritis
gyn	woman	gynecology
hem	blood	hematoma

Word Part	Definition	Example
hepat	liver	hepatitis
hist	tissue	histology
labi	lip	quadratus labii
my(o)	muscle	myology
nephr(o)	kidney	nephritis
neur(o)	nerve	neurology
ocul	eye	ocular
oss,ost(e)	bone	osteoblast
phleb	vein	phlebitis
pneum	lung	pneumonia
pod	foot	podiatrist
psych	mind	psychologist
pulmo	lung	cardiopulmonary
therm	heat	thermometer
vas	vessel	vascular

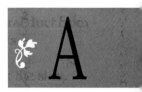

abampere (ab·AM·peer)—the cgs electromagnetic unit of electric current equivalent to 10 amperes.

abbreviate (uh·BREE·vee·ayt)—to make shorter; to reduce; make briefer.

abdomen (AB·duh·men)—the belly; the cavity in the body between the thorax and the pelvis. Contains the stomach, intestines, liver, and kidneys.

abducent (ab·DOOS·int)—drawing away from, as muscles draw away.

abducent nerve (ab·DOOS·int NURV)—the sixth cranial nerve; a small motor nerve supplying the external rectus muscle of the eye.

abductor (ab·DUK·tur)—a muscle that draws a part away from the median line (opp., adductor). Abductor muscles are located at the base of each digit.

abductor hallucis (ab·DUK·tor huh·LOO·sis)—a muscle of the foot.

ability (uh·BIL·ih·tee)—the quality or state of being able to perform.

abiogenesis (ay·by·oh·JEN·uh·sus)—the generating or springing up of living from nonliving matter; spontaneous generation.

abiosis (ab·ee·OH·sis)—absence of life.

abirritant (ab·IHR·uh·tant)—a soothing agent that relieves irritation.

abnormal (ab·NOR·mul)—irregular, contrary to the natural law or customary order.

abnormality (ab·nor·MAL·ih·tee)—the state or condition of being abnormal or unusual.

abohm (ab·OHM)—the cgs electromagnetic unit of resistance equal to one millionth of an ohm.

aboral (ah·BOHR·ul)—located or situated opposite to or away from the mouth.

abrade (uh·BRAYD)—to remove or roughen by friction or rubbing.

abrasion (uh·BRAY·zhun)—scraping of the skin; rubbing or wearing off the surface; an irritation; a scraped or scratched area of the skin.

abrasive (uh·BRAY·siv)—a substance used for smoothing, as in dermabrasion (the sanding or brushing of the skin).

abreast (uh·BREST)—in line with; side by side with; up to the mark.

abruption (uh·BRUP·shun)—a sudden breaking off.

abscess (AB·ses)—a collection or pocket of pus in any part of the body, characterized by dead tissue and inflammation.

absolute (ab·suh·LOOT)—pure, as a liquid; perfect, beyond a doubt.

absorb (ab·SORB)—to take in and make part of an existing whole; to suck up or take up; as a towel absorbs water.

absorbefacient (ab·sor·buh·FAY·shent)—substance causing or promoting absorption.

absorbent (ub·SOR·bunt)—able to absorb.

absorption (ub·SORP·shun)—assimilation of one body by another; act of absorbing; the process whereby digested nutrients are transferred to the blood and lymph to be transported to the cells.

abstract design (AB·strakt dih·ZYN)—cosmetology; a hairstyle with broken lines, planned to give a casual, relaxed effect; informal hairstyle.

absurd (ub·SURD)—inconsistent with reason.

abundance (uh·BUN·dens)—ample, plentiful quantity.

abuse (uh·BYOOS)—to misuse; to use improperly.

academic (ak·uh·DEM·ik)—pertaining to an academy, school, college, or university; scholarly.

acanthosis (ak·an·THOH·sis)—altered skin metabolism that can produce thickening of the stratum corneum.

acariasis (ak·uh·RY·uh·sus)—any condition, usually dermatitis, caused by an acarid (tick or mite).

acarid (AK·uh·rud)—any of an order of arachnids, including mites and ticks.

accelerate (ak·SELL·uh·rayt)—increase speed; hasten action.

acceleration (ak·SELL·uh·ray·shun)—an increase in speed; the process of moving or developing faster.

accelerator (ak·SELL·uh·rayt·ur)—any agent that hastens or quickens action. (*See* activator.)

accent (AK·sent)—to give special force or emphasis; to highlight or give added color tone.

accent color (AK·sent KUH·lur)—*See* color additive.

11

accentuate (ak·SEN·choo·ayt)—to emphasize; to heighten effect; in makeup; to emphasize the features of the face.

accessory (ak·SESS·uh·ree)—a person or item that aids subordinately or assists; something added.

accessory nerve (ak·SESS·uh·ree NURV)—spinal accessory nerve; eleventh cranial nerve; affects the sterno-cleido-mastoid and trapezius muscles of the neck.

accidental (ak·sih·DEN·tul)—happening by chance; not planned.

acclimate (AK·luh·mayt)—to adapt or become adapted to environment, climate, or situation.

accord (uh·KORD)—to bring into agreement or harmony.

accreditation (uh·kred·ih·TAY·shun)—the granting of approval and status to an institution by an accrediting body after its credentials are approved.

accretion (uh·KREE·shun)—growth or increase by external additions; something added; pathology: an accumulation of foreign matter in a body cavity.

acellular (ay·SEL·yuh·lur)—containing no cells, as a noncellular substance.

acentric (ay·SEN·trik)—off center; not centered; not arising centrally, as from a nerve center.

acetic (uh·SEET·ik)—pertaining to vinegar; sour.

acetic acid (uh·SEET·ik AS·ud)—a colorless, pungent, liquid acid that is the chief acid of vinegar.

acetone (AS·uh·tohn)—a colorless, inflammable liquid, miscible with water, alcohol, and ether, and having a sweetish order or burning taste; used as a solvent.

acetyl (uh·SEET·ul)—pertaining to that which is derived from acetic acid and found in compounds.

acetylated (uh·SEET·ul·ayt·ed)—any organic compound that has been heated with acetic anhydride or acetyl chloride to remove water.

acetylated lanolin (uh·SEET·ul·ayt·ed LAN·ul·un)—lanolin treated to be water resistant; used in cosmetics to reduce water loss from the skin; an emollient.

acetylcholine (uh·SEET·ul·koh·leen)—the acetic acid ester of choline, a constituent of many body tissues; used in treatment of some diseases and for lowering of blood pressure; a neurotransmitter that plays a role in muscle contraction.

ache (AYK)—a dull, distressing, and often persistent pain.

Achilles heel (uh·KIL·eez HEEL)—calcaneal tendon; a tender or vulnerable spot associated with the Achilles tendon, which joins the muscles of the calf of the leg to the bone of the heel; named for the Greek hero, Achilles.

achromasia (ak·roh·MAY·zhuh)—a condition such as albanism or vitiligo in which there is loss of normal color or lack of melanin in the skin.

acid (AS·ud)—having a sour taste; an aqueous (water-based) solution; having a pH number below 7.0. The opposite of an alkali or base; compounds of hydrogen, a non-metal, and sometimes oxygen that release hydrogen into a solution.

acid balanced (AS·ud BAL·anst)—describes a product whose pH level is stabilized; commonly used to refer to products such as shampoos and conditioners that are balanced to the pH of skin and hair which is 4.5–5.5.

acid mantle (AS·ud MAN·tul)—the natural acidity of the skin or hair that helps retard irritation or bacterial growth.

acidic (uh·SID·ik)—containing a high percentage of acid; having properties of an acid.

acidify (uh·SID·ih·fy)—to change into an acid; to lower the degree of alkalinity.

acidosis (as·ih·DOH·sus)—a condition in which there is an excess of acid products in the blood or excreted into the urine.

acid peel (AS·ud PEEL)—a skin-peeling treatment or process using a diluted acidic substance.

acid rinse (AS·ud RINS)—a solution or emulsion that has acidic properties; commonly used to close the cuticle of the hair after shampooing or chemical services.

acidulate (uh·SIJ·oo·layt)—to make acid or sour.

acidum boricum (AS·ih·dum BOR·ih·kum)—boric acid; a white crystalline compound used as a preservative and as an antiseptic.

acid wave (AS·ud WAYV)—permanent wave with lotion that has a pH of 7.0 or below and requires heat or other form of activator to speed processing.

acne (AK·nee)—a skin disorder characterized by chronic inflammation of the sebaceous glands from retained secretions; related to sebaceous overactivity and hormonal changes.

acne albida (AK·nee AL·bih·duh)—milium; whitehead.

acne artificialis (AK·nee ar·tih·fish·AL·is)—pimples due to external irritants.

acne atrophica (AK·nee uh·TROF·ih·kuh)—acne in which the lesions leave a slight amount of scarring.

acne cachecticorum (AK·nee kah·KEK·tih·kor·um)—pimples that sometimes occur when anemia or some debilitating constitutional disease is present.

acne conglobata (AK·nee kon·gloh·BAY·tuh)—a severe and stubborn form of acne that usually affects the back, buttocks, the face, and sometimes the thighs; often causes scarring.

acne cream (AK·nee KREEM)—a facial cream, containing medicinal substances or agents, used in the treatment of acne.

acne cystica (AK·nee SIS·tih·kuh)—a form of acne with lesions that are primarily cysts.

acne hypertrophica (AK·nee hy·pur·TRAHF·ih·kuh)—pimples in which the lesions on healing leave conspicuous pits and scars.

acne indurata (AK·nee in·dyoo·RAH·tuh)—deeply seated pimples with hard tubercular lesions or papules occurring chiefly on the back.

acne keratosa (AK·nee kair·uh·TOH·sus)—an eruption of papules consisting of horny plugs projecting from the hair follicles, accompanied by inflammation.

acne miliaris (AK·nee mil·ee·AIR·us)—a condition marked by excessive whiteheads (milia).

acne pits (AK·nee PITS)—pitlike scars produced by acne.

acne punctata (AK·nee punk·TAH·tuh)—acne that appears as red papules in which blackheads are usually found.

acne pustulosa (AK·nee pus·tyuh·LOH·suh)—acne in which pustular lesions predominate.

acne rosacea (AK·nee roh·ZAY·see·uh)—a form of acne usually occurring around the nose and cheeks, in which the capillaries become dilated and sometimes broken.

acne simplex (AK·nee SIM·pleks)—acne vulgaris; simple uncomplicated pimples.

acne vulgaris (AK·nee vul·GAIR·is)—acne simplex; simple uncomplicated pimples.

acoustic (uh·KOO·stik)—pertaining to the science of sound or the sense or organs of hearing.

acoustic nerve (uh·KOO·stik NURV)—eighth cranial nerve, controlling the sense of hearing.

acquire (uh·KWYR)—to receive; to attain; to master.

acquired immunity (uh·KWY·erd ih·MYOO·nih·tee)—immunity acquired after the body overcomes a disease or through inoculation.

acrolein (uh·KROH·lee·un)—a light, volatile, oily liquid that gives off an irritating vapor.

acromion process (uh·KROH·mee·on PRAH·ses)—the outward extension of the spine of the scapula, forming the point of the shoulder.

acronyx (AK·roh·niks)—an ingrowing nail.

acrylic acid (uh·KRIL·ik AS·ud)—unsaturated aliphatic acids used in the making of plastics, which are used in the manufacture of items useful to cosmetology (combs, brushes, capes, etc.).

acrylic nails (uh·KRIL·ik NAYLS)—artificial nails made by combining a liquid acrylic product with a powdered product.

actin (AK·tin)—a muscular filament that plays a role in giving muscle its contractile ability.

actinic (ak·TIN·ik)—relating to the chemically active rays of the spectrum.

actinic carcinoma (ak·TIN·ik kahr·sin·OH·muh)—a basal cell carcinoma of the face or body due to prolonged exposure to the sun.

actinic dermatosis (ak·TIN·ik der·muh·TOH·sis)—an inflammatory condition of the skin caused by strong sunlight; it may be uticarial, papular, or eczematous.

actinic ray (ak·TIN·ik RAY)—an invisible ray that produces chemical action; a ray of light beyond the violet spectrum that is capable of bringing about chemical changes.

actinodermatitis (ak·tin·oh·dur·muh·TY·tus)—dermatitis caused by overexposure to sunlight, actinic rays, or X rays.

actinomycosis (ak·tin·oh·my·KOH·sus)—a chronic, infectious disease that affects animals and people, caused by bacteria and characterized by the forming of lesions and tumors around the jaws.

actinotherapy (ak·tin·oh·THAIR·uh·pee)—the treatment of disease by use of sunlight, X rays, and ultraviolet rays.

activate (AK·tih·vayt)—to make active; to start the action of hair-coloring products.

activator (AK·tih·vay·ter)—1) a chemical agent employed to start the action of chemical products on hair. 2) an additive used to quicken the action or progress of a chemical. Another word for booster, accelerator, protenator, or catalyst.

activator machine (AK·tih·vay·ter muh·SHEEN)—a device employed in facial therapy that helps to cleanse, stimulate and firm the skin.

active electrode (AK·tiv ih·LEK·trohd)—the electrode used on the area to be treated.

active immunity (AK·tiv ih·MYOO·nih·tee)—*See* acquired immunity.

activity (AK·tiv ih··tee)—natural or normal function or operation; physical motion or exercise of force.

aculeate (uh·KYOO·lee·ut)—causing a sting as from a pin prick.

acuminate (uh·KYOO·muh·nut)—to sharpen to a point or taper.

acupressure (AK·yoo·presh·ur)—employs methods of stimulating pressure points on the body to regulate "chi" or the life force.

acupuncture (AK·yoo·punc·chur)—puncturing the skin with needles at specific points for therapeutic purposes.

acute (uh·KYOOT)—coming to a crisis quickly, as opposed to chronic: said of a disease having a rapid onset, severe symptoms and short course.

ad (AD)—a prefix denoting to, toward; addition, intensification.

adapt (uh·DAPT)—to make suitable; to alter so as to fit a new use.

adaptable (uh·DAPT·uh·bul)—capable of or given to adapting one's self to new conditions and uses.

additive (AD·ut·iv)—a substance that is to be added to another product.

adductor (uh·DUK·tur)—a muscle that draws a part toward the median line of the body or toward the axis of an extremity. Located at the base of each digit.

adenitis (ad·un·ITE·us)—inflammation of the lymph nodes.

adenoid (AD·un·oyd)—an enlarged lymphoid growth located behind the pharynx.

adenology (ad·uh·NAHL·uh·jee)—the branch of anatomy concerned with glands.

adenoma (ad·un·OH·muh)—a tumor of glandular origin.

adenoma sebaceum (ad·un·OH·muh see·BAY·see·um)—a small tumor of translucent appearance, originating in the sebaceous glands.

adenosine diphosphate (uh·DEN·uh·seen dy·FAHS·fayt)—ADP; formed when a muscle contracts and a phosphate splits from ATP, releasing energy.

adenosine triphosphate (uh·DEN·uh·seen try·FAHS·fayt)—ATP; an energy-carrying molecule that is required for muscular contractions; a substance that stores energy until it is released for muscular and other cellular activity.

adermogenesis (ay·dur·moh·JEN·uh·sus)—imperfect development or healing of the skin.

adhere (ad·HEER)—to remain in contact; to unite.

adhesive (ad·HEE·siv)—a sticky substance used for holding something fast.

adhesive patch (ad·HEE·siv PACH)—a small area of the underside of a man's hairpiece that is covered with oiled silk.

adiaphoretic (ay·dy·uh·foh·RET·ik)—any agent, drug, or cosmetic preparation that reduces, checks, or prevents perspiration.

adipic acid (ay·DIP·ik AS·ud)—hexanedioic acid; an agent derived from beets; used in hair-coloring products for its buffering and neutralizing qualities.

adipose (AD·uh·pohs)—relating to fat.

adipose tissue (AD·uh·pohs TISH·oo)—areolar connective tissue containing fat cells: subcutaneous tissue; acts to protect against heat loss and stores energy in the form of fat cells.

adjacent (ad·JAY·sent)—lying near or adjoining.

adjust (ad·JUST)—to make exact; to fit; to bring into proper relationship.

adjustable block holder (ad·JUST·uh·bul BLOK HOL·dur)—a metal bracket, which can be screwed to a work bench; used to hold the wooden or malleable head block in position while working on a hairpiece or mannequin head.

adjustable wig (ad·JUST·uh·bul WIG)—a wig designed for ready-to-wear use, constructed with an elastic insert at the back to make it easily adjustable for various head sizes.

admix (ad·MIKS)—to mix with something else.

adnata alopecia (ad·NAY·tuh al·uh·PEE·shuh)—baldness at birth.

adolescence (ad·uh·LES·ens)—state or process of growing from childhood to adulthood: the period of time encompassing that process.

adorn (uh·DORN)—to decorate a person or object.

adrenal (uh·DREEN·ul)—an endocrine gland situated on top of the kidneys.

adrenaline (uh·DREN·ul·un)—a hormone secreted under stress by the adrenal glands; it stimulates the nervous system, raises metabolism, increases cardiac pressure and output, and increases blood pressur, to prepare the body for maximum exertion.

adroit (uh·DROYT)—skillful; dexterous; having physical and mental capabilities.

adsorption (ad·SORP·shun)—the adhesion of an extremely thin layer of one substance (a gas or liquid) to the surface of a solid body or liquid with which it is in contact.

adult (uh·DULT)—grown to full age, size, or strength.

adulterate (uh·DUL·ter·ayt)—to falsify; to alter; to make impure by the addition of other substances.

advanced (ad·VANCT)—progressive; ahead of the times; beyond the elementary or introductory.

advisable (ad·VYZ·uh·bul)—proper to be done or practiced; expedient.

adynamia (ad·ih·NAY·mee·uh)—loss of physical strength; weakness.

aerate (AIR·ayt)—to supply or charge with air or gas; to oxygenate.

aeration (air·AY·shun)—exposure to air; saturating a fluid with air or gas; conversion of venous to arterial blood.

aerification (air·ih·fih·KAY·shun)—the process of converting into gas, air or vapor.

aerobe (AIR·ohb)—a microorganism that can live only in the presence of oxygen.

aerobic (air·ROH·bik)—living or occurring only in the presence of oxygen; a term applied to modern dance exercises; aerobic exercise improves cardiac fitness.

aerobic respiration (air·ROH·bik res·puh·RAY·shun)—takes place in the mitochondria of cells and is responsible for the sustained energy supply needed for synthesis of ATP.

aerosol (AIR·uh·sahl)—colloidal suspension of liquid or solid particles in a gas; container filled with liquefied gas and dissolved or suspended in ingredients that can be dispersed as a spray; used for cosmetic and food preparations.

aerotherapeutics (air·oh·thair·uh·PYOO·tiks)—a system by which disease is treated by varying the pressure or the composition of the air breathed.

Aesculapius (es·kyoo·LAY·pree·us)—combined exercise and massage to create gymnastics.

aesthetician (esthetician) (es·the·TISH·un)—a specialist in esthetics; one who works in a profession dedicated to the cleansing and maintenance of the health and beauty of the skin.

aesthetics (esthetics) (es·THET·iks)—a branch of philosophy pertaining to or dealing with the forms and nature of beauty and judgments concerning beauty; the branch of cosmetology dealing with skin care.

afferent (AF·uh·rent)—bearing or carrying toward the center; inward.

afferent nerves (AF·uh·rent NURVZ)—nerves that convey stimuli such as impulses or messages from the external sense organs to the brain.

affinity (uh·FIN·ut·ee)—attraction; in chemistry: the characteristic that impels certain atoms to unite with certain others to form compounds.

affix (uh·FIKS)—to attach, fix, or fasten.

affixative (uh·FIKS·uh·tiv)—a product, hair spray or setting lotion used in holding the finished style in place.

Afro-comb (AF·roh KOHM)—a comb designed especially for thick, curly hair; hair lifter.

Afro-lifter (AF·roh-LIFT·ur)—a fork-like comb for styling and lifting curly hair.

Afro-pick (AF·roh-PIK)—a styling tool with long fork-like prongs used to pick the hair into place.

Afro-styling (AF·roh-STYL·ing)—styling and shaping excessively curly or kinky hair in accordance with its natural tendencies and the facial features of the client.

after-image (AF·tur-IHM·uj)—an image or sensation that stays or comes back after the external stimulus has been withdrawn; e.g., seeing spots after looking at the sun.

after rinse (AF·tur RINS)—a prepared cosmetic product used to rinse hair following a hair treatment, to accomplish some special purpose; a color, cream, or finishing rinse.

agenesis (ay·JEN·uh·sus)—the imperfect development of any part of the body.

agent (AY·jent)—an active power that can produce a physical, chemical, or medicinal effect.

aggravate (AG·ruh·vayt)—to make worse; intensify, as an illness or skin condition.

aging skin (AY·jing SKIN)—skin that has lost its elasticity and has developed lines or wrinkles.

agitate (AJ·ih·tayt)—to stir up; shake; disturb.

agnail (AG·nayl)—the condition in which the cuticle splits around the nail.

agonist (AG·uh·nust)—a contracting muscle that executes movements of a part and is opposed by an antagonistic muscle.

AIDS (AYDZ)—Acquired immune deficiency syndrome; a viral disease that breaks down the body's immune system.

air purifier (AYR PYOOR·ih·fy·ur)—an apparatus that removes impure substances from the air.

air waving (AYR WAYV·ing)—a technique of rolling the hair over the fingers while air drying the hair; drying, combing and styling of the hair with a hand hair dryer.

al (UL)—a word termination denoting belonging to, of, or pertaining to.

ala (AY·luh); pl., **alae** (AY·lee)—a winglike structure, as the wing of the nose.

alae nasi (AY·lee NAY·zy)—the wing cartilage of the nose.

albida, acne (AL·bih·duh AK·nee)—whitehead; milium.

albinism (AL·buh·niz·um)—congenital leucoderma or absence of pigment in the skin, hair, and eyes; it may be partial or complete.

albino (al·BY·noh)—an individual affected with albinism; having little or no coloring pigment in the skin, hair, or iris of the eyes.

albumen (al·BYOO·men)—the white of an egg; the nutritive protein substance in germinating animal or plant cells; sometimes used in facial masks for its tightening effect.

albumin (al·BYOO·min)—any of a class of proteins naturally occurring, soluble in water, coagulated by heat, and found in eggs, milk, muscle tissue, blood, and in many vegetable tissues.

albuminous (al·BYOO·mih·nus)—relating to albumen.

albumose (AL·byuh·mohs)—a substance formed from protein during digestion; chemical compounds derived from albumins by the action of certain enzymes.

alcohol (AL·kuh·hawl)—a readily evaporating, colorless liquid with a pungent odor and burning taste; powerful stimulant and antiseptic; obtained by the fermentation of starch, sugar, and other carbohydrates.

alcohol 70% (AL·kuh·hawl)—alcohol used as a disinfectant to sanitize implements, surfaces, and metal instruments.

algae (AL·jee)—primitive plants found in fresh or salt water (seaweed, kelp, stoneworts, etc.); considered a nutrient.

algin (AL·jun)—the dried gelatinous form of various seaweeds, especially kelp, used as an emulsifier, thickening, and ripening agent.

align (uh·LYN)—to bring into place or line.

aliment (AL·uh·ment)—nourishment; food or anything that feeds or adds to a substance in natural growth.

alimentary (al·uh·MENT·uh·ree)—relating to food or nutrition; the canal that extends from the mouth to the anus.

alkali (AL·kuh·ly)—a class of compounds (hydrogen, a metal, and oxygen) that reacts with acids to form salts, turn red litmus blue, saponify fats and form soluble carbonates; having a pH number above 7.0.

alkalimeter (al·kuh·LIM·ut·ur)—an apparatus for measuring the amount of alkali in a mixture or solution and quantity of carbon dioxide in solids.

alkaline (AL·kuh·lin)—having the qualities of, or pertaining to, an alkali. An aqueous (water-based) solution having a pH greater than 7.0. Opposite of acid.

alkalinity (al·kuh·LIN·ut·ee)—the quality or state of being alkaline.

alkaloid (AL·kuh·loyd)—any organic base containing nitrogen; a substance containing alkaline properties.

alkalosis (al·kuh·LOH·sus)—excessive alkalinity of the blood, other body fluids, and tissues of the body.

alkanolamine (al·kan·uh·LAA·myn)—a substance comprised of alcohols from alkene (a saturated, fatty hydrocarbon) and amines (from ammonia); used in cosmetic creams as a solvent.

alkylation (al·kuh·LAY·shun)—the introduction of an alkyl group into an organic compound.

allantoin (al·AN·shun)—a uric acid derivative originally found in foetal allantoic fluid and in some roots, bark, and grain; used in healing and cleansing preparations.

allergic (al·UR·jik)—pertaining to having an allergy, aversion, or disagreeable sensitivity.

allergy (AL·ur·jee)—a reaction due to extreme sensitivity to certain foods, chemicals, or other normally harmless substances.

allergy test (AL·ur·jee TEST)—a test to determine the existence or nonexistence of extreme sensitivity to certain substances, foods, or chemicals that do not adversely affect most individuals; a test used before applying hair color or facial cosmetics; a test done on a small section of skin or scalp. Also known as a patch test, predisposition test, or skin test.

almond (AH·mund)—the kernal or seed of the fruit of the almond tree; used in facial and other cosmetic preparations.

almond meal (AH·mund MEEL)—pulverized, blanched almonds; a powder used in the manufacture of cosmetics and some fragrances.

almond oil (AH·mund OYL)—emolient; natural vegetable oil pressed from almonds and having penetrating and softening powers; used in some cosmetic preparations.

aloe (AL·oh)—any member of a genus of plants of the lily family; used in some cosmetic preparations and as a cathartic.

aloe vera (AL·oh VAIR·hu)—a juice extracted from the South African aloe plant leaf; contains water, amino acids, and carbohydrates; used in some cosmetic and medicinal preparations.

alopecia (al·uh·PEE·shuh)—deficiency of hair; baldness; abnormal hair loss.

alopecia adnata (al·uh·PEE·shuh ad·NAY·tuh)—baldness at birth.

alopecia areata (al·uh·PEE·shuh ay·reh·AH·tuh)—baldness in spots or patches.

alopecia cicatrisata (al·uh·PEE·shuh sih·kah·trih·SAH·tah)—baldness in uneven patches caused by atrophy of the skin.

alopecia dynamica (al·uh·PEE·shuh dy·NAM·ih·kuh)—loss of hair due to destruction of the hair follicle by ulceration or some disease process.

alopecia follicularis (al·uh·PEE·shuh fol·ik·yoo·LAIR·is)—loss of hair due to inflamed hair follicles.

alopecia localis (al·uh·PEE·shuh loh·KAY·lis)—loss of hair occurring in patches on the course of a nerve at the site of an injury.

alopecia maligna (al·uh·PEE·shuh muh·LIG·nuh)—a term applied to the form of alopecia that is severe and persistent.

alopecia prematura (al·uh·PEE·shuh pree·muh·TOO·ruh)—baldness beginning before middle age.

alopecia seborrheica (al·uh·PEE·shuh seb·or·EE·ih·kah)—baldness caused by diseased sebaceous glands.

alopecia senilis (al·uh·PEE·shuh seh·NIL·is)—baldness occurring in old age.

alopecia syphilitica (al·uh·PEE·shuh sif·il·IT·ih·kuh)—loss of hair resulting from syphilis, occurring in the second stage of the disease.

alopecia traction (al·uh·PEE·shuh TRAK·shun)—hair loss caused by holding the hair tight and under tension for long periods of time.

alopecia universalis (al·uh·PEE·shuh yoo·nih·vur·SAA·lis)—a condition manifested by general falling out of body hair.

alpha (AL·fuh)—beginning or first of anything; alpha and omega, the first and last or beginning and the end.

alpha helix (AL·fuh HEE·liks)—the spiral of the polypeptide chains within the hair cortex in the first or unstretched position.

alphosis (al·FOH·sis)—pertaining to lack of skin pigmentation, as in albinism.

alternate (AWL·tur·nayt)—to do by turns; being one of two or more choices.

alternating (AWL·tur·nayt·ing)—occurring in reciprocal succession.

alternating current, AC (AWL·tur·nayt·ing KUR·rent)—a current that rises and falls in strength of flow, alternating in opposite directions at regular intervals.

alternating rod (AWL·tur·nayt·ing RAHD)—a permanent waving technique recommended for fine or weak hair; this method alternates rods having two different circumferences.

alternator (AWL·tur·nayt·ur)—a generator giving an alternating current of electricity.

alum, alumen (AL·um, uh·LOO·men)—an aluminum salt; sulphate of potassium and aluminum; an astringent; used as a styptic and in mouthwashes, shave lotions, etc.

aluminum (uh·LOO·mih·num)—silver·white metal with low specific gravity, noted for its lightness and resistance to oxidation; often used in the manufacture of combs, rollers, etc.

aluminum acetate solution (uh·LOO·mih·num AS·uh·tayt suh·LOO·shun)—a solution diluted with water and used as an antiseptic and astringent.

aluminum chloride (uh·LOO·mih·num KLOHR·yd)—a crystalline powder, soluble in water; used as an astringent, antiseptic, or deodorant.

aluminum sulfate (uh·LOO·mih·num SUL·fayt)—cake alum; used in antiseptics, astringents, and in some deodorant preparations.

alveola (al·VEE·oh·lah); pl., **alveolae** (·lee)—a small hollow alveolae border; the portion of the jaws bearing the teeth; branch of the internal maxillary artery.

alveolar ducts (al·VEE·oh·lar DUKTS)—air passages in the lungs branching from the respiratory bronchioles leading to the alveolar sacs.

alveolar nerve (al·VEE·oh·lar NURV)—a nerve servicing the teeth.

alveolar process (al·VEE·oh·lar PRAH·ses)—the ridge of bone in the maxilla and in the mandible, containing the alveolar of the teeth.

alymphia (ay·LIM·fee·uh)—absence or deficiency of lymph.

amber (AM·bur)—a fossil resin of pine trees found in northern Europe; it becomes negatively electrified in friction: the oil is sometimes used as a stimulant.

amber color (AM·bur KUL·ur)—a yellow-brown color resembling amber.

ambergris (AM·ber·gris)—an opaque, grayish secretion from the sperm whale; used in perfumery.

ambidextrous (am·bih·DEK·strus)—able to use both hands equally well.

amines (AM·eenz)—compounds that are the basic ingredients of proteins.

amino acids (uh·MEE·noh AS·udz)—the chemical building blocks of all proteins that make up the body, including skin and hair; amino acids are used in some shampoos and hair conditioners to recondition damaged hair.

amino dye (uh·MEE·noh DY)—a synthetic, organic tint produced from a coal tar derivative known as analine.

amitosis (ay·my·TOH·sus)—cell multiplication by direct division of the nucleus in the cell.

amma (AM·uh)—the ancient Chinese technique of massage.

ammonia (uh·MOH·nee·uh)—a colorless gas composed of hydrogen and nitrogen, with a pungent odor; very soluble in water.

ammonia water (uh·MOH·nee·uh WAW·tur)—ammonia gas dissolved in water. Used in cosmetology to swell the cuticle. When mixed with hydrogen peroxide, activates the oxidation process on melanin and allows the melanin to decolorize.

ammonium bisulfide (uh·MOH·nee·um by·SUL·fyd)—a chemical used in cosmetology products, such as hair relaxers in permanent waving.

ammonium hydroxide (uh·MOH·nee·um hy·DRAHKS·yd)—an alkaline base formed from ammonia and water; used in products such as permanent hair color, lightener preparations, hair relaxers, and cleansing solutions.

ammonium persulfate (uh·MOH·nee·um pur·SUL·fayt)—ammonium salt; soluble in water; used as an oxidizer and bleach in some hair and skin cosmetics; an ingredient used in some disinfectants and deodorants.

ammonium stearate (uh·MOH·nee·um STEER·ayt)—stearic acid; ammonium salt; powder used as a texturizer in some cosmetic creams such as vanishing creams.

ammonium sulfide (uh·MOH·nee·um SUL·fyd)—a combination of ammonia and sulfur.

ammonium sulfite (uh·MOH·nee·um SUL·fyt)—a combination of ammonia and salt of sulfuric acid.

ammonium thiocyanate (uh·MOH·nee·um thy·oh·SY·uh·nayt)— a combination of ammonia and thiocyanic acid.

ammonium thioglycolate (uh·MOH·nee·um thy·oh·GLY·kuh·layt)—a combination of ammonia and thioglycolic acid; reducing agent used primarily in permanent waving and hair-relaxing solutions and creams.

amotile (ay·MOH·tul)—incapable of movement, as a muscle; opposite of motile, to move.

amp (AMP)—amperage; the strength of an electric current.

ampere (AM·peer)—the unit of measurement of strength of an electric current.

amphetamine (am·FET·uh·meen)—an acrid, colorless liquid compound used as an inhalant or stimulant for relief of colds.

amphiarthrotic joints (am·fee·arth·RAH·tik JOYNTS)—joints such as the sacroiliac and symphis pubis that have limited motion.

ampholytic surfactant (AM·foh·lih·tik sur·FAK·tent)—a base surfactant found in shampoos; does not sting eyes; behaves as an anionic or cationic substance depending on the pH of the solution.

amphoteric (am·fuh·TAIR·ik)—having the characteristics of both an acid and an alkali; a substance used in cleaning agents.

ampule (AM·pyool)—a small glass container used for one application of a product; a glass attachment for vacuuming.

amyl acetate (AM·ul AS·uh·tayt)—banana oil; a colorless, aromatic, and inflammable liquid employed as a solvent in making nail polishes.

amyl alcohol (AM·ul AL·kuh·hawl)—a colorless, strong smelling alcohol, obtained by the fermentation of starchy substances; found naturally in oranges; used as a solvent in nail polish.

amylase (AM·uh·lays)—an enzyme that helps to change starch into sugar; found in pancreatic secretions; used as a texturizer in cosmetics; also used in some medications to reduce inflammation.

amylopectin (am·uh·loh·PEK·tin)—amioca; a substance derived from starch, almost insoluble; used as a texturizer in cosmetics.

anabolism (uh·NAB·uh·liz·um)—constructive metabolism; the process of assimilation of nutritive matter and its conversion into living substance; the process of building up of larger molecules from smaller ones.

anaerobic respiration (AN·uh·roh·bik res·puh·RAY·shun)—consists of breaking down of glucose, releasing energy for synthesis of ATP and production of lactic acid.

anagen phase (AN·uh·jen FAYZ)—the phase during which new hair is synthesized; the early productive phase of the hair cycle in a follicle.

analgesic (an·ul·JEE·sik)—a drug for the alleviation of pain.

analine derivative tint (AN·ul·un duh·RIV·uh·tiv TINT)—a synthetic, organic hair tint produced from a coal tar product. (*See* amino dye.)

analogous (an·AL·uh·gus)—similar or comparable in certain respects.

analysis (uh·NAL·uh·sis)—the process by which the nature of a substance is recognized and its chemical or physical composition is determined.

analysis, hair (uh·NAL·uh·sis HAYR)—examination to determine the conditon and natural color of the hair prior to a hair treatment. (*See* consultation, condition.)

analyze (AN·uh·lyz)—to make an analysis.

anaphase (AN·uh·fayz)—a stage in cell division which two coiled strands called chromatids are separated and again called chromosomes.

anaphoresis (an·uh·for·EE·sis)—the use of the negative pole to force, or push, a netatively charged substance (an alkaline pH solution) into the skin.

anaplastic (AN·uh·plas·tik)—pertaining to the restoration of lost or absent parts, as in reconstructive surgery.

anaplasty (an·uh·PLAS·tee)—an operation for the restoration of lost parts; plastic surgery.

anaplerosis (an·uh·pluh·ROH·sis)—plastic surgery; replacement of defective parts of the body, caused by injury or disease.

anatomy (uh·NAT·uh·mee)—the study of the gross structure of the body that can be seen with the naked eye and what it is made of; the science of the structure of organisms, or of their parts.

androgen (AN·druh·jen)—any of various hormones that control the development of masculine characteristics.

androsterone (an·DRAHS·tuh·rohn)—a male sex hormone.

anemia, anaemia (uh·NEE·mee·uh)—a condition in which the blood is deficient in or produces inadequate amounts of red corpuscles or is deficient in hemoglobin, or both.

anesthesia, anaesthesia (an·us·THEE·zhuh)—a state of insensibility, local or general, with or without loss of consciousness.

anesthetic, anaesthetic (an·US·thet·ik)—substance producing anesthesia.

anesthetize (uh·NES·thuh·tyz)—to render insensible by use of an anesthetic; to make unable to feel sensation, such as pain, cold, or extreme heat.

anethole (an·uh·THOHL)—a colorless crystaline compound from anise and fennel oils, used in perfumery.

aneurosa (an·yuh·ROH·suh)—a localized dilation of a blood vessel.

angelica (an·JEL·ih·kuh)—an herb of the parsley family used in fragrances, mouthwash, toothpastes, and medicinal preparations.

angiectid (an·jee·EK·tid)—abnormal dilation of the blood vessels causing tension and tenderness in the skin.

angiodermatitis (an·jee·oh·dur·muh·TY·tus)—inflammation of the blood vessels of the skin.

angiology (an·jee·AHL·uh·jee)—the science of the blood vessels and lymphatic system.

angioma (an·jee·OH·muh)—a tumor formed of blood vessels or lymphatic vessels.

angiorhexis (an·jee·oh·REK·sus)—rupture of a blood vessel.

angle (ANG·gul)—the space between two lines or surfaces that intersect at a given point; in haircutting, the hair is held away from the head to create elevation; degree of elevation used to determine base relationship in setting the hair.

angora (ang·GOR·uh)—long, silky hair from the angora goat; used in some mannequin heads for its superior white, glossy finish.

angstrom (ANG·strum)—a unit of measurement for the wave length of light.

angular artery (ANG·yoo·lur ART·ur·ee)—the terminal part of the facial artery that supplies the lacrimal sac, the eye muscles, and the sides of the nose.

angular chelitis (ANG·yoo·lur KEE·ly·tus)—an acute or chronic inflammation of the skin around the corners of the mouth.

anhidrosis (an·hy·DROH·sis)—partial or complete lack of perspiration.

anhydration (an·hy·DRAY·shun)—dehydration; removal of water; lacking moisture.

anhydrous (an·HY·drus)—without water; not hydrated.

anidrosis (an·ih·DROH·sis)—a deficiency in producing perspiration.

aniline (AN·ul·un)—a colorless liquid with a faint characteristic odor, obtained from coal tar and other nitrogenous substances; combined with other substances, it forms the aniline colors or dyes derived from coal tar.

aniline dye (AN·ul·un DY)—any dye produced synthetically from coal tar; used in the manufacture of hair-coloring products and fragrances.

animal-human hair (AN·ih·mul-HYOO·mun HAYR)—a blend of animal and human hair that is used in the manufacture of wigs.

anion (AN·eye·on)—the ion that carries a charge of negative electricity; the element that, during electrolysis of a chemcial compound, appears at the positive pole or anode.

anionic (an·eye·AHN·ik)—a base surfactant found in shampoos, producing rich foam that rinses easily.

anise (AN·is)—the fragrant seed of the anise plant, used in medicine, cookery, and in some cosmetic preparations.

ankle (ANG·kul)—the joint connecting the foot and the leg.

ankle bone (ANG·kul BOHN)—the talus; the proximal bone of the foot.

annular (AN·yuh·lur)—ringlike.

annular finger (AN·yuh·lur FING·gur)—the ring finger or third finger of the left hand.

anode (AN·ohd)—the positive terminal of an electric source; a positive electrode.

anodermous (an·uh·DUR·mus)—lacking skin.

anomalous (uh·NAHM·uh·lus)—abnormal; unusual; irregular.

anoxia (uh·NAHK·see·uh)—condition of inefficient oxygen supply to body tissues.

antacid (ant·AS·ud)—a substance that relieves or neutralizes acidity.

antagonist (an·TAG·uh·nust)—in anatomy, a muscle that acts counter to another muscle.

antalkali (ant·AL·kuh·ly)—any substance able to neutralize alkalis.

anterior (an·TEER·ee·ur)—situated before or in front of; the ventral side of the body.

anterior auricular artery (an·TEER·ee·ur aw·RIK·yuh·lur ART·uh·ree)—artery that supplies blood to the anterior part of the ear.

anterior auricular muscle (an·TEER·ee·ur aw·RIK·yuh·lur MUS·ul)—the muscle in front of the ear.

anterior auricular nerve (an·TEER·ee·ur aw·RIK·yuh·lur NURV)—nerve found in the skin anterior to the external ear.

anterior cardiac vein (an·TEER·ee·ur KARD·ee·ak VAYN)—vein located anterior (in front of) the right ventricle; vein affecting the heart.

anterior facial veins (an·TEER·ee·ur FAY·shul VAYNZ)—veins located on the anterior sides of the face; draw into the internal jugular vein located on the sides of the neck.

anterior interosseous artery (an·TEER·ee·ur in·tur·AHS·ee·us ART·uh·ree)—supplies blood to the anterior part of the forearm.

anterior jugular vein (an·TEER·ee·ur JUG·yuh·lur VAYN)—vein located near the midline of the neck that drains into the external jugular or subclavian veins.

anthrax (AN·thraks)—a disease found in man and some animals; has characteristic carbunclelike lesions.

anti (AN·ty)—prefix meaning against or opposed to.

antibacterial (ant·ih·bak·TEER·ee·ul)—destructive to or preventing the growth of bacteria.

antibiotic (ant·ih·by·AHT·ik)—a drug, such as penicillin, made from substances derived from mold or bacterium, that inhibits the growth of bacteria.

antibody (ANT·ih·bahd·ee)—a substance in the blood that builds resistance to disease.

anticatalyst (an·tih·KAT·uh·list)—a substance that stops or inhibits a chemical reaction.

anticathode (an·tih·KATH·ohd)—the electrode in an electron or X-ray tube that receives and reflects rays emitted from a cathode.

antidote (ANT·ih·doht)—an agent preventing or counteracting the action of poison.

antifungal (ant·ih·FUN·gal)—pertaining to a substance that stops or inhibits the growth of fungi.

antigen (ANT·ih·jin)—any of several substances such as toxins, enzymes, or foreign proteins, that stimulates the development of antibodies.

antioxidant (ant·eye·AHK·sih·dent)—preservative that prevents fats from spoiling; that which prevents oxidation.

antiperspirant (ant·ih·PUR·spih·rent)—a strong astringent liquid or cream used to stop the flow of perspiration in the region of the armpits, hands, or feet.

antiphlogistic (ant·ih·fluh·JIS·tik)—reducing or preventing fever or inflammation.

antisepsis (ant·uh·SEP·sis)—a method by which a substance, item, or organism is kept sterile, by preventing the growth of pathogenic bacteria.

antiseptic (ant·uh·SEP·tik)—a chemical agent that may kill, retard, or prevent the growth of bacteria.

antisepticize (an·tuh·SEP·tih·syz)—to make antiseptic by treating with antiseptic preparations.

antitoxin (ant·ih·TAHK·sun)—a substance in serum that binds and neutralizes toxin (poison).

antixerotic (an·tuh·zuh·RAHT·ik)—preventing dryness of the skin.

antripsis (an·TRIP·sis)—in masage, the art of rubbing upward.

anus (AY·nus)—the lower opening of the digestive tract, through which fecal matter is extruded.

aorta (ay·ORT·uh)—the main arterial trunk leaving the heart and carrying blood to the various arteries throughout the body.

aortic semilunar valve (ay·ORT·ik SEM·ih·loo·nur VALV)—heart valve that permits the blood to be pumped from the left ventricle into the aorta.

apex (AY·peks)—the summit or extremity; the upper end of a lung or the heart; the high part of the arch of the eyebrow.

apocrine glands (AP·uh·krin GLANZ)—sweat glands that produce a characteristic odor; found in the underarms and pubic areas of the body.

aponeurosis (ap·uh·noo·ROH·sus)—a broad, flat tendon that serves to connect muscle to the part that it moves.

apparatus (ap·uh·RAT·us)—a collection of instruments or devices adapted for a specific purpose.

appendage (uh·PEN·dij)—an outgrowth attached to an organ or part of the body and dependent on it for growth; a limb or limblike structure.

appendicular skeleton (ap·pen·DIK·yoo·lur SKEL·uh·tun)—consists of bones of the shoulder, upper extremeties, hips, and lower extremities.

appendix (uh·PEN·diks)—the vermiform appendix, a small appendage of the intestine.

apple blossom (AP·ul BLAH·sum)—essence of flowers from the apple tree; used in fragrances.

appliance (uh·PLY·ens)—a device or implement used for a certain purpose.

applicator (AP·lih·kay·tur)—an instrument or item used to apply products; as brushes, combs, spatulas, containers, etc.

apposition (ap·uh·ZISH·un)—the act of fitting together or being fitted together.

apprentice (uh·PREN·tis)—one who learns a trade by working and studying under the direction of others who are already skilled in that trade.

appropriate (uh·PROH·pree·ut)—suitable; fitting.

approximately (uh·PRAHK·sih·mat·lee)—about; nearly.

apricot (AP·rih·kot)—a yellow, juicy fruit similar to a peach; its kernel produces an oil used in some cosmetic preparations; a pinkish-orange color.

aptitude (AP·tih·tood)—natural or acquired ability that makes one suited to pursue a specific activity or career.

aptitude test (AP·tih·tood TEST)—a test designed to determine the ability of an individual to engage in certain activities or to pursue specific career goals.

aqueous (AY·kwee·us)—watery; pertaining to water. Descriptive term for water solution or any medium that is largely composed of water.

arc (ARK)—part of the circumference of a circle; an incomplete circle; in hairstyling, the first half of a shaping is referred to as base direction and the last half of the shaping is called the arc.

arch (ARCH)—a curved or archlike part of the body, such as the arch of the foot; dental arch.

area (AY·ree·uh)—an open space; a limited extent of surface.

areata, alopecia (ay·reh·AH·tuh, al·uh·PEE·shuh)—baldness appearing in spots or patches.

areola (uh·REE·uh·lah)—any small ringlike discoloration; the pigmented ring surrounding the nipple of the breast.

areolar tissue (uh·REE·uh·lar TISH·oo)—loose connective tissue with many interspaces; binds skin to underlying tissues and fills spaces between muscles.

arm (ARM)—the part of the human anatomy from the shoulder joint to the wrist.

arnica (AR·nih·kuh)—an aromatic plant containing astringent and healing qualities; used in cosmetic and medicinal preparations.

aroma (uh·ROH·muh)—a distinctive flavor, fragrance, or odor.

aromatherapy (uh·ROH·muh·THAIR·uh·pee)—the use of aromatic fragrances to induce relaxation; used in the practice of esthetics; facial and body treatments using aromatic oils.

aromatic (air·uh·MAT·ik)—pertaining to or containing aroma; fragrant.

aromatic bitters (air·uh·MAT·ik BIT·urz)—obtained from bitter herbs such as ginger and cinnamon; used in the manufacture of fragrances.

arrectores pilorum (ah·REK·tohr·eez py·LOR·um)—the minute involuntary muscle fiber in the skin attached to the base of the hair follicles.

arrector pili (uh·REK·tor PY·ly) (plural of arrectores pilorum)— small involuntary muscle fibers in the skin attached to the base of the hair follicles.

arrowroot (AIR·oh·root)—named for its use in healing wounds caused by arrows; the root of a starchy plant; used in the manufacture of dusting powders and hair, coloring products.

arsenical compound (ar·SEN·ih·kul KOM·pownd)—a compound used in some hair products and skin medications; it can have a highly caustic action on the skin.

art (ART)—skill; dexterity or facility in performing any operation, intellectual or physical, acquired by experience or study, as the art of hairdressing or hairstyling.

arterial (ar·TEER·ee·ul)—pertaining to an artery.

arteriole (ar·TEER·ee·ohl)—a minute artery; a terminal artery continuous with the capillary network.

arteriosclerosis (ar·teer·ee·oh·skluh·ROH·sus)—an abnormal condition of the arteries marked by loss of elasticity; hardening and thickening of the arterial walls.

artery (AR·tuh·ree)—a muscular and elastic vessel that conveys oxygenated blood from the heart to other parts of the body.

artherosclerosis (ar·thuh·roh·skluh·ROH·sus)—an accumulation of fatty deposits on the inner walls of the arteries.

arthritic (ar·THRIT·ik)—pertaining to or affected with arthritis; inflammation of a joint.

articular (ar·TIK·yuh·lur)—pertaining to the junction of two or more skeletal parts, or to the muscle or ligament associated with a joint. Articular cartilage provides smooth shock absorbing surface where two bones meet to form a joint.

articulate (ar·TIK·yoo·layt)—divided into individual points; made up of distinctive parts.

articulation (ar·tik·yoo·LAY·shun)—in anatomy, the junction of two or more skeletal parts.

artificial (ar·tih·FISH·ul)—not natural; imitation.

artifical eyelashes (ar·tih·FISH·ul EYE·lash·ez)—eyelashes made from synthetic or human hair to be glued to or in place of one's own lashes.

artificial hair (ar·tih·FISH·ul HAYR)—manufactured hairlike fiber made of dynel, nylon, etc., which is employed in the construction of lower-priced wigs and hair pieces.

artificialis, acne (ar·tih·fish·AL·is AK·nee)—a papular eruption caused by external irritants such as tar.

artificial nails (ar·tih·FISH·ul NAYLZ)—plastic nails formed and hardened on the fingers, or premanufactured and then glued to the natural nails.

artist (AR·tist)—one who is skilled in fine arts; in cosmetology, one skilled in the artistry of hairstyling and/or makeup application.

ascertain (as·UR·TAYN)—to acquire an accurate knowledge of.

ascorbic acid (uh·SKOR·bik AS·ud)—chemical component of vitamin C; scurvy-preventing vitamin found in fruits and vegetables.

asepsis (ay·SEP·sis)—a condition in which pathogenic bacteria are absent.

aseptic (ay·SEP·tik)—free from pathogenic bacteria.

ash (ASH)—a drab shade containing no red or gold tones; dominated by greens, blues, violets, or grays. May be used to counteract unwanted warm tones.

ash blond (ASH BLAHND)—whitish-gray light hair color with no red or gold tones.

Asiatic hair (ay·zhih·AT·ik HAYR)—human hair from Eastern nations; dark, straight, coarse hair generally used in inexpensive wigs and hair pieces.

asperation (as·per·AY·shun)—a mechanical method used to remove dead surface cells from the skin.

asphyxia (as·FIK·see·uh)—a lack of oxygen or excess of carbon dioxide in the body causing unconsciousness.

asphyxic skin (as·FIK·sik SKIN)—skin lacking oxygen.

aspirator (AS·pih·ray·tur)—an appliance for drawing fluids from the body by suction.

assimilate (uh·SIM·ih·layt)—to absorb; to incorporate into the body; to digest.

assimilation (uh·sim·ih·LAY·shun)—the incorporation of materials prepared by digestion of food, into the tissues of the body.

asteatosis (as·tee·ah·TOH·sis)—dry and scaly skin due to a deficiency or absence of the sebaceous secretion, called sebum.

asthma (AZ·muh)—a condition characterized by coughing and difficulty in breathing.

astrictive (uh·STRIK·tiv)—astringent; styptic.

astringent (uh·STRIN·jent)—a substance in cosmetics and medicines that causes contraction of the tissues and checks secretions.

asymmetric (ay·sih·MET·rik)—lacking symmetrical balance; off center.

asymmetrical (ay·sih·MET·rih·kul)—off center; unbalanced; unequal in proportion; a hairstyle that has unequal proportions designed to balance facial features.

ataxia (uh·TAK·see·uh)—a term used in physical therapy pertaining to irregularity in bodily functions or muscular movements; inability to coordinate voluntary movements.

athlete's foot (ATH·leets FOOT)—a fungal foot infection; ringworm; medical name, epidermophytosis.

atlas (AT·lis)—in anatomy, the first cervical vertebra in the spinal column.

atmosphere (AT·mus·feer)—the whole mass of air surrounding the earth; the effect produced by decor, furnishings, or the environment.

atom (AT·um)—the smallest particle of an element that can exist and still retain the chemical properties of the element; particles that all substances are composed of.

atomize (AT·uh·myz)—to reduce to minute particles or to a fine spray.

atomizer (AT·uh·myz·ur)—a container used to spray a fine liquid mist of perfume, hairspray, or other product.

atrichia (uh·TRIK·ee·uh)—absence of hair; congenital or acquired.

atrium (AY·tree·um)—the auricle or upper chamber of the heart.

atrophy (A·truh·fee)—a wasting away of the tissues of the body or of a part of the body from lack of nutrition or because of injury or disease.

attachment (uh·TACH·ment)—the physical connection by which one thing is fastened to another.

attenuate (uh·TEN·yoo·ayt)—to make thin; to increase the fluidity or thinness of the blood or other secretions; to lessen the effect of an agent.

attolens aurem (AT·uh·lenz OH·rem)—auricularis superior; muscle that elevates the ear slightly.

attrahens (AT·ruh·henz)—a muscle that draws or pulls forward.

attrahens aurem (AT·ruh·henz OH·rem)—a muscle that pulls the ear forward.

attune (uh·TOON)—to bring into harmony with.

auburn (AW·burn)—a reddish-brown color.

auditory nerve (AWD·uh·tohr·ee NURV)—eighth cranial nerve, controlling the sense of hearing.

aurantiosis cutis (oh·ran·TY·uh·sus KYOO·tis)—a condition of the skin that renders it a golden yellow; sometimes caused by excessive intake of carotene.

auricle (AW·rih·kul)—the external ear; one of the upper cavities of the heart.

auricular (aw·RIK·yuh·lur)—pertaining to the ear or cardiac auricle.

auricular anterior artery (aw·RIK·yuh·lur an·TEER·ee·ur ART·uh·ree)—artery that supplies blood to the anterior part of the ear.

auricularis, anterior (aw·rik·yuh·LAIR·is, an·TEER·ee·ur)—the anterior auricularis; the muscle in front of the ear that draws the ear forward.

auricularis, posterior (aw·rik·yuh·LAIR·is poh·STEER·ee·ur)—the muscle behind the ear that draws the ear backward.

auricularis, superior (aw·rik·yuh·LAIR·is soo·PEER·ee·ur)—muscle, above the ear that draws the ear upward.

auricular nerve (aw·RIK·yuh·lur NURV)—nerve that receives stimuli from the skin around the ear.

auricular posterior artery (aw·RIK·yuh·lur poh·STEER·ee·ur ART·ur·ee)—posterior artery that supplies blood to the scalp and paratid gland.

auriculotemporal nerve (aw·RIK·yuh·loh·TEM·puh·rul NURV)—sensory nerve affecting the temple and external ear; up to the top of the skull.

auto (AW·toh)—denoting self; acting upon one's self, or by itself.

autoclave (AW·toh·klayv)—a vessel or chamber producing steam for the sterilization of instruments.

auto condensation (AW·toh kon·den·SAY·shun)—a method of applying high-frequency current for therapeutic purposes by making the patient part of the condenser.

autolysis (aw·TAHL·uh·sis)—the disintegration of cells and tissues by the action of enzymes already present; self-digestion of tissues within a living body.

automatic (aw·toh·MAT·ik)—acting from forces within; self-acting; largely or entirely involuntary.

autonomic; autonomous (aw·toh·NAHM·ik; aw·TAHN·uh·mus)—independent in origin, action, or function; self-governing.

autonomic nervous system (aw·toh·NAHM·ik NURV·us SIS·tum)—the part of the nervous system that controls the involuntary muscles; regulates the action of glands, smooth muscles, and the heart.

avitaminosis (ay·vyt·uh·muh·NOH·sus)—a disease that results from lack of vitamins in the diet, such as scurvy (vitamin C) or rickets (vitamin D).

avocado (ah·vah·KAH·doh)—a pear-shaped, green pulpy fruit; its oils are used in some cosmetics and in facial masks to cleanse and moisturize the skin.

axial skeleton (AK·see·ul SKEL·uh·tun)—bones of the skull, thorax, vertebral column, and hyoid bone.

axilla (ag·ZIL·uh)—armpit; the region between the arm and the thoracic wall bounded by the pectoralis major muscle and the latissimus dorsi muscle.

axillary (AK·suh·lair·ee)—pertaining to the axilla or armpit.

axillary artery (AK·suh·lair·ee AR·tur·ee)—artery associated with the region of the muscles of the upper arm, chest, shoulder, and the skin of the pectoral region.

axillary glands (AK·suh·lair·ee GLANZ)—the axillary lymph nodes.

axillary nerves (AK·suh·lair·ee NURVZ)—nerves located in the shoulder and armpit regions that stimulate deltoid muscles.

axillary veins (AK·suh·lair·ee VAYNZ)—veins located within the regions of the armpits.

axiom (AK·see·um)—an established principal or rule.

axis (AK·sis)—the line around which a body turns or rotates, or around which parts are arranged.

axon (AK·sahn)—a long nerve fiber extending from the nerve cell body that sends messages to other neuron, glands, and muscles.

azo dye (AY·zoh DYE)—a group of synthetic dyes derivable from azobenzene; used in some hair-coloring products.

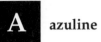

azuline (AZH·oo·leen)—an intensely blue liquid hydrocarbon found in the oil of chamomile flowers; used as a coloring agent and in some shampoos.

azure (AZH·oor)—pertaining to the color of a clear, blue sky; sky blue.

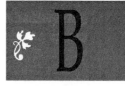

babassu (bahd·uh·SOO)—the oil from nuts produced by the Brazilian palm tree; widely used in making soap and similar products.

baby fine hair (BAY·bee FYN HAYR)—a hair fiber that is extremely fine due to its very small cortex diameter and delicate construction.

baby oil (BAY·bee OYL)—a product made of mild, soothing oils such as lanolin, vegetable, or mineral oils.

bacillus (bah·SILL·us); pl., **bacilli** (-eye)—rod-shaped bacterium that cause diseases such as tetanus (lockjaw), influenza, typhoid fever, tuberculosis.

back (BAK)—the rear or posterior part of the body or head; the part of the body nearest the spine.

backbone (BAK·bohn)—the spinal or vertebral column.

back brushing (BAK BRUSH·ing)—a method used in styling hair; while holding the ends of hair strands up and outward, the strands are brushed back toward the scalp to create a look of softness and bulk in some hair designs.

back combing (BAK KOHM·ing)—combing small sections of hair from the ends toward the scalp, causing shorter hair to mat at the scalp, forming a cushion or base; also called teasing.

back design (BAK dih·ZYN)—design of the hairstyle at the back of the head.

backhand (BAK·hand)—a movement made with the back of the hand turned in the direction of the movement; used in barbering techniques.

back of head (BAK UV HED)—the area of the head behind the ears.

backsweep (BAK·sweep)—sweeping the hair backward with comb or brush; also upsweep: hair is swept upward into the desired style.

backward curls (BAK·ward KURLZ)—curls wound in a counterclockwise direction on the left side of the head; curls wound in a clockwise direction on the right side of the head; curls with stems directed toward the back of the head.

backward direction (BAK·ward dih·REK·shun)—movement used when brushing, combing, winding, or wrapping the hair away from the face.

bacteria (bak·TEER·ee·ah); pl., **bacterium** (bak·TEER·ee·uhm)—widely distributed unicellular microorganisms with both plant and animal characteristics; the three varieties are bacillus, coccus, and spirillum; some are harmful; some are harmless; commonly known as microbes or germs.

bacterial (bak·TEER·ee·ul)—pertaining to bacteria.

bactericide (bak·TEER·uh·syd)—an agent that destroys bacteria.

bacteriology (bak·teer·ee·AHL·uh·jee)—the science that deals with microorganisms called bacteria.

bacterium (bak·TEER·ee·uhm); pl., **bacteria** (bak·TEER·ee·ah)—unicellular vegetable microorganism.

bakelite shield (BAYK·lyt SHEELD)—a shield made of a substance that strongly resists chemicals; used as a scalp protector.

balance (BAYL·uns)—harmony or proportion created in a hairstyle by the proper degree of height and width.

baldness (BALLD·nes)—a deficiency of hair; hair loss.

balm (BALL·m)—an aromatic resinous substance used as a medicine or fragrance.

bal masque makeup (BAl MASK MAYK·up)—a fantasy makeup applied with exaggerated colors and designs; makeup based on a fantasy theme as an added attraction at hairdressing and cosmetology shows, or in makeup competitions.

balneology (bal·nee·AHL·uh·jee)—the science of treating disease by baths in the waters of mineral springs.

balneotherapy (bal·nee·oh·THAYR·uh·pee)—the science of treating disease, burns, emotional disorders, or skin diseases by use of therapeutic baths.

balsam of Peru (BAl·sum UV PUR·oo)—a thick, dark brown, oily fluid exuded from the cut bark of Tolurfera pereirae; used as an antiseptic and astringent.

banana oil (buh·NAH·nuh OYL)—oil from the fruit of the banana (isoamye acetole) used in cosmetics and medicinal preparations.

band (BAND)—a narrow strip of hair that is discolored; a narrow strip of material placed around the hairline when giving facials or applying makeup; elastic fastener on permanent wave rod.

bandeau hair piece (BAND·oh HAYR·pees)—hair piece sewn to a headband covering the hairline; band wig.

band wig (band WIG)—bandeau-style hair piece.

bang (BAYNG)—front hair cut so as to fall over the forehead; often used in the plural, as to "wear bangs."

bang frame (BAYNG FRAYM)—the shaping of bangs so as to frame the face.

banker's pin (bayn·KURS PIN)—also called a "T" pin. It resembles the letter T and is used to secure a hair piece to the styling block.

barba (BAR·ba)—the growth of beard hair of either men or women.

barber (BAR·bur)—one whose occupation includes haircutting, hairdressing, shaving and trimming beards, and related services.

barber chair (BAR·bur CHAYR)—a specially designed chair for barber clients; a hydraulic, reclining chair with adjustable footrest and headrest.

barber comb (BAR·bur KOHM)—a comb of plastic or hard rubber with a 3/4-inch wide set of teeth tapering to a narrow end about 1-inch wide with a set of fine teeth; an implement for combing and styling the hair.

barber science (BAR·bur SY·ens)—the study of the beard and hair and their treatment.

barber shop (BAR·bur SHOP)—the place of business where the barber's clients receive services.

barber's itch (BAR·burz ITCH)—tinea sycosis; ringworm of the beard; chronic inflammation of the hair follicles.

barbiturate (BAR·bich·yoo·it)—a sedative or sleeping pill; a drug thatcan interfere with healthy body metabolism when taken in excess.

barium sulfide (BAYR·ee·um SUL·fyd)—a yellowish powder that decomposes in water with liberation of hydrogen sulfide gas; used in dipilatory preparations.

barrel (BAYR·ul)—the part of a thermal heating iron or curling iron that contains the heating element.

barrel curl (BAYR·ul KURL)—a curl, wound in croquignole fashion, with large center opening and fastened to the head in a standing position; a pin curl technique used in place of rollers.

barrette (bar·ET)—a small bar with a clasp used to pin the hair in place.

basal (BAY·zul)—foundation; located at the base which is the lowest or supporting part of anything; lowest or least.

basal layer (bay·ZUL LAY·ur)—the layer of cells at the base of the epidermis closest to the dermis.

base (BAYS)—a cosmetic preparation applied to the face to form a foundation upon which to apply other cosmetics such as powder and cheek color; in wiggery, the foundation upon which the hair is attached to form a wig; in hairstyling, the portion of a curl that is attached to the scalp; in chemistry, the chief substance of a compound; an electropositive element that unites with an acid to form a salt.

base coat (BAYS KOHT)—a clear liquid similar to nail enamel that is applied to fingernails before the application of colored polish; also used as a protective top coat.

base cream (bays creem)—an oily cream used to protect the scalp during a hair straightening process.

base direction (BAYS dy·REK·shun)—a line of motion from the starting point or foundation created in setting the hair.

base of a curl (BAYS UV UH KURL)—that portion of the hair strand being curled that isnearest the scalp.

base part (BAYS PART)—the working part of the hair toward which the curl is rolled.

base, protective (BAYS proh·TEK·tiv)—in hairdressing: a petroleum base applied to the entire scalp to protect it from the active agents contained in the chemical hair relaxer.

base substance (BAYS SUB·stans)—a supporting or carrying ingredient in a preparation that serves as a vehicle for active ingredients in some medicinal and cosmetic preparations.

basic (BAYS·ik)—pertaining to the fundamental or foundation knowledge and skills of any craft, skill, or profession.

basify (BAYS·if·eye)—to change into a base by chemical means; to make alkaline.

basil (BAY·zil)—any of certain aromatic plants of the mint family; used in cookery and in some cosmetics.

basilar plexis vein (BAY·zil·lar PLEX·is VAYN)—vein located at the base part of the occipital bone.

basilic vein (bay·ZIL·ic VAYN)—the large vein on the inside of the arm.

basin (BAYS·in)—a shallow vessel with sloping sides used to hold liquids, such as a shampoo bowl or a small vessel for manicures or pedicures.

bath (BATH)—to wash or dip in water or other liquid.

bath lotion (BATH LOH·shun)—a fragrant emollient applied after the bath.

bath oil (BATH OYL)—emulsifying oil; a fragrant oil, usually vegetable or mineral oil used after the bath or in the bath water to soften and soothe the skin.

bath powder (BATH POW·dur)—dusting powder, usually of scented talcum powder to which boric, starch, and zinc may have been added.

bath salts (BATH SAWLTS)—rock salt to which fragrances and color are usually added; used to soften water and aid in cleansing the skin.

battery (BAT·ur·ee)—an apparatus containing two or more cells for generating electricity.

bayberry plant (BAY·bair·ee PLANT)—the leaves of myrcia acris that yield oil of bay used to make bay rum.

bayberry wax (BAY·bair·ee WAKS)—wax from the bayberry shrub used in some hair tonics and soaps.

bay rum (BAY RUM)—an after-shave lotion; a tonic and astringent.

beaker (BEE·kur)—a vessel of glass with a lip for pouring; used in chemical analyses and in mixing preparations.

beard (BEERD)—the hair on a man's face, especially on the chin (the hair over the upper lip is usually called a mustache, which may be a part of a full beard).

beat (BEET)—to whip or stir rapidly.

beautician (byoo·TISH·un)—a term used to describe one skilled in the art of beautifying the appearance of a person; licensed to perform cosmetology services.

beauty clinic (BYOO·tee KLIN·ik)—a space set aside in a cosmetology school where students can practice their skills on clients before becoming employed in a salon.

beauty culture (BYOO·tee KUL·chur)—pertaining to cosmetology; the study and practice of the improvement of personal appearance; personal grooming performed on another person.

beauty operator (BYOO·tee OP·ur·ay·tur)—a term, considered outdated, used to describe one who works as a hairdresser and cosmetologist.

beauty parlor (BYOO·tee PAR·lur)—an outdated term used to describe the place of business of a hairdresser or cosmetologist; also called a beauty shop or beauty salon.

beauty salon (BYOO·tee sah·LAHN)—the term used to describe the place of business of a cosmetologist or hairdresser (also called hairdressing or facial salon); a full-service salon supplies all cosmetology services, such as care of hair, skin, or nails; a facial salon supplies facial services, such as massage, treatments, and makeup.

beauty spot (BYOO·tee SPAHT)—a small patch or mark put on the face as an accent; a mole or other natural mark that is accented; originally, a small patch of fabric used to cover a blemish.

bed hair (BED HAYR)—hair that has separated from the papilla and lies loosely in the follicle.

beehive (BEE·hyv)—a hairstyle shaped like a beehive, popular in the 1960s; the hair was teased, pulled back, and formed into the desired shape.

beer (BEER)—a fermented beverage made from grain and hops; used as a hair rinse to add body.

beeswax (BEEZ·waks)—wax given out by bees, from which they make their honeycomb; used in making of hair pieces to add strength to sewn parts; also used to dress unruly ends.

beige (BAYZH)—a color term used to describe hair that is pale yellow-gray or pale gray-brown; a type of blond.

belly (BEL·ee)—the abdomen; the prominent part of the bulging muscle.

benign (bih·NYN)—mild in character; in relation to tumors, the opposite of malignant; characterizing any growth not likely to reoccur after removal.

bentonite (BENT·un·yt)—a porous clay from volcanic ash; used as a facial mask to absorb oil on the face; used in a variety of cosmetic products to thicken lotions, emulsify oils, and suspend pigments.

benzine (BEN·zeen)—an inflammable liquid derived form petroleum and used as a cleaning fluid.

benzoic acid (BEN·zoh·ik AS·ud)—a preservative and antiseptic substance used in mouthwashes, after-shave lotions, deodorants, and creams.

benzoin (BEN·zuh·wun)—a balsamic resin used as a stimulant and also as a perfume.

benzoldehyde (ben·ZAHL·duh·hyd)—a liquid with an odor similar to that of almonds; used in the dye and perfume industries.

benzoyl peroxide (BEN·zoyl puh·RAHK·syd)—an ingredient used in cosmetic preparation and used to treat skin eruptions such as acne.

bergamot oil (BUR·guh·mant OYL)—oil extracted from the rind of citrus fruits; used in some perfumes and lotions.

beriberi (BAIR·ee BAIR·ee)—a deficiency disease characterized by weakness, anemia, etc.; due to lack of vitamin B1 in the diet.

berloque dermatitis (ber·LOK der·mah·TYT·us)—a skin eruption characterized by red patches on the face and neck, generally caused by a reaction to a chemical (bergapten) found in some perfumes and other liquid cosmetics.

beta helix (BAY·tuh HEE·liks)—term indicating that the spiral of the body of the poly peptide chains within the cortex of the hair is in the second position; the spiral is stretched but can return to its alpha or first position when released.

bevel (BEV·ul)—to slope the edge of a surface; in haircutting, to taper the ends of the hair.

bevel cut (BEV·ul KUT)—haircutting technique of rolling a strand of hair upward before cutting so that top of strand is slightly shorter, encouraging the hair to turn upward.

beveling (BEV·ul·ing)—a technique for creating fullness in a haircut; cutting the ends of the hair at a slight taper.

bi (BY)—a prefix denoting two, twice, double.

bias (BY·us)—a diagonal or slanted line; to cut on the bias.

bib (BIB)—an item of plastic or cloth placed across the client's chest and shoulders and around the back to protect clothing; a neutralizing bib has a pocket hem to catch solution.

bicarbonate of soda (by·KAR·buh·nayt UV SOH·duh)—baking soda; relieves burns, itching, urticarial lesions, and insect bites; is often used in bath powders as an aid to cleansing oily skin; adding baking soda to the water in which instruments are to be boiled will keep them bright.

biceps (BY·seps)—a muscle having two heads or points of attachment, as the biceps brackic, which rotates and flexes the forearm, and the biceps femores, which flexes the knee and extends the hip joint.

bichloride (by·KLOHR·yd)—a compound having two parts or equivalents of chlorine to one of the other elements.

bicipital (by·SIP·ut·ul)—pertaining to the biceps.

bicuspid valve (by·KUS·pid VALV)—heart valve allowing blood to flow from the left atrium to the left ventricle.

bigoudi (big·OO·dee)—a small wooden curler employed in the formation of wigs for the winding of curls.

bilateral (by·LAT·uh·rul)—pertaining to or affecting two sides.

bile (BYL)—a bitter alkaline fluid, greenish yellow to brown, secreted by the liver; it aids in the remulsification, digestion, and absorption of fats.

bi-level haircut (by·LEV·ul HAYR·kut)—a style that divides the head into two separate design lines.

binder (BYND·ur)—a substance such as gum arabic, glycerin, and sorbitol with the ability to increase consistency and hold ingredients together; used in compact powders, toothpaste, and like cosmetics.

binding (BYND·ing)—in wiggery, ribbon used at the edges of the netting to secure the edges and to connect two pieces together; also used for reinforcement; tubular binding is used to contain wire and springs.

binocular (bin·OK·yuh·lur)—referring to the use of both eyes; a binocular optical instrument.

biocatalyst (by·oh·KAT·ul·est)—a substance that acts to promote or modify some physiological process, especially an enzyme, vitamin, or hormone.

biochemistry (by·oh·KEM·is·tree)—the chemistry of living animals and plants; the study of chemical compounds and processes occurring in living organisms.

biodegradable (by·oh·dee·GRAYD·uh·bul)—the ability of a substance to decay organically or naturally.

bioelectricity (by·oh·ee·lek·TRIHS·ih·tee)—electric phenomena occurring in living tissues; effects of electric current on living tissues.

bioesthegenics (by·oh·es·thuh·JEN·iks)—scientific study of the skin as an organ; relating to organic skin care.

bioflavonoid (by·oh·FLAY·vuh·noyd)—a biologically active flavonoid; also called vitamin P; considered an aid to healthy skin and found most abundantly in fruits of the citrus variety.

biology (by·AHL·uh·jee)—the science of life and living things.

biorhythm (BY·oh·rith·um)—any regular pattern or change of cycle in an organism, such a speriodic variations in body temperature, blood pressure, etc.

biostimulant (by·oh·STIM·yoo·lant)—an agent used to stimulate activity in living tissue.

biotin (BY·uh·tihn)—a vitamin B complex, found in small amounts in plant and animal tissue.

biphosphate (by·FAHS·fayt)—a salt of phosphoric acid in which one of the three hydrogen atoms of the acid is replaced by a base.

bipolar (by·POH·lar)—of or having two poles; characterized by opposite natures.

bipolarity (by·poh·LAIR·ih·tee)—the use of two electrodes in the stimulation of muscles or nerves; the condition of having two processes extending from opposite poles.

birchwood stick (BURCH·wood STIK)—a thin stick used as a swab or stirring implement, similar to an orangewood stick, which is used as a manicure implement.

birthmark (BURTH·mark)—any mark on the face or body that is present at birth, usually lasting; a form of nevus.

bisulfate (by·SUL·fayt)—an acid sulfate.

bisulfide (by·SUL·fyd)—a compound containing two atoms of sulfur; a disulfide.

bisulfite (by·SUL·fyt)—an acid sulfite.

biterminal (by·TUR·mih·nul)—two terminals or poles of an electric source.

black (BLAK)—a neutral hue having no brightness or color; the maximum degree of darkness in hair coloring; a term used to describe dark skin and hair; the opposite of white.

blackhead (BLAK·hed)—a comdone; a plug of hardened sebaceous matter that has darkened upon contact with air.

bladder (BLAD·ur)—a membranous sac that serves as a reservoir for holding urine.

bland (BLAND)—pertaining to nonirritating substances such as a bland, mild diet free of roughage or irritating spices; a smooth mild facial.

blastema (bla·STEE·muh)—the hypothetical lymph or fluid from which cells and organs are formed; the formative cellular matrix from which an organ, tissue, or part is derived.

bleach (BLEECH)—a chemical preparation used to remove the color from hair; also used in some preparations to lighten skin pigmentation.

bleached hair (BLEECHT HAYR)—hair from which the color has been wholly or partially removed by means of a bleaching or lightening agent.

bleaching solution (BLEECH·ing suh·LOO·shun)—hydrogen peroxide with the addition of ammonia.

bleach pack (BLEECH PAK)—a bleach formula prepared in a thick consistency.

bleb (BLEEB)—a blister of the skin filled with watery fluid.

bleeding (BLEED·ing)—seepage of tint/lightener from foil or cap due to improper application.

blemish (BLEM·ish)—a mark, spot, or defect on the skin.

blemish cover (BLEM·ish KUV·ur)—a cosmetic in stick or cream form, based on alcohol, oil, wax and pigments; used to conceal minor blemishes.

blend (BLEND)—to meet or join; in hair coloring: to mix or blend colors to achieve various hair colors; in haircutting: to graduate from shorter to longer lengths; in makeup: to mix together so there is no line of demarcation.

blending (BLEND·ing)—the physical act of merging one tint of tone with another during hair color and lightening applications; mixing of makeup colors; connection between two or more shapes in hair design.

blepharoplasty (BLEF·uh·roh·plas·tee)—plastic surgery of the eyebrows and/or eyelids.

blister (BLIS·tur)—a vesicle; a collection of serous fluid causing an elevation of the skin.

block (BLAHK)—to mark off or indicate sections in an outline to be followed when subsectioning the hair.

blockhead (BLAHK·hed)—a head-shaped form usually made of canvas-covered cork, to which a wig is secured for fitting, cleaning, and styling.

block holder (BLAHK HOLD·ur)—a clamping device used to hold a blockhead form to a table.

blocking (BLAHK·ing)—the act of dividing the hair into sections to work on smaller parts.

block point (BLAHK POYNT)—headless steel pin used to attach hair pieces or other materials to the head block.

blond on blond (BLAHND on BLAHND)—two shades (colors) used to create light and darker strands of hair to achieve a natural sun-bleached look.

blonde; blond (BLAHND)—a person with fair complexion, light hair, and eyes; a term used to describe hair shades and tints that range from light yellowish-brown to platinum or silver white.

blonding (BLAHND·ing)—the process of lightening the hair, sometimes in preparation for the application of a toner, and sometimes as an end result in itself.

blood (BLUD)—the nutritive fluid circulating through the body (heart, veins, arteries, and capillaries) to supply oxygen and nutrients to cells and tissues.

blood platelets (BLUD PLAYT·lehts)—blood cells smaller than red or white corpuscles that aid in the formation of clots.

blood poisoning (BLUD POY·zun·ing)—an infection which gets into the bloodstream. (*See* septicemia.)

blood pressure (BLUD PREHSH·ur)—the pressure exerted by the circulatory blood on the walls of the blood vessels or heart.

blood stream (BLUD STREEM)—the flow of blood in its circulation through the body.

blood vascular system (BLUD VAS·kyoo·lur SIS·tum)—the group of structures: the heart, arteries, veins, and capillaries that distribute blood throughout the body.

blood vessel (BLUD VES·ul)—an artery, vein, or capillary.

blotch (BLAHCH)—a spot or eruption on the skin.

blouse (BLOWS)—in hairstyling, a loose fitting at the base of a pin curl or wound perm rod; to push up to create fullness or puffiness.

blow-dry (BLOH-dry)—to use a blow-drying machine to dry and style the hair in a single process, usually without presetting; a service performed after a haircut and shampoo when a soft style is desired.

blower (BLOH·ur)—a small hand-held hair dryer used when styling and blow-drying the hair.

blow-out (BLOH-owt)—a term used to describe styling of the hair when it is done with a blower and brush; the process in which hair is styled with a blower and brush.

blow-out perm (BLOH-out PURM)—a permanent wave that is styled with a blow-dryer, brush, and comb; a permanent wave that does not require setting with rollers or pin curls.

blow-style (BLOH·styl)—a hairstyle created with the blow-dryer, brush, and comb.

blue (BLOO)—the color of a clear sky, between green and violet in the spectrum; a primary color; the color of venous blood that shows through the skin as in a bruise.

blue light (BLOO LYT)—a therapeutic lamp used to soothe the nerves.

blue nails (BLOO NAYLZ)—nail condition caused by poor blood circulation or a heat disorder.

blue nevus (BLOO NEE·vus)—a nevus (birthmark) composed of spindle-shaped pigmented melanocytes usually in the middle and lower portions of the dermis.

bluing rinse (BLOO·ing RINS)—a temporary coloring used to neutralize the unbecoming yellowish tinge in gray or white hair.

blunt (BLUNT)—having a thick or rounded edge or end.

blunt cutting (BLUNT KUT·ing)—cutting straight across a strand of hair without thinning or tapering. (*See* club cutting.)

blusher (BLUSH·ur)—a powdered substance, also called "rouge," used to add color or highlights to the cheeks or to shade areas of the face.

boar bristle brush (BOR BRIS·ul BRUSH)—a brush made with the short, stiff hairs from a wild boar; considered to be less damaging to hair than other types of bristle; also called "natural bristle brush."

boardwork (BORD·wurk)—the art of making hairpieces.

boardworker (BORD·wur·kur)—one who makes hair pieces.

bob (BAHB)—pertaining to a short, blunt haircut for women and children; to cut long hair to shoulder length or shorter.

bobby pin (BAHB·ee PIN)—a long "U"-shaped clamp or clasplike pin with the ends pressing close together, used to hold the hair in place in a style or hair set.

body (BAHD·ee)—in anatomy: the human or animal frame and its organs; in cosmetology: the consistency or solidarity of texture or quality of liveliness and springiness the hair possesses.

body brushing (BAHD·ee BRUSH·ing)—a treatment for the body that benefits circulation and removes dead surface cells from the epidermis.

body cream (BAHD·ee KREEM)—a creamy substance used for smoothing and softening the skin of the entire body.

body image (BAHD·ee IM·ij)—the conscious and unconscious concept a person has of his or her body as it may be perceived by others.

body lotion (BAHD·ee LOH·shun)—a smooth liquid to be used on the body following the bath or a skin treatment; a lotion applied after the removal of superfluous hair from any part of the body.

body perm (BAHD·ee PURM)—a permanent wave given to impart body rather than curl or visible wave to the hair.

body surface area (BAHD·ee SUR·fus AIR·ee·uh)—the area covered by a person's skin, expressed in square meters.

body wave (BAHD·ee WAYV)—a large wave pattern created by a permanent wave as a foundation for a style.

body wrap (BAHD·ee RAP)—a wrapping treatment used to treat cellulite, the condition of fatty deposits; the substances used and the wrapping technique have a diuretic effect that sometimes aids weight reduction.

boil (BOYL)—a furuncle; a subcutaneous abscess caused by bacteria that enter through the hair follicles.

boiling point (BOYL·ing POYNT)—212°F (fahrenheit) or 100°C (Celsius); the temperature at which a liquid begins to boil.

bond (BAHND)—the attractive force that binds one atom to another in a molecule, resulting from the transfer or sharing of one or more electrons, often represented in formulas by a line or dot.

bond breaker (BAHND BRAYK·ur)—a substance that has the ability to disrupt or destroy the bond units of chemical compounds.

bone (BOHN)—the hard tissue forming the framework of the body.

bone tissue (BOHN TISH·oo)—the substance forming the layers of bone and dentine of the teeth.

bonnet (BAHN·et)—in hairstyling: a head covering made of rubber or plastic with perforations used for frosting, highlighting, or glazing strands of hair. Also called a frosting or highlighting cap.

book end wrap (BOOK END RAP)—technique of protecting hair ends with porous paper by folding single end paper over the hair strands like an envelope; conducive to the use of concave rods.

boom boom iron (BOOM BOOM EYE·urn)—also called bop iron. A thermal curling iron with oversized rod and groove.

booster (BOOST·ur)—oxidizer added to hydrogen peroxide to increase its chemical action. (*See* activator.)

borax (BOR·aks)—sodium tetraborate; a white powder used as an antiseptic and cleansing agent.

borderline (BOR·dur·lyn)—pertaining to being neither normal nor abnormal; doubtful; difficult to classify; a line of demarcation; between.

boric acid (BOR·ik AS·ud)—acidum boricum; used as a mild antiseptic dusting powder and in liquid form as an eyewash or healing agent.

bouffant (boo·FAHNT)—the degree of fullness, height, and width in a particular hairstyle; a wide, full, teased hairstyle popular in the 1960s and early 1970s.

boutique (boo·TEEK)—a specialty shop or department that may be situated within a salon, in which cosmetics or accessories are sold.

brachial artery (BRAY·kee·ul ART·uh·ree)—the main artery of the upper arm.

brachialis (bray·kih·AY·lis)—the muscle that flexes the elbow joint.

brachioradialis (bray·kih·oh·ray·dih·AL·us)—a flexor muscle of the radial side of the forearm.

brachium (BRAY·kih·um)—the part of the arm above the elbow.

bracing (BRAYS·ing)—the cotton that holds a hair piece foundation in the proper position on the wooden block during the process of manufacture.

braid (BRAYD)—three interwoven strands of hair that form a repetitive pattern; a braided or coiled hair switch that is used to create different hairstyles; a three-stemmed switch joined with a loop at the top; to weave, entwine, or interlace hair strands.

brain (BRAYN)—that part of the central nervous system contained in the cranial cavity, and consisting of the cerebrum, the cerebellum, the pons, and the medulla oblongata; controls sensation, muscles, glandular activity, and the power to think and feel.

brain stem (BRAYN STEM)—intricate masses of nerve fiber that relay and trasmit impulses from one part of the brain to another.

brassy tone (BRAS·ee TOHN)—in hair coloring; a harsh color quality exhibiting excess red, orange, or gold.

breakage (BRAYK·ij)—a condition in which hair splits and breaks off; caused by damage to the hair.

breastbone (BREST·bohn)—the sternum; the narrow, flat bone located in the middle of the chest.

brewer's yeast (BROO·urz YEEST)—a yellowish substance consisting of small plants or cells that grow rapidly in a liquid containing sugar; a natural source of vitamin B complex and protein.

brightening (BRYT·un·ing)—adding highlights and luster to the hair by lightening or toning the natural shade.

brilliantine (BRIL·yun·teen)—an oily preparation that imparts luster to the hair.

bristle (BRIS·ul)—the short, stiff hair of a brush; short, stiff hair of an animal used in brushes.

brittle hair (BRIT·ul HAYR)—hair that is dry and fragile and is easily broken.

broad (BRAWD)—wide; having great breadth as distinguished from length; having much width or breadth; not narrow.

bromide (BROH·myd)—a compound that is formed by the replacement of the hydrogen in hydrobromic acid by a metal or organic radical; such substances are used to allay nervous excitement and are employed as sedatives.

bromidrosis (broh·mih·DROH·sis)—excretion of perspiration (sweat) that has an unpleasant odor.

bromo-acid (broh·moh-AS·ud)—a soluble dye used to impart a red indelible color in lipsticks and similar cosmetics.

bromoderma (broh·moh·DUR·muh)—a skin eruption due to the ingestion of bromides.

bronchial (BRAHNG·kee·ul)—pertaining to or involving the bronchi and their branches.

bronchus (BRAHNG·kus); pl., **bronchi** (-kee)—the main branch of the windpipe.

bronze powder (BRAHNZ POW·dur)—fine flakes of a metal such as copper alloy or aluminum; used as a pigment in cosmetics to impart a "frost" or sheen.

brow (BROW)—the upper anterior portion of the head; the forehead; the supraorbital ridge; the hair above the eyes called the eyebrows.

bruise (BROOZ)—a superficial injury without laceration caused by a blow or impact with an object, which produces capillary hemorrhage beneath the surface of the skin causing a bluish discoloration; to injure.

bruised fingernails (BROOZD FING·ur·naylz)—bluish spots underneath the nails caused by a blow or other injury.

brunet, brunette (broo·NET)—a person having brown or olive skin, brown or black hair and dark eyes; term used to describe dark hair color.

brush (BRUSH)—a grooming tool with a handle and rows of bristles embedded in the other end.

brush blow-drying (BRUSH BLOH·dry·ing)—the use of a hand-held blow-dryer and a brush to style the hair.

brush combing (BRUSH KOHM·ing)—back combing the hair with a brush.

brush-curl (BRUSH-KURL)—to turn, bend, or form the hair into ringlets by means of a hairbrush and the fingers.

brush dryer (BRUSH DRY·ur)—a hand-held hair dryer or blower with a brush attachment.

brush electrode (BRUSH ih·LEK·trohd)—an electrode resembling a brush that is used for the application of electricity.

brushing machine (BRUSH·ing muh·SHEEN)—a machine with a facial brush attachment that rotates at varied speeds and is used for facial and body treatments to increase circulation.

brushless shaving cream (BRUSH·les SHAYV·ing KREEM)—a cream for shaving that does not have the lathering action of soap; brushless creams usually contain lanolin or mineral oil, stearic acid, gums, and thickeners.

brush-out (BRUSH-OWT)—the use of a brush and comb to achieve the opening and blending of the hair set (its curls and waves) into the finished coiffure.

brush roller (BRUSH ROL·ur)—wire or plastic mesh hair roller with fine brush bristles to hold the hair to the roller while it is rolled into place.

brush waves (BRUSH WAYVZ)—a series of alternating rows of pin curls that are then brushed into waves.

bubble bath (BUB·ul BATH)—crystals or powders that form surface bubbles when used in bath water; usually contain sodium lauryl sulfate, sodium chloride, alcohol, and fragrance.

bubo (BOO·boh)—an inflammatory condition causing enlargement of the lymph nodes.

bucca (BUK·uh)—the hollow part of the cheek.

buccal artery (BUK·ul ART·uh·ree)—the artery that supplies blood to the buccinator muscle located in the mucus membrane of the cheeks.

buccal nerve (BUK·ul NURV)—a motor nerve affecting the buccinator and the orbicularis-oris (mouth) muscle; the sensory branch of the modular nerve of the cheek.

buccinator (BUK·sih·nay·tur)—the thin, flat muscle of the cheek, shaped like a trumpet.

buckle (BUK·ul)—distortion of a curl caused by a bend in its formation.

buffer (BUF·ur)—a manicuring implement used with powdered polish or buffering cream to impart a sheen to the nails and to improve circulation of blood to the nail area; a system that resists changes in pH.

buffer activity (BUF·ur ak·TIV·ih·tee)—the action of a buffer solution that has a tendency to resist changes in its pH when treated with strong acids or bases.

buildup (BILD·up)—repeated coatings on the hair shaft. In hairstyling: an accumulation of excess foreign matter deposited in the hair shaft; in manicuring" an accumulation of substance to create artificial nails.

buildup cut (BILD·up KUT)—to cut hair so that it appears fuller.

bulb (BULB)—the lowest area or part of a hair.

bulbous (BUL·bus)—pertaining to or like a bulb in shape and structure.

bulk (BULK)—in haircutting and hairstyling: the density, thickness, textured length, and volume of the hair.

bulky (BUL·kee)—pertaining to hair that is thick and heavy; having great thickness and weight.

bulla (BULL·uh)—a large blister containing watery fluid.

bullous pemphigoid (BULL·us PEM·fih·goyd)—a chronic skin disease characterized by large bulla that heal without leaving scars.

bump (BUMP)—an area of raised, swollen tissue.

bun (BUN)—a roll of hair shaped like a bun or small roll of bread.

bundle (BUN·dul)—a structure composed of a group of fibers, muscular or nervous.

bunion (BUN·yun)—a swelling of a bursa of the foot, generally affecting the joint of the great (big) toe.

burdock root (BUR·dok ROOT)—a coarse, biennial weed used as an ingredient in some hair and skin care products formulated to control excess oil secretions.

burn (BURN)—the tissue reaction or injury resulting from application of extreme heat, cold, friction, electricity, radiation, or caustic substances.

burrowing hair (BUR·oh·ing HAYR)—a condition in which the hair does not emerge from the skin but grows beneath the surface and may become infected.

bursae (BUR·see)—fibrous sacs lined with synovial membrane and lubricated with synovial fluid.

bursitis (bur·SY·tis)—inflammation and swelling of the bursae.

butter (BUT·ur)—in cosmetology: a substance that is solid at room temperature but melts at body temperature; cocoa butter and lip lubricants are examples and are manufactured in stick or molded forms: cosmetic butters usually contain hydrogenated oils, lanolin, wax, preservative, and coloring ingredients.

butterfly clamp (BUT·ur·fly KLAMP)—a clamping device designed to hold the hair in place while sectioning, ;or during other procedures. Also referred to as a jaw clamp.

butyl alcohol (BYOOT·ul AL·kuh·hawl)—any of four isomeric alcohols obtained from petroleum products; used as a clarifying agent in shampoos.

butylene glycol (BYOOT·ul·een GLY·kawl)—a substance made from acetylene formaldehyde and hydrogen, used in hair sprays and hair setting preparations.

butyl stearate (BYOOT·ul STEE·uh·rayt)—stearic acid; butyl ester; used in nail polish, lipstick, creams, and bath oils.

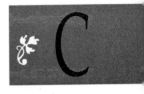

cabinet sanitizer (KAB·ih·net SAN·ih·ty·zur)—an airtight cabinet containing an active fumigant.

cacao (kuh·KOW)—the seeds or beans from the theobroma cacao; used in making cocoa butter that is used to relieve dryness and tautness of the skin.

cachecticorum, acne (kah·KEK·tih·kor·um, AK·nee)—pimples occurring in subjects of anemia or some debilitating constitutional disease.

cadmium sulfide (KAD·mee·um SUL·fyd)—a yellow-orange powder, insoluble in water, used in shampoo for the treatment of scalp diseases.

cake makeup (KAYK MAYK·up)—a shaped, solid mass usually containing finely ground pigment, kaolin, zinc, titanium oxide, calcium carbonate, iron oxide, lanolin or other oils, sorbital and fragrance; a moistened cosmetic sponge is used to apply the makeup to the face; gives good coverage.

cake mascara (KAYK mas·KAIR·uh)—a makeup for the eyelashes applied with a moistened brush or applicator; comes in dry molded form or a more liquid product in a cylinder or tube: ingredients usually used in mascara are carnauba wax, paraffin, lanolin, carbon black, triethanolamine stearate, and propylparaben.

caking (KAYK·ing)—the process in which small particles cling and form a thick or hardened mass such as caking of powder or lipstick when applied.

calamine (KAL·uh·myn)—zinc carbonate; a pinkish powder of zinc oxide and ferric oxide used to treat skin ailments.

calamine lotion (KAL·uh·myn LOH·shun)—zinc carbonate in alcohol used as a mild astringent and healing lotion, especially for skin irritations.

calcaneal nerve (kal·KAY·nee·ul NURV)—nerve that receives stimuli from the skin of the heel.

calcaneus (kal·KAY·nee·us)—the heel bone; the large tarsal bone.

calcified tumor (KAL·sih·fyd TOO·mur)—any cutaneous neoplasm containing calcium.

calcium (KAL·see·um)—a silvery-white metal; in compounds, a component of bone.

calcium carbonate (KAL·see·um KAHR·guh·nayt)—chalk; a tasteless, odorless, absorbent powder that occurs in coral, limestone, and marble; used as a whitener in cosmetics and as a buffer in face powders; also used in toothpaste or powders, in deodorants and some medicinal preparations.

calcium propionate (KAL·see·um PROH·pee·oh·nayt)—propanoic acid; calcium salt; used as a preservative in cosmetics.

calefacient (kal·uh·FAY·shunt)—a substance that produces a sensation of heat and warmth; ingredients used in a facial mask or body wrap.

calendula (kah·LEN·juh·luh)—commonly known as the marigold plant; used in some skin care preparations as a softening agent.

caliber, calibre (KAL·ih·bur)—the diameter of a tube, such as the esophagus, urethra, or artery.

calibrate (KAL·ih·brayt)—to correct, graduate, or adjust the scale of a measuring instrument, such as a pH meter.

caliper (KAL·uh·pur)—an instrument used for measuring diameters, thickness, and distance between surfaces; often used to measure facial proportions.

callosity (ka·LAHS·ut·ee)—a portion of skin that has been thickened by persistent friction or pressure, caused by hypertrophy of the horny layer of the epidermis; dry, hard, calloused skin.

callous, callus (KAL·us)—hardened skin usually appearing on the feet and palms of the hands.

callus remover (KAL·us ree·MOOV·ur)—an implement, usually rounded or cylinder-shaped and covered with emery paper, used to smooth and remove calluses during a manicure or pedicure.

calomel (KAL·uh·mul)—a white powder, insoluble in water; used in ointment form as an antibacterial.

calor (KAL·ur)—pertaining to heat; one of four classic signs of inflammation: color, heat; dolar, pain; rubor, redness; and tumor, swelling.

calorie (KAL·uh·ree)—a measurement of heat or energy; the amount of heat necessary to raise the temperature of water from zero to one degree centigrade; a unit of heat used to express the heat-energy producing content of foods. (*See* kilogram; calorie.)

calvaria (kal·VAIR·ee·uh)—the upper part of the skull.

calvities (kal·VISH·eye·eez)—baldness; baldness of the anterior and upper part of the head.

camomile, chamomile (KAM·uh·meel)—an herb with leaves that produce an oily substance used in lotions for the skin; used in concentrated form as a hair lightener; a soothing tea.

camphor (KAM·fur)—oil distilled from the bark and wood of the camphor tree; used with other ingredients, such as castor oil and wax, to produce a product that is healing to chapped skin; it is slightly anaesthetic and cooling.

canaliculas (kan·uh·LIK·yoo·lus)—a small canal or groove, as in a bone.

cancellous (kan·SEL·us)—pertaining to bone; having a porous or spongy structure.

cancer (KAN·sur)—a malignant tumor.

candida (KAN·dih·duh)—a very sensitive AIDS-related rash that can spread upon contact from one part of the body to another. When resistance is low, candida can appear in the mouth; this is called thrush.

candlestick curl (KAN·dul·stik KURL)—a hair-setting technique in which rollers are placed vertically; elongated, spiral wound curls; also called "long" or "poker" curls.

caninus (kay·NY·nus)—the levator anguli oris muscle that lifts the angle of the mouth.

canitics (kuh·NIT·iks)—the study of canities; the graying of the hair.

canities (kah·NIT·eez)—loss of natural hair pigment causing grayness or whiteness of the hair.

canities, accidental (kah·NIT·eez ak·sih·DEN·tul)—grayness of hair caused by fright.

canities, congenital (kah·NIT·eez kahn·JEN·uh·tul)—a type of grayness or whiteness of the hair that is hereditary.

canities, premature (kah·NIT·eez pree·muh·CHOOR)—graying of the hair before the usual age for this occurrence.

canities senile (kah·NIT·eez SEN·yl)—grayness of hair that is associated with advanced age.

canities unguium (kah·NIT·eez UN·gwee·um)—abnormal whiteness or white spots on nails.

canker (KANG·kur)—an ulceration usually affecting the mucous membranes of the mouth.

cantharides (kan·THAR·uh·deez)—a powerful counterirritant.

canthus (KAN·thus)—the corner of each side of the eye where the upper and lower lids meet.

cap (KAP)—the netting and binding of a hair piece that form the base to which the hair is attached.

cap coiffure (KAP kwah·FUR)—a caplike haircut that is short and closely trimmed at the nape line.

cape (KAYP)—a sleeveless garment of cloth or plastic used to protect the client's clothing during cosmetology services.

capillarectasia (kap·ih·lahr·ik·TAY·zee·uh)—dilation of the capillaries.

capillaritis (kap·ih·lair·EYE·tis)—a progressive pigmentary disorder of the skin that has no inflammation but causes dilation of the capillaries.

capillarity (kap·uh·LAIR·ut·ee)—elevation or depression of liquids in narrow tubes due to the surface tension that exists between the molecules of the liquid and those of the solid tube.

capillary (KAP·uh·lair·ee)—any one of the minute blood vessels that connect the arteries and veins; hairlike blood vessels.

capillary hemangioma (KAP·uh·lair·ee hee·man·jee·OH·muh)—a benign vascular tumor made up largely of capillaries.

capilli (KAP·uh·lee)—hair of the head.

capillurgy (kap·ih·LUR·jee)—the art of destroying superfluous hair.

capitate (KAP·uh·tayt)—shaped like or forming a head as the rounded end of a bone; the large bone of the wrist; the largest carpal bone.

capsicum (KAP·sih·kum)—an herb of the nightshade family, including varieties of red pepper, used in condiments for food and in medical preparations as gastric stimulants.

capsule (KAP·sool)—a membranous or saclike structure enclosing a part of an organ; a small case to enclose substances of disagreeable taste.

caput (KAY·put)—a head or headlike part.

caramel (KAIR·uh·mul)—burnt sugar used to color and flavor foods; in cosmetology, used as a soothing agent in skin lotions.

carbohydrate (kahr·boh·HY·drayt)—a substance containing carbon, hydrogen, and oxygen, the two latter in proportion to form water; sugars, starches, and cellulose belong to class of carbohydrates.

carbolic acid (kahr·BAHL·ik AS·ud)—phenol; a caustic and corrosive poison found in coal tar used in dilute solution as an antiseptic.

carbomer (KAHR·boh·mur)—a polymer of acrylic acid; when cross-linked with other agents, it forms a substance that is used for preparing suspensions and emulsifiers.

carbon (KAHR·bun)—an element in nature that predominates in all organic compounds and occurs in three distinct forms: black lead, charcoal, and lamp black (soot); the symbol for carbon is the capital letter C.

carbona (kahr·BOH·nuh)—a trade name for a cleaning fluid containing carbon tetrachloride, which is sometimes used in giving a dry shampoo and for cleaning wigs.

carbon arc lamp (KAHR·bun ARK LAMP)—an instrument that produces ultraviolet rays.

carbonate (KAHR·buh·nayt)—a compound of carbonic acid and a base; to charge with carbon dioxide.

carbon dioxide (KAHR·bun dy·AHK·syd)—carbonic acid gas; product of the combustion of carbon with a free supply of air.

carbonic acid (kahr·BAHN·ik AS·ud)—an acid formed by the union of carbon dioxide and water.

carbon monoxide (KAHR·bun mahn·AHK·syd)—a colorless, odorless, and poisonous gas; its toxic action being due to its strong affinity for hemoglobin.

carbon tetrachloride (KAHR·bun tet·ruh·KLOHR·yd)—a nonflammable, colorless liquid used as a solvent in cleaning mixtures.

carbuncle (KAHR·bung·kul)—a large circumscribed inflammation of the subcutaneous tissue caused by staphylococci, similar to a furuncle (boil) but more extensive.

carcinogen (kahr·SIN·uh·jin)—a cancer-causing agent or substance.

carcinoma (kahr·sin·OH·muh)—a malignant tumor.

carcinomatous dermatitis (kahr·sin·OH·mut·us der·mah·TYT·us)—reddening of the skin associated with carcinoma; inflammatory carcinoma.

card (KARD)—a device, mounted on a workbench, consisting primarily of sharp, steel prongs; the instrument used for disentangling hair to be used in a hair piece; also used to direct all the hair imbrications in one direction to prevent tangling.

cardiac (KAHRD·ee·ak)—pertaining to the heart.

cardiac cycle (KAHRD·ee·ak SY·kul)—the rhythmic cycle of contraction, dilation, and relaxation of all four chambers of the heart, both atris, and ventricles.

cardiac glands (KAHRD·ee·ak GLANZ)—the glands of the cardia of the stomach.

cardiac muscle (KAHR·ee·ak MUS·ul)—the involuntary muscle that makes up the heart.

cardiac nerves (KAHRD·ee·ak NURVZ)—nerves affecting the heart.

carnation (kahr·NAY·shun)—a bright pink or red flower used in some cosmetics and as a fragrance in perfumery.

carotene (KAIR·uh·tun)—any of three orange-colored isomeric hydrocarbons found in carrots and similar vegetables; used as a coloring material for cosmetics; used in the manufacture of vitamin A.

carotid artery (kuh·RAHT·ud ART·uh·ree)—the artery that supplies blood to the head, face, and neck; the principal artery on either side of the neck.

carotid nerves (kuh·RAHT·ud NURVZ)—sympathetic nerves associated with glands and smooth muscles of the head.

carpal (KAHR·pul)—pertaining to the wrist or carpus.

carpus (KAHR·pus)—the wrist; the group of eight bones between the metacarpals and the radius and ulna, held together by ligaments.

carrot (KAIR·ut)—the long, orange root used as a vegetable and source of vitamin A; carrot oil is used in some cosmetics to treat skin blemishes.

cartilage (KAHRT·ul·ij)—gristle; a nonvascular connective tissue softer than bone; tough, elastic substance that cushions the bones at the joints, prevents jarring between bones in motion, and gives shape to external features such as ears and nose.

carve (KARV)—in hairsetting, to pick up or slice a strand of hair from a shaping.

carved curl (KARVD KURL)—a pin curl, sliced from a shaping and formed without lifting the hair from the head.

cascade (kas·KAYD)—a hair piece with an oblong-shaped base, worn primarily at the back of the head where it falls (cascades) like a waterfall.

cascade curl (kas·KAYD KURL)—a strand of hair held directly up from the scalp and wound with a large center opening, in croquignole fashion; the curl is fastened to the head in a standing position to allow the hair to flow upward and then downward.

casein (kay·SEEN)—a phosphoprotein found in milk and constituting the principal ingredient in cheese; used in the manufacture of plastics and resins.

cassia oil (KASH·uh OYL)—oil made from a variety of cinnamon that is used in some skin care preparations to speed surface circulation of the blood.

Castile soap (kas·TEEL SOHP)—a hard, white soap containing olive oil and other oils; originally from the region of Castile, Spain.

castor oil (KAS·tur OYL)—oil obtained from the castor bean; used as a lubricant and in some laxative preparations.

casual (KAZH·oo·ul)—in dress or hairstyling, informal, natural, and relaxed.

catabolism (kuh·TAB·uh·liz·um)—the phase of metabolism that involves the breaking down of complex compounds within the cells into smaller ones, often resulting in the liberation of energy.

catagen faz (KAT·uh·jen FAYZ)—the brief transitional period between growth and inactive stage of a hair follicle.

catalysis (kuh·TAL·uh·sus)—an increase in the rate of a chemical reaction, caused by the presence of a substance that is not altered by the reaction.

catalyst (KAT·ul·est)—any substance that increases the reaction time of physical and chemical processes and remains unchanged.

cataphoresis (kat·uh·fuh·REE·sus)—the forcing of substances into the deeper tissues, using the galvanic current from the positive toward the negative pole; the use of the positive pole to introduce an acid pH product, such as an astringent solution, into the skin.

cathode (KATH·ohd)—the negative pole or electrode of a constant electric current; the negatively charged electrode from an outside source of current during electrolysis.

cathodermia (kath·oh·DUR·mee·uh)—a process in which the skin acts as a cathode or negative electrode.

cation (KAT·eye·un)—an ion carrying a charge of positive electricity; during electrolysis of a chemical compound, the element appears at the negative pole or cathode.

cationic (kat·eye·AHN·ik)—having a positive charge.

cationic detergent (kat·eye·AHN·ik dee·TUR·jent)—a detergent, such as a quaternary ammonium salt, in which the cleansing action is inherent in the cation process.

catnip (KAT·nip)—an aromatic, minty herb used in some cosmetic preparations to reduce puffiness around the eyes; also used as an antiseptic ingredient for dandruff control.

Caucasian (kaw·KAY·zhun)—a member of the Caucasoid division of the human species; relating to the white race as defined by physical characteristics.

Caucasoid (KAW·kah·zoyd)—pertaining to a major ethnic division of the human race; characterized by skin color ranging from light to brown and hair varying from light to dark and curly to straight.

caul (KAWL)—a type of netting with an open weave that is strong, soft, and flexible; used in the crown area of some wigs.

causative (KAWZ·uh·tiv)—being or acting as a cause.

caustic (KAW·stik)—an agent that damages proteins or tissues by burning; capable of eating away by chemical action.

caustic potash (KAW·stik PAHT·ash)—potassium hydroxide.

caustic soda (KAW·stik SOH·duh)—sodium hydroxide.

cauterize (KAWT·uh·ryz)—to burn or sear with a caustic.

cautery (KAWT·uh·ree)—pertaining to the destruction of growths on the skin by use of a caustic substance or a cauterizing implement.

cava (KAH·vuh); pl. **cavum** (KAH·vum)—vena cava; any cavity or hollow of the body.

cavity (KAV·it·ee)—a hollow space.

cayenne (ky·EN)—a biting powder made from seeds and fruit of a pepper plant; used as a condiment and in some medicine preparations.

celery seed (SEL·ah·ree SEED)—seed of the celery plant noted for its diffusive power in the manufacture of perfume; also used in cookery.

cell (SELL)—a minute mass of protoplasm forming the structural unit of every organized body; capable of performing all the fundamental functions of life.

cell division (SELL dih·VIZH·un)—the reproduction of cells by the process of each cell dividing in half and forming two cells.

cell membrane (SELL MEM·brayn)—a delicate protoplastic material that encloses a living plant or animal cell and permits soluble substances to enter and leave the cell; cell wall.

cellular (SEL·yuh·lur)—consisting of or pertaining to cells; having a porous texture.

cellular pathology (SEL·yuh·lur puh·THAHL·uh·jee)—the study of changes in cells as the basis of disease.

cellular physiology (SEL·yuh·lur fiz·ee·AHL·uh·jee)—the physiology of individual cells as compared with entire tissues or organisms.

cellulite (SEL·yoo·lyt)—a word coined in European esthetics to describe the gel-like lumps composed of fat, water, and residues of toxic substances beneath the skin, usually around the hips and thighs of overweight people.

cellulitis (sel·yuh·LYT·us)—a diffuse inflammation of connective tissues, especially the subcutaneous tissues.

cellulose (SEL·yuh·lohs)—the principal carbohydrate constituent of the cell membranes of plants; absorbent cotton is a pure form of cellulose.

cellulose paper (SEL·yuh·lohs PAY·pur)—a transparent, insoluble paper used to confine the ends of the hair in croquignole permanent waving.

Celsius (SEL·see·us)—in metric measurement, a temperature scale in which the freezing point of water at normal atmospheric pressure is zero degrees and the boiling point is 100 degrees; the centigrade scale.

centrigrade (SENT·uh·grayd)—consisting of 100 divisions or degrees; pertaining to a temperature scale in which the freezing point of water is zero degrees and the boiling point is 100 degrees.

centrigrade scale (SENT·uh·grayd SKAYL)—a temperature scale in which the freezing point of water is zero degrees and the boiling point is 100 degrees.

centigram (SENT·ih·gram)—in the metric system, the hundredth part of a gram.

centimeter (SENT·ih·mee·tur)—in the metric system, the hundredth part of a meter.

central nervous system (SEN·tril NUR·vus SIS·tum)—that part of the nervous system in vertebrates that consists of the brain and spinal cord.

centric (SEN·trik)—relating to or having a center; of or relating to a nerve center.

centrifugal movement (sen·TRIF·ih·gul MOOV·ment)—movement directed away from the center part or point; in massage, the directing of massage movement away from the heart; moving outward from a nerve center.

centriole (SEN·tree·ohl)—a minute structure enclosed within the centrosome of the cell, considered to be the division center of the cell.

centripetal movement (sen·TRIP·ut·ul MOOV·ment)—movement directed toward a center; in massage, a movement directed toward the heart; afferent; toward the central nervous system.

centrosome (SEN·truh·sohm)—a small, round body in the cytoplasm near the cell nucleus, that affects the reproduction of the cells.

cephalic (suh·FAL·ik)—pertaining to the head; directed toward, at, on, or near the head.

cephalic vein (suh·FAL·ik VAYN)—the vein of the upper arm.

cerebellum (sair·uh·BEL·um)—the posterior and lower part of the brain controlling body balance, coordination of voluntary muscles, and smooth muscular movements.

cerebral (suh·REE·brul)—pertaining to the brain or the cerebrum.

cerebral allergy (suh·REE·brul AL·ur·jee)—symptoms of cerebral disturbances associated with certain allergies.

cerebral hemisphere (suh·REE·brul HEM·ih·sfeer)—one of the two halves of the brain.

cerebrospinal system (suh·ree·broh·SPYN·ul SIS·tum)—consists of the brain, spinal cord, spinal nerves, and the cranial nerves.

cerebrovascular (suh·ree·broh·VAS·kyoo·lur)—pertaining to the blood vessels of the cerebrum (brain).

cerebrum (suh·REE·brum)—the upper part of the brain, considered to be the seat of consciousness controlling speech, sensation, communication, memory, reasoning, will, and emotions.

ceresin (SAIR·ee·sin)—a white or yellow waxy substance made of naturally occurring hydrocarbons, soluble in alcohol, benzine, chloroform, and naptha and insoluble in water; used in the manufacture of some cosmetics.

certificate (sur·TIF·ih·kit)—an official document certifying that one has fulfilled the requirements set forth and may practice or work in a particular field.

certification (sur·tih·fih·KAY·shun)—the act of certifying or guaranteeing certain facts; a written statement verifying something, such as completion of a course of study.

certified color (SUR·tih·fyd KUL·ur)—a commercial coloring product permitted in foods, drugs, and cosmetics by the FDA (Federal Food and Drug Administration) by meeting certain standards for purity.

cerumen (suh·ROO·mun)—the waxy substance found within the ear; earwax.

cervical (SUR·vih·kul)—pertaining to the neck or the neck of any organ or structure.

cervical artery (SUR·vih·kul ART·uh·ree)—deep cervical artery that supplies blood to the deep muscles of the neck and the spinal cord.

cervical cutaneous nerve (SUR·vih·kul kyoo·TAY·nee·us NURV)—the nerve that receives stimuli from the front and sides of the neck as far down as the breastbone.

cervical glands (SUR·vih·kul GLANZ)—the lymph nodes of the neck.

cervical nerves (SUR·vih·kul NURVZ)—motor sensory nerves affecting the neck muscles and skin, muscles and skin of the upper back, and diaphragm.

cervical vertebrae (SUR·vih·kul VURT·uh·bray)—the seven bones of the top part of the vertebral column, located in the neck region.

cervico facial (SUR·vih·kol FAY·shul)—pertaining to the face and neck.

cervix (SUR·viks)—the neck; any necklike structure.

cetyl alcohol (SEET·ul AL·kuh·hawl)—a fatty alcohol soluble in water, used as an emollient in lotions and ointments. Also used as a stabilizer for emulsion systems and in hair color and cream developer as a thickener.

cetyl ammonium (SEET·ul uh·MOH·nee·um)—an ammonium compound, fungicide, and germicide used in a wide range of cosmetic products, chiefly in creams and deodorants.

cetyl lactate (SEET·ul LAK·tayt)—cetyl alcohol and lactic acid; an emollient used in cosmetic preparations to improve its texture.

chafe (CHAYF)—to irritate the skin by friction.

chamomile, camomile (KAM·uh·myl)—a plant having strongly scented foliage and flowers that are used in some skin care products, as a brightening rinse for hair, and as a healthful tea.

chancre (SHANG·kur)—a sore; the primary lesion of syphilis (a venereal disease) or sporotrichosis; a fungus infection.

channel (CHAN·ul)—in anatomy, a passage for liquids such as blood and lymph channels.

chapped (CHAPT)—pertaining to a skin condition characterized by rough, red, and cracked areas, generally caused by exposure to cold wind and moisture.

characterize (KAIR·ak·tur·yz)—to indicate, delineate, or describe the nature or qualities of a person or object.

character makeup (KAIR·ak·tur MAYK·up)—makeup and prosthetics used to create an appearance suitable for the portrayal of a certain character or personality type.

charcoal (CHAR·kohl)—a black, porous substance used in pencils or pieces for drawing; a term used to describe a color of lead used in cosmetic eye makeup.

chartreuse (shahr·TROOZ)—a bright, yellowish-green color used in some articles of clothing and in decor.

check (CHEK)—in cosmetology, to test, examine, or compare; to give a final inspection or examination of a completed hairstyle, makeup, or other service.

cheek (CHEEK)—the fleshy part of the sides of the face, below the eyes and above the sides of the mouth.

cheekbone (CHEEK·bohn)—zygomatic bone.

cheek color (CHEEK KUL·ur)—a cream or powder cosmetic used to color the cheek and the skin beneath the cheek bones; also called rouge.

cheilitis (KEE·ly·tis)—dermatitis of the lips usually caused by dyes found in lipsticks; dry, chapped lips.

cheiroplasty (KY·roh·plas·tee)—plastic surgery of the hand.

chelating stabilizer (KEE·layt·ing STAY·buh·ly·zur)—a molecule that binds metal ions and renders them inactive.

chemabrasion (keem·uh·BRAY·zhun)—a medical process that removes superficial layers of the epidermis and upper layer of the dermis by applying a chemical agent to the skin; used to remove scars and other skin imperfections.

chemical (KEM·uh·kul)—relating to chemistry; a substance of chemical composition.

chemical action (KEM·uh·kul AK·shun)—the molecular change produced in a substance through the action of electricity, heat light, or another chemical.

chemical blow-out (KEM·uh·kul BLOH·owt)—a chemical hair, relaxing technique; a combination of chemical hair straightening and hairstyling for overcurly hair.

chemical bond (KEM·uh·kul BAHND)—the force exerted by shared electrons that holds atoms together in a molecule.

chemical cauterization (KEM·uh·kul KAWT·uh·ryz·ay·shun)—the process by which tissue is destroyed by use of a caustic substance.

chemical change (KEM·uh·kul CHAYNJ)—alteration in the chemical composition of a substance in which a new substance or substances are formed, having properties different from the original.

chemical composition (KEM·uh·kul kom·poh·ZIH·shun)—the balance and proportion of elements that make up a given substance; the formation of compounds.

chemical compound (KEM·uh·kul KOM·pownd)—a combination of elements chemically united in definite proportions; compounds formed by the chemical combination of the atoms of one element and the atoms of another element or elements.

chemical damage (KEM·uh·kul DAM·ihj)—the destruction of the protein structure of the hair produced by reactive chemicals during the process of permanent waving, coloring, or bleaching of the hair.

chemical dye remover (KEM·uh·kul DYE ree·MOOV·ur)—a dye remover containing a chemical solvent.

chemical hair processing (KEM·uh·kul HAYR PRAHS·es·ing)—the process of straightening overcurly hair by the use of chemical agents.

chemical hair relaxer (KEM·uh·kul HAYR ree·LAKS·ur)—also called straightener; a chemical agent that is employed to straighten overcurly hair.

chemical peeling (KEM·uh·kul PEEL·ing)—a technique for improving the appearance when wrinkles of the skin are present.

chemical sterilizer (KEM·uh·kul STAIR·ih·ly·zur)—an apparatus that contains chemical agents that sterilize implements by the destruction of living microorganisms.

chemistry (KEM·uh·stree)—the science that deals with the composition, structures, and properties of matter and how matter changes under different chemical conditions.

cherry bark (CHAIR·ee BARK)—the bark of a cherry tree, used as a soothing astringent and as an ingredient in some hair conditioners to add body to the hair.

chestnut (CHES·nut)—a color resembling that of a chestnut; a reddish brown.

chevron (SHEV·run)—in hairstyling, the inverted V shape that forms the base curve of the hair shaping.

chi (KY)—the vital force of growth and change.

chiaroscuro (kee·ahr·uh·SKOOR·oh)—a technique of using contrasts of light and dark makeup to emphasize the contours of the face.

chic (SHEEK)—stylish; a term used to describe a fashionable, well-groomed appearance.

chickweed (CHIK·weed)—an herb used in some cosmetics for its strong cleansing qualities.

chigger (CHIG·ur)—a red larva of mites that attach to the skin, whose bites produce a painful, itching wheal.

chignon (SHEEN·yahn)—a knot or coil of hair worn at the crown of the head or nape of the neck.

chin (CHIN)—the anterior prominence of the lower jaw below the mouth; the lower part of the face between the mouth and neck.

chin bone (CHIN BOHN)—the anterior part of the human mandible; the bone beneath the fleshy part of the chin.

chiropody (kuh·ROP·ud·ee)—the art of treating minor diseases of the hands and feet.

chirurgy (KY·rur·jee)—healing with the hands.

chloasma (kloh·AZ·muh)—characterized by increased pigmentation; large brown irregular patches on the skin, such as liver spots.

Chlorazene (KLOH·ruh·zeen)—a trade name; a chemical used for preparing an antiseptic or disinfectant.

chloride (KLOHR·yd)—a compound of chlorine with another element.

chlorinate (KLOHR·uh·nayt)—to treat or combine with chlorine.

chlorine (KLOHR·een)—greenish-yellow gas with a disagreeable, suffocating odor; used in combined form as a disinfectant and bleaching agent.

chlorophyll (KLOHR·uh·fil)—the green coloring matter of plants by which photosynthesis is accomplished; preparations of water-soluble chlorophyll derivatives are used in deodorants, in some medicinal preparations and as coloring agents.

cholesterin; cholesterol (koh·LES·tur·in; koh·LES·tur·awl)—a waxy alcohol found in human and animal tissues and their secretions that is important in metabolism; present in lanolin and used as an emulsifier and ingredient in some cosmetics; a constituent of animal fats and oils.

choline (KOH·leen)—a vitamin of the B complex group and a component of lecithin found in animal and vegetable tissues; essential to proper liver function.

chop (CHAHP)—to cut hair in an irregular pattern; to cut abruptly so a line of demarcation can be seen.

choroid (KOR·oyd)—the membrane of the eyeball lying between the sclera (outer membrane) and the retina.

chromatic colors (kroh·MAT·ik KUL·urz)—all colors other than the achromatic (neutral) colors: black, white, and gray.

chromatics (kroh·MAT·iks)—the science of color.

chromatic vision (kroh·MAT·ik VIZH·un)—vision pertaining to the color sense.

chromatologist (kroh·muh·TAHL·uh·jest)—a person who specializes in the technology of hair coloring.

chromatology (kroh·muh·TAHL·uh·jee)—the science of colors; chromatics.

chromidrosis (kroh·mih·DROH·sus)—the excretion of colored sweat. (*See* chromhidrosis.)

chromosome (KROH·muh·sohm)—any of several bodies in the cell nucleus that transmit hereditary characteristics during cell division.

chromotherapy (kroh·moh·THAIR·uh·pee)—treatment of disease by use of various colored lights or colors in the surroundings.

chronic (KRAHN·ik)—long; continued; the opposite of acute.

chrysarobin (kris·uh·ROH·bun)—a powerful parasiticide indicated in various forms of tinea (skin disease).

chuck (CHUK)—in massage, to strike vigorously.

chucking (CHUK·ing)—a massage movement (primarily for use on arms) accomplished by grasping the flesh firmly in one hand and moving the hand up and down along the bone, while the other hand keeps the arm in a steady position.

chunky (CHUNK·ee)—a term used to describe a blunt haircut that creates weight; also called a club cut.

chyle (KYL)—a creamy mixture of fat and lymph formed in the small intestine during digestion.

cicatrix (SIK·uh·triks); pl., **cicatrices** (sik·uh·TRY·seez)—the skin or film that forms over a wound, later contracting to form a scar.

cilia (SIL·ee·uh)—the eyelashes; microscopic, hairlike extensions that assist bacteria in locomotion.

cinnamon oil (SIN·uh·mun OYL)—oil of cassia; yellowish-brown oil from the leaves and stems of the cinnamon shrub; used as a flavoring and as a fragrance in cosmetics.

circle (SUR·kul)—a geometric curvature shape, bounded by a circumference having equal radii from the point of origin.

circle design (SUR·kul dee·ZYN)—a design that is created by the equal distribution of straight or curved lines from a center point.

circle end (SUR·kul END)—the circular part of a pin curl, which determines the size and tightness of the curl.

circle technique (SUR·kul TEK·neek)—pertaining to inner or outer circles, a technique in hair setting of expanding a circle by a second row of rollers or pin curls.

circuit (SUR·kit)—the path of an electric current.

circuit breaker (SUR·kit BRAYK·ar)—a switch that automatically interrupts an electric circuit.

circuit, broken (SUR·kit, BROH·ken)—a circumstance in which the current is diverted from its regular circuit.

circuit, closed (SUR·kit, KLOHZD)—a circuit in which current is continually flowing.

circuit, complete (SUR·kit, kum·PLEET)—the path of an electric current in actual operation.

circuit, short (SUR·kit, SHORT)—a term used when electrical current is diverted from its regular circuit.

circular movements (SUR·kyoo·lur MOOV·ments)—in massage, movements (circulatory friction) employed to increase circulation and glandular activity of the skin.

circulation (sur·kyoo·LAY·shun)—the passage of blood throughout the body.

circulation, general (sur·kyoo·LAY·shun, JEN·ur·ul)—blood circulation from the heart throughout the body and back again.

circulation, pulmonary (sur·kyoo·LAY·shun, PUL·muh·nair·ee)—blood circulation from the heart to the lungs and back to the heart.

circulatory system (SUR·kyoo·luh·tohr·ee SIS·tum)—the system that carries blood from the heart to all parts of the body and back to the heart, circulating oxygen and nutrients for and wastes from the entire body.

circulatory vessels (SUR·kyoo·luh·tohr·ee VES·ulz)—the blood vessels of the circulatory system consisting of the large arteries (muscular), small arteries (arterioles), capillaries, and veins.

circumference (sur·KUM·fur·ens)—the outside boundary of a circle.

citral (SIH·tral)—a liquid aldehyde, found in citrus fruits, oil of lemon, oil of lime, and grapefruit; used in fragrances and cosmetic products for its pleasant odor.

citric acid (SIT·rik AS·ud)—acid found in fruits such as lemons, limes, oranges, and grapefruit, and often added to finishing rinses to smooth tangles and increase the sheen of the hair.

civet (SIV·it)—the yellowish, fatty substance with a musklike scent secreted by a gland of the genitalia of the civet cat; used as a fixative in perfumes.

civet cat (SIV·it KAT)—a large catlike animal with yellowish, spotted fur and valued for its civet; generally, the civet cat is found in Africa and India.

clamp (KLAMP)—a small device used to hold a wave in place; in medicine, a surgical instrument for holding or compressing.

clamp (KLAMP), **table top**—a device employed to hold another object, such as a mannequin head, or for compressing something within its parts; used in wig styling to hold or steady the wood or canvas wig block.

clapping (KLAP·ing)—a movement in body massage accomplished by striking the area of skin with the palm of the hand slightly cupped.

clasp (KLASP)—a bar with a catch or hook used to hold the hair in place, similar to a barrette; a catch or hook used to hold two parts together, such as an opening in a garment.

classic (KLAS·ik)—belonging to a first class or highest rank; approved; accepted as in good taste; standard of excellence; as a classic hairstyle.

classic style (KLAS·ik STYL)—a hairstyle that is universally accepted and continues to be used.

clavicle (KLAV·ih·kul)—collarbone joining the sternum and scapula.

clay (KLAY)—an earthy substance containing kaolin; used for facial masks and packs.

clay mask (KLAY MASK)—also called a clay pack; a colloidal clay preparation used in facial treatments to stimulate circulation and temporarily contract the pores of the skin; usually recommended for oily and blemished skin.

clean (KLEEN)—the quality of being free from dirt, pollution, or other offensive substances.

clean-cut (KLEEN-KUT)—neatly groomed; in hairstyling, hair that is sharply defined; to cut smooth and even.

cleaning solution (KLEEN·ing suh·LOO·shun)—a liquid cleaning product especially formulated for wigs and hair pieces; both wet and dry cleaning solutions are used to clean various wig types.

cleanse (KLENZ)—to clean or purify.

cleansing cream (KLENZ·ing KREEM)—a light-textured cream used primarily to dissolve makeup and soil quickly.

cleansing lotion (KLENZ·ing LOH·shun)—a lotion formulated to remove makeup and soil.

clear (KLEER)—free of blemishes; transparent or translucent; without cloudiness or murkiness.

cleido (KLY·doh)—a prefix meaning pertaining to the clavicle.

clinic (KLIN·ik)—pertaining to an establishment where patrons can receive services, such as the cosmetology school clinic; medical clinic: an establishment where patients are received and treated.

clip (KLIP)—a metal or plastic lever-type device used to secure pin curls, waves, or hair rollers.

clipper (KLIP·ur)—a haircutting implement with a fine, medium, or coarse tooth-cutting edge; hand or electric clippers.

clipper oil (KLIP·ur OYL)—a lubricant that reduces friction, heat, and wear when used between the two blades of a hair clipper.

clipping (KLIP·ing)—the act of cutting split hair ends with the shears or the scissors; the operation of removing the hair by the use of hair clippers.

clockwise (KLOK·wyz)—the movement of hair, in shapings or curls, in the same direction as the hands of a clock.

clog (KLAHG)—to obstruct; to hamper; fill up, as a clogged pore.

closed end (KLOHZD END)—the rounded (convex) end of a shaping or wave.

clot (KLAHT)—a mass or lump of coagulated blood.

clotting (KLAHT·ing)—forming into a mass of coagulated fluid or soft matter such as blood or cream; in blood, caused by exposure of the blood's fibrinogen to oxygen; in cream, the separating of the whey from the coagulated curd as certain bacteria colonies develop.

cloudy (KLOWD·ee)—not clear; dull in color; murky.

clove (KLOHV)—an herb used in some astringents and antiseptics; an herb (spice) used in cookery.

club cutting (KLUB KUT·ing)—cutting the hair straight off without thinning, slithering, or tapering; a technique used to cut bangs and to cut ends the same length.

club hair (KLUB HAYR)—a condition caused by the root of the hair being surrounded by an enlarged substance made up of keratinized cells that occurs before normal hair loss.

cluster (KLUS·tur)—to gather in a mass or group.

cluster curls (KLUS·tur KURLZ)—artificial curls that can be pinned singly or in groups to the wearer's own hair.

coagulant (koh·AG·yuh·lunt)—a substance that produces coagulation.

coagulate (koh·AG·yuh·layt)—to clot; to convert a fluid into a soft jellylike solid.

coal tar (KOHL TAR)—a black, thick, opaque liquid obtained from bituminous coal and used to make cosmetic colors.

coarse (KORS)—rough or thick in texture; not delicate.

coarse hair (KORS HAYR)—a hair fiber that is relatively large in diameter or circumference.

coated hair (KOHT·ud HAYR)—hair covered with a substance that interferes with and retards the action of chemicals upon the hair fiber.

coating (KOHT·ing)—residue left on the hair shaft; coating conditioner that does not penetrate into the hair but coats the hair shaft.

cocci bacteria (KOK·sye bak·TEER·ee·uh)—a form of pathogenic bacteria; disease-causing bacteria.

coccus (KOK·us); pl., **cocci** (KOK·sye)—spherical cell bacterium appearing singly or in a group.

coccyx (KAHK·siks)—the last bone in the vertebral column; tailbone.

cocoa butter (KOH·koh BUT·ur)—a hard, yellowish fatty substance obtained from cocoa seeds; used in the manufacture of some soaps and cosmetics.

coconut oil (KOH·kuh·nut OYL)—the oil extracted from the meat of the coconut, used in the manufacture of soaps and shampoos because of its high lathering quality.

coif (KWAHF)—a close-fitting cap; a hairstyle; to arrange or style the hair.

coiffeur (kwah·FUR)—French term; a male hairdresser.

coiffeuse (kwah·FYOOS)—French term; a female hairdresser.

coiffure (kwah·FYOOR)—an arrangement, styling, or dressing of the hair; a finished hairstyle.

coil (KOYL)—to twist or wind the hair spirally; the spiral duct from the sweat (sudoriferous) gland to the epidermis.

cold cream (KOLD KREEM)—a cleansing ointment for the skin.

cold pack (KOLD PAK)—wet wrappings placed around the body as a form of therapy.

cold sore (KOLD SOR)—an eruption or sore around the mouth or nostril, often occurring during a cold or fever; medical name, herpes labialis.

cold waving (KOLD WAYV·ing)—a system of permanent waving involving the use of chemicals rather than heating equipment.

cold waving lotion (KOLD WAYV·ing LOH·shun)—a chemical solution that breaks S-bonds (sulphur) so that curl may be formed in hair wrapped around rods.

collagen (KAHL·uh·jen)—a protein forming the chief constituent of the connective tissues and bones; used in some cosmetics, such as face creams.

collapse (kuh·LAPS)—an abnormal sinking or retraction of the walls of an organ.

collarbone (KAHL·ur BOHN)—the clavicle; the bone connecting the shoulder blade and breastbone.

collodion (kuh·LOHD·ee·un)—a thick viscous substance used to dress wounds.

colloid (KAHL·oyd)—a substance consisting of particles having a certain degree of fineness and possessing a sticky consistency.

cologne (kuh·LOHN)—a toilet water consisting of alcohol scented with aromatic oils; a lighter fragrance than perfume.

color (KUL·ur)—visual sensation caused by light; any tint or hue distinguished from white; achromatic colors include black, white, and the range of grays in between; chromatic colors are all other colors.

color additive (KUL·ur AD·ih·tiv)—a concentrated color product that can be added to hair color to intensify or tone down the color. Another word for concentrate.

color base (KUL·ur BAYS)—the combination of dyes that makes up the tonal foundation of a specific hair color.

color blender (KUL·ur BLEND·ur)—a preparation that cleanses, highlightss and blends gray hair.

color blind (KUL·ur BLYND)—partial or total inability to distinguish one or more chromatic colors.

color builder (KUL·ur BIL·dur)—a color filler employed on damaged or overporous hair so it can take and hold color evenly.

color catalyst (KUL·ur KAT·uh·lest)—a chemical preparation added to hair tint to aid penetration of the product and improve coverage; helps to eliminate a harsh, reddish, brassy cast.

color chart (KUL·ur CHART)—a chart of colors produced by manufacturers of haircoloring products to serve as a guide in selecting appropriate colors; the color is shown as it would appear after application to white hair.

color developer (KUL·ur dee·VEL·up·ur)—an oxidizing agent, usually hydrogen peroxide, which is added to coloring agents before application to develop the color during processing.

color etching (KUL·ur ECH·ing)—a technique of highlighting the hair by combing a frosting product through the hair.

colorfast (KUL·ur·fast)—resistant to fading or running.

colorfast shampoo (KUL·ur·fast sham·POO)—a shampoo especially prepared to cleanse the hair and protect the color stability of hair that has been lightened or tinted.

color filler (KUL·ur FIL·ur)—a preparation used to revitalize and correct abused or damaged hair, to equalize porosity and deposit a base color prior to tinting.

colorful (KUL·ur·ful)—vivid; full of color, especially constrasting colors.

colorimeter (KUL·uh·RIM·ut·ur)—an apparatus for determining color and color intensity.

colorist (KUL·ur·ist)—a cosmetologist who specializes in the application of hair color.

colorless (KUL·ur·less)—lacking color; dull, uninteresting.

color lift (KUL·ur LIFT)—the amount of change natural or artificial color pigment undergoes when lightened or removed by a substance.

color lifter (KUL·ur LIFT·ur)—a chemical designed to remove artificial color from the hair. Also called a color remover or dye solvent.

color, makeup (KUL·ur MAYK·up)—color used in makeup; eye color, lip color, cheek color; foundation color, etc.

color mixing (KUL·ur MIKS·ing)—combining two or more colors together to obtain some in-between shade or tint, creating a custom color.

color palette (KUL·ur PAL·et)—a selection of colors arranged on a kidney-shaped board or in a flat container; used by artists and makeup artists.

color pencil (KUL·ur PEN·sul)—a temporary hair color in the shape of a pencil used to add color to the scalp where the hair is thin; a pencil with colored lead used as a makeup item.

color, personal (KUL·ur, PUR·sun·ul)—an individual's hair, eye, and skin colors.

color pigment (KUL·ur PIG·ment)—the organic coloring matter of the body; substances that impart color to animal or vegetable tissues, as chlorophyll and melanin.

color pigment, hair (KUL·ur PIG·ment, HAYR)—pigment found in the cortex layer of the hair.

color pigment, skin (KUL·ur PIG·ment, SKIN)—coloring matter of the skin: melanin, hemoglobin (oxygenated and reduced), and carotenes.

color priming (KUL·ur PRYM·ing)—the process of adding pigments to prepare the hair for the application of a final color formula.

color psychology (KUL·ur sy·KAHL·uh·jee)—the science of color as it affects the emotions.

color refresher (KUL·ur ree·FRESH·ur)—1) color applied to mid-shaft and ends of hair to give more uniform color appearance. 2) color applied by a shampoo-in method to enhance the natural color. Also called color wash, color enhancer.

color remover (KUL·ur ree·MOOV·ur)—a prepared commercial product designed to move artificial pigment from the hair. Dye solvent, color lifter.

color rinse (KUL·ur RINS)—a rinse that gives a temporary tint to the hair.

color shampoo (KUL·ur sham·POO)—a preparation that colors the hair permanently without requiring presoftening treatment.

color stick (KUL·ur STIK)—a crayon used to color new hair growth temporarily between permanent color treatments.

color swatch (KUL·ur SWAHCH)—a small sample of hair or cloth used to determine matching colors.

color test (KUL·ur TEST)—a method of determining the action of a selected tint on a small strand of hair; also called strand test. The process of removing or wiping product from a hair strand to monitor the progress of color development during tinting or lightening.

color tone (KUL·ur TOHN)—a shade, tint, or degree of a particular color, or a slight modification of a color, as blue with a green undertone or red with an orange tone.

color value (KUL·ur VAL·yoo)—the degree of shading, lightness, or darkness of a color.

color vision (KUL·ur VIZH·un)—the ability to see and distinguish colors.

color wash (KUL·ur WASH)—*see* color refresher.

color wheel (KUL·ur WHEEL)—a chart, usually circular, used as a tool for selecting and formulating colors for hair, makeup, clothing and decorating; the arrangement of primary, secondary, and tertiary colors in the order of their relationship to each other; shows harmonizing and contrasting colors.

coltsfoot (KOLTS·fut)—an herb bearing yellow flowers used for medicinal purposes.

comb (KOHM)—a toothed strip of plastic, metal, bone, or other material used to groom and hold the hair in place; decorative combs are often used to enhance a hairstyle.

comb and brush cleaner (KOHM AND BRUHSH KLEEN·ur)—a powdered or liquid substance, usually diluted in water and used to clean combs and brushes.

comb out (KOHM OWT)—the opening and blending of the hair setting, curls, or waves, into the finished style, using a hairbrush and/or comb.

combustion (kum·BUS·chen)—the rapid oxidation of any substance, accompanied by the production of heat and light.

comedo (KAHM·uh·doh); pl., **comedones** (kahm·uh·DOH·neez)— blackhead; a wormlike mass in an obstructed sebaceous duct.

comedone extractor (KAHM·uh·dohn eks·TRAK·tur)—an instrument sometimes used as an aid in removing blackheads.

comfrey (KUM·free)—an herb whose root contains tannin; used as a tea to aid bodily functions, and in some cosmetic preparations for its astringent, soothing, and healing qualities.

common carotid artery (KAHM·un kuh·RAHT·ud ART·uh·ree)—the artery that supplies blood to the face, head, and neck.

communicable (kuh·MYOO·nih·kuh·bul)—able to be communicated; transferable by contact from one person to another as a communicable disease.

commutator (KAHM·yuh·tayt·ur)—an instrument for automatically interrupting or reversing the flow of electric current.

comose (KOH·mohs)—having soft hair.

compact (KAHM·pakt)—closely united; dense; solid; a container, usually having a mirror on one side and a space for a cosmetic such as powder, eye, or lip makeup.

compact bone (KAHM·pakt BOHN)—hard bone tissue that forms the outer covering of a bone.

compact tissue (KAHM·pakt TISH·oo)—a dense, hard type of bony tissue.

complement (KAHM·pluh·ment)—something that completes or makes perfect.

complementary (kahm·pluh·MEN·tur·ee)—serving as a complement; to fill out or complete.

complementary colors (kahm·pluh·MEN·tur·ee KUL·urz)—a primary and secondary color positioned opposite each other on the color wheel. When these two colors are combined, they create a neutral color. Combinations are as follows: blue/orange, red/green, yellow/violet.

complex (kahm·PLEKS)—complicated; intricate; difficult to analyze.

complexion (kum·PLEK·shun)—hue or general appearance of the skin, especially the face.

compliment (KAHM·plih·ment)—an expression of admiration, praise, or congratulation.

complimentary (kahm·plih·MEN·tur·ee)—given free as a favor or courtesy.

component (kahm·POH·nent)—one of the parts of a whole; a constituent part; an ingredient.

composition (kahm·poh·ZISH·un)—the kind and number of atoms constituting the molecule of a substance.

compound (KAHM·pownd)—a substance formed by a chemical union of two or more elements, and different from any of them.

compound henna (KAHM·pownd HEN·uh)—Egyptian henna to which has been added one or more metallic preparations.

comprehend (kahm·pree·HEND)—to grasp mentally; to understand.

compress (KAHM·pres)—a folded strip of cotton or cloth forming a pad that is pressed upon the face or a part of the body; cotton compress as used in facial treatments.

compressor (kahm·PRES·ur)—a muscle that presses; an instrument for applying pressure on a blood vessel to prevent loss of blood.

compressor nasi (kahm·PRES·ur NAY·zye)—the muscle that compresses the nostrils.

concave (kahn·KAYV)—hollow and round or curving inward; concave profile; a face having a prominent forehead and chin with other features receded inward; the opposite of convex.

concave rod (kahn·KAYV RAHD)—a cold wave rod that has a smaller circumference in the center and increases to a larger circumference at both ends.

conceal (kahn·SEEL)—to cover; hide; keep from sight; as to conceal a blemish with cosmetics.

concentrate (KAHN·sen·trayt)—a strong or undiluted substance or solution; to make less dilute. (*See* color additive.)

concentrated (KAHN·sen·trayt·ud)—condensed; increased the strength by diminishing the bulk.

concentric (kahn·SEN·trik)—having a common center, such as curls, waves, and other movements of the hair that radiate from a common center.

concentric contraction (kahn·SEN·trik kahn·TRAK·shun)—a type of isotonic muscle contraction when the distance between a contracting muscle decreases.

concha (KAHNG·kuh)—a structure comparable to a shell in shape, as the auricle or pinna of the ear or a turbinated bone in the nose.

concise (kahn·SYS)—brief and comprehensive.

condensation (kahn·den·SAY·shun)—act of changing a gas or vapor to a liquid; reduction to a denser form.

condition (kun·DIH·shun)—to protect or restore the natural strength and body of the hair; the existing state of health of the hair, in reference to elasticity, strength, texture, porosity, and evidence of previous treatments.

conditioner (kun·DIH·shun·ur)—a special chemical agent applied to the hair to help restore its strength and give it body to protect it against possible breakage.

condition filler (kuh·DIH·shun FIL·ur)—a cosmetic preparation used to recondition and correct damaged hair.

conditioning (kun·DIH·shun·ing)—the application of special chemical agents to the hair to help restore its strength and to give it body to protect it against possible breakage; descriptive of conditioning shampoos and rinses that help to normalize the condition of the hair.

conducting cords (kahn·DUKT·ing KORDZ)—insulated copper wires that convey the current from the wall plate to the patron and the cosmetologist who is performing the service.

conductivity (kahn·duk·TIV·ut·ee)—the capacity to transmit sound, heat, or electricity.

conductor (kahn·DUK·tur)—any substance, material, or medium that conducts electricity, heat, or sound.

condyle (KAHN·dyl)—a rounded articular surface at the extremity of a bone.

condyloid (KAHN·duh·loyd)—relating to or resembling a condyle.

cone-shaped curl (KOHN-SHAYPT KURL)—a curl formed to be smaller at the end of the hair shaft and larger at the scalp.

congeal (kun·JEEL)—to change from a fluid to a solid condition as by freezing or curdling to change to a jellylike substance.

congenital (kahn·JEN·uh·tul)—pertaining to a condition existing at birth.

congestion (kuh·JES·chun)—excessive or abnormal accumulation of fluid in the vessels of an organ or body part; usually blood, but occasionally bile or mucus; this condition occurs in some diseases, infections, or injuries.

conical (KAHN·ih·kul)—resembling the shape of a cone; as a cone-shaped curl or hair piece.

conical hair roller (KAHN·ih·kul HAYR ROHL·ur)—a cone-shaped hair roller.

connect (kahn·EKT)—to join or fasten together; link; associate.

connecting (kahn·EKT·ing)—in fingerwaving,the joining of a ridge of wave from one side of the head with the ridge of a wave from the opposite side of the head.

connecting cords (kahn·EKT·ing KORDZ)—the insulated strands of copper wires which join the apparatus and the commercial electric current.

connecting line (kahn·EKT·ing LYN)—a line blending two circular shapes of clockwise and counterclockwise forces; also referred to as a blending; connection between two or more shapes, referred to as blending, dovetailing, and dividing.

connective tissue (kuh·NEK·tiv TISH·oo)—fibrous tissue that unites and supports the various parts of the body, such as bone, cartilage, or tendons.

connective tissue massage (kuh·NEK·tiv TISH·oo muh·SAHZH)—massage directed toward the subcutaneous connective tissue for the treatment of circulatory or visceral disease.

consistency (kun·SIS·ten·see)—the degree of density, solidity, or firmness of either a solid or a fluid.

constant base factor (KAHN·stant BAYS FAK·tur)—in hair coloring, the factor that enhances warm tones and adds depth to dark shades; an ingredient in color formulation that neutralizes and balances color and prevents brassy tones.

constituent (kun·STICH·uh·wunt)—a necessary part or element of something; that which composes or makes up something.

constitutional (kahn·stih·TOO·shun·ul)—belonging to or affecting the physical or vital powers of an individual.

constrict (kun·STRIKT)—to make narrow; pressing together.

constructive (kun·STRUK·tiv)—promoting improvement or development.

consultant (kun·SUL·tent)—one who gives professional advice.

consultation (kahn·sul·TAY·shun)—verbal communication with a client to determine desired result. (*See* analysis [hair].)

consumer (kun·SOO·mur)—one who uses materials or services; one of the buying public.

contact (KAHN·takt)—to bring together so as to touch.

contagion (kun·TAY·jen)—transmission of specific diseases by direct or indirect contact.

contagiosa (kohn·tay·jee·OH·suh)—impetigo; a form of impetigo marked by flat vesicles that first become pustular, then crusted.

contagious (kun·TAY·jus)—transmittable by contact.

contagium animatum (kun·TAY·jee·um AN·ih·may·tum)—any living or animal organism that causes the spread of an infectious disease.

contaminate (kun·TAM·uh·nayt)—to make impure by contact; to taint or pollute.

contamination (kun·tam·uh·NAY·shun)—pollution; soiling with infectious matter.

contemporary (kun·TEM·puh·rair·ee)—belonging to the same age; living or occurring at the same time.

contemporary style (kun·TEM·puh·rair·ee STYL)—a current style in dress, hairstyle, makeup, etc., that is accepted and worn at the present time; modern.

contiguous (kun·TIG·yuh·wus)—in contact; touching; adjoining.

contour (KAHN·toor)—the outline of a figure or body, particularly one that curves; to shape the outline or shape something to fit the outline.

contour coloring (KAHN·toor KUL·ur·ing)—to shade or highlight the contours of a hairstyle with hair color; to use makeup to create shading or highlighting on the contours of the face.

contouring (KAHN·toor·ing)—a makeup technique that utilizes the principles of light and shadow to sculpt or contour the face; used in theatrical and corrective makeup.

contour makeup (KAHN·toor MAYK·up)—a cream or powdered makeup used to create optical illusions by the shading and highlighting of facial features.

contour of hairstyle (KAHN·toor UV HAYR·styl)—the outline of the finished hairstyle.

contra (KAHN·tra)—a prefix denoting against, opposite, contrary.

contract (kun·TRAKT)—to draw together; to acquire a disease by contagion.

contractible (kun·TRAK·tih·bul)—having the ability to contract.

contractility (kahn·trak·TIL·ut·ee)—the property of muscles to contract or shorten thereby exert force.

contraction (kun·TRAK·shun)—the act of shrinking or drawing together; the shortening and thickening of a functioning muscle.

contrary (KAHN·trair·ee)—in opposition.

contrast (KAHN·trast)—a striking difference that appears by comparison.

contributing pigment (kun·TRIB·yoot·ing PIG·ment)—the current level and tone of the hair affecting the final color result. Refers to both natural underlying pigment and decolorized (or lightened) contributing pigment. (*See* undertone.)

control (kun·TROHL)—to direct, regulate, or influence; in experiments, a standard by which experimental observations may be studied and evaluated, as in determining safe or unsafe ingredients in products.

control brushing (kun·TROHL BRUSH·ing)—in hairstyling, a comb-out technique to relax the setting pattern; hair is brushed with one hand while the palm of the other hand molds the hair into design lines.

controller (kun·TROHL·ur)—a magnetic device for the regulation and control of an electric current.

contusions (kun·TOO·zhunz)—common bruises.

convalesce (kahn·vuh·LES)—to recover health and strength gradually after illness.

conventional (kun·VEN·shun·ul)—growing out of established customs; lacking in originality or spontaneity.

converge (kun·VURJ)—to come together at a particular point.

conversion (kun·VUR·zhun)—the act of converting or being converted in condition, substance, form, or function.

conversion layer (kun·VUR·zhun LAY·ur)—a cutting technique used to increase length; hair is directed opposite the area of the desired length increase.

converter (kun·VUR·tur)—an apparatus used to convert direct current to alternating current or alternating current to direct current.

convertible cut (kun·VUR·tih·bul KUT)—a haircut that can be styled in a variety of ways.

convex (kahn·VEKS)—curving outward like an exterior segment of a circle; in a convex profile, the forehead and chin recede.

convolve (kun·VAHLV)—to roll together; to coil, wind, or twist as in braiding the hair.

convulsion (kun·VUL·shun)—an abnormal, violent, involuntary muscular contraction or series of contractions.

coolant (KOOL·unt)—a substance, usually liquid, used as a cooling agent.

cool colors (KOOL KUL·urz)—colors suggesting coolness; in hair colors, white, gray platinum, silver gray, steel gray, ash blond, blue gray; in clothing, blue, green, and violet.

cooling period (KOOL·ing PIHR·ee·ud)—a waiting period, generally ten minutes, before removing permanent wave rods from the hair following the neutralizing process.

cool tones (KOOL TOHNZ)—*see* ash.

coordinate (koh·OR·dih·nayt)—to bring into harmonious relationship, as to harmonize hair, makeup, and clothing colors.

copious (KOH·pee·us)—large in amount.

copper (KAHP·ur)—a metallic element that is a good conductor of heat and electricity.

copper color (KAHP·ur KUL·ur)—a reddish-gold color of hair resembling the color of copper.

coracoid (KOR·uh·koyd)—a projecting part of the shoulder blade.

core (KOR)—the central or most vital part of anything.

corium (KOH·ree·um)—the dermis or true skin; the layer of the skin deeper than the epidermis, consisting of a dense bed of vascular connective tissue; also called cutis vera.

corkscrew curl (KORK·skroo KURL)—strands of hair having the form of a corkscrew spiral.

corn (KORN)—a horny, thickened, small area of skin, usually on the toes, caused by pressure or friction.

corner (KOR·nur)—in haircutting and styling, a point where the direction or outline changes; the point formed where two lines meet.

corneum (KOR·nee·um)—the horny layer of the skin; the stratum corneum.

cornflower (KORN·flow·ur)—an herb used in some cosmetic preparations for its astringent, moisturizing, and softening qualities.

cornification (kor·nuh·fuh·KAY·shun)—the process of becoming a horny substance or tissue.

corn oil (KORN OYL)—a concentrated oil from corn used in shampoo and in some skin preparations; also used in cookery.

corn rowing (KORN ROH·ing)—a technique used in creating a hairstyle incorporating intricate braiding and braided patterns; strands of hair are woven to create narrow rows of braids that lie close to the scalp.

corn silk (KORN SILK)—the soft silky strands on an ear of corn that are commonly used in facial masks and powdered makeup.

cornstarch (KORN·starch)—a very fine flour obtained from corn, used as a thickening agent in some cosmetics and foods.

corona (kuh·ROH·nuh)—a crownlike structure as the top of the head, or a crownlike braid of hair.

coronal plane (KOR·un·ul PLAYN)—divides body into front and back.

coronal suture (KOR·un·ul SOO·chur)—the line of junction of the frontal bone with the two parietal bones of the skull.

coronary (KOR·uh·ner·ee)—relating to a crown; a term applied to vessels, nerves, or attachments that encircle a part or an organ; pertaining to either of two arteries of the aorta that supply blood to the heart muscle.

coronoid (KOR·uh·noyd)—crown-shaped, as the process of the large bone of the forearm or of the jaw.

corpus (KOR·pus)—a body; the human body.

corpuscle (KOR·pus·ul)—a small mass or body; a minute cell; a cell found in the blood.

corpuscle, red (KOR·pus·ul RED)—cells in blood whose function is to carry oxygen to the cells.

corpuscle, white (KOR·pus·ul WHYT)—cells in the blood whose function is to destroy disease germs.

corrective coloring (kor·EK·tiv KUL·ur·ing)—the process of altering or correcting an undesirable color.

corrective makeup (kor·EK·tiv MAYK·up)—a procedure using a makeup product such as a cream or stick to cover blemishes or birthmarks and to bring uneven facial features into balance.

corrode (kuh·ROHD)—to eat away or destroy gradually, usually by chemical action.

corrosive (kuh·ROH·siv)—having the power to corrode; a substance that eats away or destroys.

corrugated (KOR·uh·gayt·ud)—formed or shaped in wrinkles or folds or alternate ridges and grooves.

corrugations, nail (kor·uh·GAY·shuns, NAYL)—ridges caused by uneven growth of the nail, usually the result of illness or injury.

corrugator supercilli (KOR·uh·gayt·ur SOO·pur·sil·eye)—muscle that draws eyebrows inward and downward.

cortex (KOR·teks)—the second or middle layer of the hair shaft; a fibrous protein core of the hair fiber, containing melanin pigment; gives strength and elasticity to hair; the external portion of the adrenal glands.

cortical (KORT·ih·KUL)—pertaining to or consisting of the outer portion; the bark, rind, or outer layer (cortex) of the hair.

cortical fibers (KORT·ih·KUL FY·burz)—fibers that make up the cortex of the hair.

cortisol (KOR·tih·sawl)—a hormone that acts as an anti-inflammatory and anti-allergenic.

cortisone (KOR·tih·sohn)—a powerful hormone extracted from the cortex of the adrenal gland and also made synthetically; used in the treatment of disease and some diseases of the skin.

corynebacterium (kor·uh·nee·bak·TEER·ee·um)—pathogenic bacterium that spreads infection and is usually present in acne lesions along with other bacteria.

coryza (kuh·RY·zuh)—an acute condition affecting the nasal mucous membranes associated with the common cold, causing a discharge from the nostrils.

cosmetic (kahz·MET·ik)—any external preparation intended to beautify the skin, hair, or other areas of the body.

cosmetic acne (kahz·MET·ik AK·nee)—a skin disorder caused by hormonal changes in the body during puberty; acne that becomes activated by improper cleansing and improper use of cosmetics.

cosmetic chemistry (kahz·MET·ik KEM·is·tree)—scientific study of cosmetics.

cosmetic dermatology (kahz·MET·ik der·mah·TAHL·uh·jee)—a branch of dermatology devoted to improving the health and beauty of the skin and its appendages.

cosmetician (kahz·muh·TISH·un)—one trained in the use and/or art of selling and demonstrating the application of cosmetics.

cosmetic surgery (kahz·MET·ik SUR·juh·ree)—plastic surgery performed to correct and beautify the face or body.

cosmetic therapy (kahz·MET·ik THAIR·uh·pee)—a term used by some state boards to designate the practice of cosmetology; cosmetic treatments for skin, hair, or nail disorders.

cosmetologist (kahz·muh·TAHL·uh·jist)—one skilled in the science and practice of cosmetology.

cosmetology (kahz·muh·TAHL·uh·jee)—the art or science of beautifying and improving the skin, nails, and hair; the study of cosmetics and their application.

cosmopolitan (kahz·muh·PAHL·it·un)—common to all the world; not limited to one area or locality.

costal (KAHS·tul)—pertaining to a rib or riblike structure.

cotton (KAHT·un)—a soft, fibrous material, usually white or light yellow, of high cellulose content, from the seed of the cotton plant; used widely as a textile.

cotton cleansing pads (KAHT·un KLENZ·ing PADZ)—small round or square pads made of beautician's cotton; used as eye pads and for cleansing during facial treatments.

cotton compress mask (KAHT·un KAHM·prehs MASK)—strips of cosmetologist's cotton moistened in water and applied to the face to aid in the removal of a treatment mask.

cotton mitts (KAHT·un MITZ)—strips of cotton wrapped around the fingers and used to remove cosmetic products following cleansing or a facial treatment.

cottonseed oil (KAHT·un·seed OYL)—a pale yellow, odorless, oily liquid pressed from the seed of the cotton plant; used in creams, lotions, soaps, lubricants, and polish remover.

counteract (kown·tur·AKT)—to neutralize or make ineffective; to act in opposition.

counterclockwise (kown·tur·KLAHK·wyz)—the movement of hair, in shapings or curls, in the opposite direction to the hands of the clock.

counter-irritant (KOWN·tur·IHR·ih·tent)—a substance that produces inflammation of the skin to relieve a more deep-seated inflammation.

couperose (KOO·per·ohs)—a word used by estheticians to describe a skin condition caused by dilated or broken capillaries.

couvette (koo·VET)—a specially designed bowl used during the spraying procedure of a facial treatment.

coverage (KUV·ur·ej)—the degree to which gray or white hair has been covered by the coloring process; also references the ability of a color product to conceal gray, white, or other colors of hair; the degree of concealment provided by a cosmetic product, foundation, or coverage stick.

cowlick (KOW·lik)—a tuft of hair that stands up.

cradle cap (KRAY·dl KAP)—an oily type of dandruff characterized by heavy, greasy crusts on the scalp of an infant.

cranial (KRAY·nee·ul)—of or pertaining to the cranium.

cranial index (KRAY·nee·ul IN·deks)—a method of measuring the skull.

cranial nerves (KRAY·nee·ul NURVZ)—any pair of nerves arising from the lower surface of the brain.

cranium (KRAY·nee·um)—the bones of the head, excluding the bones of the face; bony case of the brain.

crayon (KRAY·ahn)—a temporary hair coloring, massaged or brushed on with a lipsticklike applicator.

cream (KREEM)—a semi-solid cosmetic preparation such as cleansing cream and other skin care creams.

crease (KREES)—a line or slight depression in the skin, such as grooves across the palms of the hands, at the wrist, or where there are folds of skin.

create (kree·AYT)—to bring into being, specifically to produce something that has not existed before, such as a new hairstyle or work of art.

creatine phosphate (KREE·uh·teen FAHS·fayt)—a cellular substance that has a high-energy phosphate bond, which is required for the formation of ATP.

creme (KREEM)—a thick liquid or lotion.

creme bleach (KREEM BLEECH)—a chemical preparation of thick consistency, used to remove color from hair.

creme rinse (KREEM RINS)—a colorless, usually acidic preparation applied to the hair to neutralize the effects of the shampoo; it assists in removing tangles from the hair and increases its manageability.

creosol (KREE·uh·sawl)—a colorless, oily liquid obtained from creosote.

creosote (KREE·uh·soht)—an oily liquid obtained from beechwood tar and used in antiseptics.

crepe wool (KRAYP WUHL)—in wiggery, wool made from sheep wool and used to confine ends in winding or to fill in bulk.

crepey skin (KRAYP·ee SKIN)—skin resembling a thin fabric, usually silk, and having a crinkled surface.

crepon (KRAYP·ahn)—a woven hair piece frontlet; usually dressed in pomadour style and extending in length to the top of the ears.

crescent shape (KREHS·ent SHAYP)—in manicuring, a term referring to the small, white area at the base of the nail; a shape like that of the moon when less than half of it is visible.

cresol (KREE·sul)—a liquid obtained from coal tar and used as a powerful antiseptic and disinfectant; used to sterilize instruments and other objects.

crest (KREST)—in hairdressing, tuft of hair; the high ridge of a finger wave; a line or thin mark made by folding or doubling over, as the crest between two waves, where one begins and the other ends.

crew cut (KROO KUT)—a very short men's haircut that leaves a bristlelike surface over the entire head.

crimping rod (KRIMP·ing RAHD)—a flat, plastic clamplike rod, designed to produce hairstyles that have a tightly waved, fluffy appearance.

crimp perm (KRIMP PURM)—a perm given with a unique crimping tool to produce small waves resembling waves created by braiding the hair.

crimpy (KRIM·pee)—having a crimped, frizzy appearance; very curly or wavy.

crimson (KRIM·zun)—a deep red color having a tinge of blue.

crinkle (KRING·kul)—to form wrinkles; a wrinkle or fold.

crisscross (KRIS·kraws)—to pass back and forth, through or over; to mark with intersecting lines, as the crisscross movement of the fingers while giving a facial.

criterion (kry·TIHR·ee·un)—a standard on which a judgment may be based; a rule or test.

croquignole (KROH·ken·yohl)—winding of hair strands from the ends to the scalp.

croquignole curl (KROH·ken·yohl KURL)—any curl that is wound from the ends of the hair toward the scalp.

croquignole heat curling (KROH·ken·yohl HEET KURL·ing)—the process of curling the hair with a hot iron by winding the hair under in a special manner, as the hair strand is clicked into the iron until the ends disappear.

croquignole marcel wave (KROH·ken·yohl MAR·sel WAYV)—a wave in the hair produced by the use of a marcel iron and winding the hair croquignole fashion.

croquignole winding (KROH·ken·yohl WYND·ing)—the process of winding the hair from hair ends toward the scalp.

cross bonds (KRAWS BAHNDZ)—the bonds holding together the long chains of amino acids that compose hair.

crown (KROWN)—the topmost part of the skull or head.

crude (KROOD)—in a natural or unrefined state; imperfect; unfinished.

crust (KRUST)—a coating of dried blood; dead cells that form over a wound or blemish while it is healing; also called a scab; an accumulation of serum and pus, mixed perhaps with epidermal matter.

cryosurgery (kry·uh·SUR·jur·ee)—a skin treatment done with the use of liquid nitrogen, usually in case of nodular and cystic forms of acne.

crypt (KRIPT)—a small cavity on the skin; a small sac or follicle; a glandular tubule.

cubic (KYOO·bik)—shaped like a cube; having three dimensions.

cubical (KYOO·bih·kul)—any small room or partitioned area, as a facial service cubical.

cucumber (KYOO·kum·bur)—a cylindrically shaped, dark green fruit, cultivated as a vegetable; contains a certain hormone said to retain smoothness of the skin; used as a natural facial mask and as an ingredient in some cosmetics.

cuneiform (kyuh·NEE·uh·form)—wedge-shaped; a bone of the wrist or corpus.

cupful (KUP·fuhl)—a measure of eight ounces; a half pint; in metric measure, one metric cup liquid equals approximately 236 milliliters.

curative (KYOOR·uh·tiv)—having the power to cure.

curd (KURD)—a soap residue found on the hair after an unsatisfactory shampoo, usually as the result of nonlathering of soap in hard water.

curd soap (KURD SOHP)—a white soap of curdy texture, usually containing free alkali.

cure (KYOOR)—to heal or restore to a sound, healthy condition.

curl (KURL)—to form hair into curves, spirals, or ringlets; a lock of hair that curves or coils.

curl, barrel (KURL, BAIR·ul)—a curl made in a similar manner to the standup curl and used where there is insufficient room to place a roller.

curl base (KURL BAYS)—the stationary or immovable foundation of the curl, which is attached to the scalp.

curl, cascade (KURL, kahs·KAYD)—a standup curl that is wound from the hair ends to the scalp.

curl clip (KURL KLIHP)—a pronged device used to secure a curl in place.

curl direction (KURL dih·REK·shun)—the placement of the hair so that it moves or curls toward or away from a certain point.

curler (KURL·ur)—that which curls anything.

curler, electric iron (KURL·ur, uh·LEK·trik EYE·urn)—a curling iron heated by electricity; thermal iron; electric vaporizing thermal iron.

curling (KURL·ing)—a process of hair waving.

curling, brush (KURL·ing, BRUSH)—tightly winding a damp strand of hair around the index finger, brushing with a stiff brush, pinning to the scalp with wire pins, and drying the hair with artificial heat.

curling iron (KURL·ing EYE·urn)—an implement with a long tube-like base over which a top piece can be raised, the hair placed between the two and curled while it is dry; thermal iron.

curling, paper (KURL·ing PAY·pur)—produced by dividing the hair into small strands that are formed into flat ringlets and held in place by means of a folded piece of paper and heated between the prongs of a pressing iron.

curling pin (KURL·ing PIN)—the forming of hair ringlets by winding the hair in a series of concentric circles, fastened in place with hair pins.

curling, round (KURL·ing ROWND)—curls produced by twisting the hair tightly and evenly around a heated curling iron.

curl, overlapping (KURL oh·vur·LAP·ing)—a strand of wet hair wound around the finger in a spiral movement with the hair ends on the outside; also known as maypole or post curl.

curl paper (KURL PAY·pur)—a fine porous tissue paper around which a lock of hair is wound for curling.

curl placement (KURL PLAYS·ment)—the positioning of a curl in a predetermined location.

curl, ridge (KURL, RIJ)—a curl placed behind and close to the ridge of a finger wave and pinned across its stem.

curl, roller (KURL, ROHL·ur)—a curl formed over a specially made roller.

curl stem (KURL STEM)—that part of the pin curl between the base and the first arc of the circle.

curl styles (KURL STYLZ)—various kinds of curls such as pin curl, sculptured curl, standup curl, and cascade curl.

curl, thermal (KURL THUR·mul)—a curl formed with thermal irons.

curly (KUR·lee)—tending to curl; full of curves, twists, ripples, ringlets.

curly hair (KUR·lee HAYR)—hair that has a curved or spiral shape; the opposite of straight.

curly head (KUR·lee HED)—pertaining to a person who has curly hair.

current, alternating (KUR·ent AWL·tur·nayt·ing)—an interrupted current of electricity.

current D'arsonval (KUR·ent DAR·sun·vahl)—a high-frequency current of low voltage and high amperage.

current, direct (KUR·ent dih·REKT); **DC**—an uninterrupted and even-flowing current of electricity.

current, electric (KUR·ent ih·LEK·trik)—electricity in motion or moving within a conductor.

current, faradic (KUR·ent fuh·RAD·ik)—an induced, interrupted current whose action is mechanical.

current, galvanic (KUR·ent gal·VAN·ik)—a direct, constant current, having a positive and negative pole and providing a chemical action.

current, high frequency; tesla (KUR·rent HY FREE·kwen·see; TES·luh)—an electric current of medium voltage and medium amperage.

current, sinusoidal (KUR·ent sy·nuh·SOYD·ul)—an induced interrupted current somewhat similar to faradic current.

current strength (KUR·ent STRENGTH)—the relation of the electromotive force to the resistance of the circuit.

current style[e] (KUR·ent STYL)—a style that is worn or in favor at the present time.

curriculum (kuh·RIK·yuh·lum)—the course of study in a college or university; a particular course of study.

curvalinear (kur·vuh·LIN·ee·ur)—in hairdressing, formed, bounded, or characterized by curved lines.

curvature (KUR·vuh·chur)—the state of being curved.

curvature lines (KUR·vuh·chur LYNZ)—shaping of the hair and combing out into a series of curved lines running inward and outward.

curve (KURV)—the continuous bending of a line as an arc or circle.

cushioning (KOOSH·un·ing)—a form of back combing or back brushing in the scalp area in order that the tapered hairs interlock and form a foundation to support the longer lengths of hair.

cushion wrap (KOOSH·un RAP)—end paper used to prevent hair from expanding against a perm rod during the processing procedure of permanent waving.

custom made (KUS·tum MAYD)—a wig or hair piece that has been specially measured and constructed for a specific individual.

cut (KUT)—in hair cutting, to reduce or shorten by removing the ends with an instrument such as a scissor or razor; a haircut; to style the hair by cutting.

cutaneous (kyoo·TAY·nee·us)—pertaining to, involving, or affecting the skin and its appendages.

cutaneous appendage (kyoo·TAY·nee·us uh·PEN·dij)—an organ or structure of ectodermal origin attached to or embedded in the skin; examples are: hair, nails, sebaceous, and sudoriferous glands.

cutaneous colli (kyoo·TAY·nee·us KOH·lih)—a nerve of the skin of the neck.

cutaneous diphtheria (kyoo·TAY·nee·us dif·THEER·ee·uh)—an ulcerlike infection of the skin.

cutaneous gland (kyoo·TAY·nee·us GLAND)—any gland of the skin.

cutaneous horn (kyoo·TAY·nee·us HORN)—a small growth resembling a miniature horn commonly found on the face, scalp, or chest.

cutaneous muscle (kyoo·TAY·nee·us MUS·ul)—a muscle having an insertion into the skin or origin and insertion in the skin.

cutaneous nerves (kyoo·TAY·nee·us NURVZ)—nerves affecting the skin.

cutaneous reaction (kyoo·TAY·nee·us ree·AK·shun)—any reaction of the skin such as a rash or change in appearance as the result of disease, drugs, sunburn, allergy, etc.

cutaneous reflex (kyoo·TAY·nee·us REE·fleks)—the response of the skin to irritation or sensations, such as goose bumps on the skin as a reaction to cold.

cutaneous sensation (kyoo·TAY·nee·us sen·SAY·shun)—pertaining to the skin's receptors for sensing touch, temperature changes, pain, or irritation.

cutaneous test (kyoo·TAY·nee·us TEST)—a test involving the skin; skin test.

cuticle (KYOO·tih·kul)—the very thin translucent protein outer layer of the skin or hair; the epidermis; the cresent of toughened skin around the base of fingernails and toenails; any fine covering.

cuticle nippers (KYOO·tih·kul NIP·urz)—a small cutting tool used in manicuring or pedicuring to nip or cut excess cuticle (epidermis); the tool is characterized by its double handle and short clipping blades.

cuticle of hair (KYOO·tih·kul UV HAYR)—the outer keratinized layers of the hair shaft that surround the polypeptide change; made of transparent, overlapping, protective cells. The cuticle layers of hair may differ in various ethnic groups. Example: Itis thought that Caucasian hair has approximately 6 layers, Negroid (black) hair 12 layers, and Oriental hair approximately 15 to 20 cuticle layers.

cuticle oil (KYOO·tih·kul OYL)—a special oil used to soften and lubricate the cuticle (epidermis) around fingernails and toenails.

cuticle pusher (KYOO·tih·kul POOSH·ur)—an implement used in manicuring or pedicuring to loosen and push back the cuticle around the fingernails or toenails; the implement is shaped to conform with the shape of the nails.

cuticle remover (KYOO·tih·kul re·MOOV·ur)—a solution of alkali, glycerine, and water used to soften and remove dead cuticle from around the nail.

cuticle scales (KYOO·tih·kul SKAYLZ)—the overlapping formation of the outer layer of the hair (the cuticle); also referred to as imbrications.

cuticle scissors (KYOO·tih·kul SIZ·urz)—a small implement designed to trim excess cuticle (epidermis) around the fingernails or toenails. It is distinguished by the long shank and short, sharp cutting blades.

cuticle softener (KYOO·tih·kul SAW·fuh·nur)—a substance used in manicuring and pedicuring to soften the cuticle (epidermis) around the fingernails and toenails prior to removing the excess cuticle.

cuticolor (kyoo·tih·KUL·ur)—simulating the color of the skin as color in some cosmetics and medicines.

cuticularization (kyoo·TIK·uh·lur·ih·zay·shun)—the growth of new skin over a wound or blemish.

cutis (KYOO·tis)—the derma or deeper layer of the skin.

cutis marmorata (KYOO·tis mahr·moh·RAY·tuh)—blue or purple spots on the skin due to exposure to cold air.

cutis rhomboidalis nuchae (KYOO·tis rahm·boy·DAY·lus NOO·kee)—a skin condition characterized by furrows and a leathery appearance; usually caused by overexposure to the sun, wind, and weather.

cutis verticis gyrata (KYOO·tis VER·tih·sus jy·RAY·tuh)—hypertrophy and looseness of the skin or scalp resulting in folds.

cutting lotion (KUT·ing LOH·shun)—a wetting agent used to control the hair during a haircut.

cuvette (kyoo·VET)—a specially designed bowl used to protect the client's body from spray during a facial treatment.

cyanosis (sy·uh·NOH·sus)—a condition of circulation due to inadequate oxygenation of the blood, causing the skin to take on a bluish cast.

cycle (SY·kul)—a complete wave of an alternating current.

cyclical (SIK·lih·kul)—pertaining to or moving in a circle; having parts arranged in a ring or closed chain structure.

cycloid (SY·kloyd)—arranged in circles; something circular.

cylinder (SIL·in·dur)—a long circular body, solid or hollow, uniform in diameter.

cylindrical (sih·LIN·drih·kul)—pertaining to, or having the form of a cylinder.

cylindrical hair roller (sih·LIN·drih·kul HAYR ROHL·ur)—a roller made of lightweight metal or plastic, in various sizes, lengths and circumferences, around which strands of hair are wound to create a specific style.

cylindrical-shaped curl (sih·LIN·drih·kul SHAYPT KURL)—a curl that is formed to be about the same circumference along its entire shaft from the ends to the scalp.

cypress oil (SY·press OYL)—oil from the buds of the cypress tree, used in astringent preparations and in some fragrances.

cyst (SIST)—a closed, abnormally developed sac, containing fluid, semi-fluid, or morbid matter, above or below the skin.

cysteic acid (SIS·tee·ik AS·ud)—a chemical substance in the hair fiber, produced by the interaction of hydrogen peroxide on the disulfide bond (cystine).

cysteine (SIS·tuh·een)—the naturally occurring amino acid responsible for the development of pheomelanin (red/yellow pigment) in the hair.

cystic acne (SIS·tik AK·nee)—acne that is distinguished by cysts.

cystine (SIS·teen)—sulfur-containing amino acid that is present in hair in the form of cross bonds (links) joining adjacent polypeptide chains; an amino acid component of many proteins, especially keratin.

cystine links (SIS·teen LINKS)—the cross bonds formed from the amino acid, cystine.

cystoma (sis·TOH·muh)—a tumor containing cysts of pathogenic origin.

cytochemistry (sy·toh·KEM·ih·stree)—the science dealing with the chemistry of cells.

cytocrine theory (SY·tuh·krin THEE·uh·ree)—the theory that pigment granules are transferred from melanocytes directly into the cells of the epidermis.

cytogenesis (cy·toh·JEN·uh·sis)—the formation of cells.

cytolysis (sy·TAHL·uh·sus)—the dissolution of cells.

cytoplasm (sy·toh·PLAZ·um)—all the protoplasm of a cell except that in the nucleus; the watery fluid that contains food materials necessary for growth, reproduction, and self-repair of the cell.

cytoplasmic organelles (SY·toh·plaz·mik or·guh·NELZ)—structures that perform specific functions necessary for cell survival.

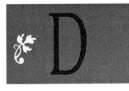

dab (DAB)—to pat or apply with a light towel; a small amount.

damage (DAM·ij)—to injure or harm; loss.

damaged hair (DAM·ijd HAYR)—a hair condition characterized by one or more of the following: high porosity, brittleness, split ends, dryness, rough, lifeless, feeling, matting, sponginess when wet, lacking gloss and elasticity.

damp (DAMP)—moist, not saturated with liquid.

D&C colors (D and C KUL·urz)—colors selected from a certified list approved by the Food and Drug Administration for use in drug and cosmetic products.

dandelion (DAN·duh·ly·un)—a green plant that provides high vitamin A and C in cosmetic substances for skin and hair.

dander (DAN·dur)—scales from animal skin, hair, or feathers; may act as an allergen.

dandricide (DAN·drih·syd)—a chemical substance; counteracts the effects of dandruff.

dandruff (DAN·druf)—pityriasis; scurf or scales formed in excess upon the scalp; greasy or dry keratotic material shed from the scalp.

dandruff conditioner (DAN·druf kun·DIH·shun·ur)—a product containing ingredients formulated to improve or eliminate a dandruff condition of the scalp.

dandruff lotion (DAN·druf LOH·shun)—a lotion applied to the scalp to aid in loosening and removing dandruff scales.

dandruff ointment (DAN·druf OYNT·ment)—a specially formulated salve or unguent to be applied to the scalp to treat a dandruff condition.

dandruff rinse (DAN·druf RINS)—a liquid applied to the hair and scalp following a treatment or shampoo to control and eliminate a dandruff condition.

dandruff shampoo (DAN·druf sham·POO)—a commercially prepared product designed to control and eliminate dandruff.

dark (DARK)—a deep shade of color; dark skin; brunette in complexion, not fair; dark hair; almost black.

darken (DARK·en)—to make a deeper color; to darken hair; to use a darker shade of makeup in contour shading of the face.

dark skin spot (DARK SKIN SPAHT)—commonly called "age" or "liver" spots; spots or splotches on the skin indicative of melanosis or melanoderm, a condition in which dark pigment is deposited in the skin and tissues.

D'arsonval current (DAR·sun·vahl KUR·ent)—high frequency of low voltage and high amperage; a biterminal current.

dart (DART)—the folding and sewing together of a curved section of material to form a tapered seam; used in wiggery to reduce the size of a wig cap.

data (DAY·tuh)—facts, figures, and various forms of information from which measurements and statistics can be drawn; record keeping.

data processing (DAY·tuh PRAHS·es·ing)—the converting by computers of information into a form for use or storage; a technique for keeping and storing all kinds of records and for ease in retrieving information when needed.

daub (DAWB)—to smear or coat with a greasy or sticky substance without exercising skill.

daylight bulb (DAY·lyt BULB)—an electric bulb made of special glass that produces light similar to daylight.

daylight makeup (DAY·lyt MAYK·up)—a choice of colors in makeup products to give the face a natural appearance for daylight wear.

de (DEE)—a prefix denoting from; down or away.

deacidify (dee·uh·SID·uh·fy)—to remove acid from a substance.

dead (DED)—lacking life; not responsive; lacking sensation; in skin care, dead surface cells; in hair care, hair that is dull, dead, lifeless.

debility (dih·BIL·ut·ee)—weakness; loss of strength.

debris (duh·BREE)—remains; rubbish; excess matter.

decade (DEK·ayd)—a period of ten years.

decalvant (duh·KAL·vunt)—a substance used to remove or destroy hair.

decay (dee·KAY)—decomposition of matter by the action of bacteria.

decimeter (DES·uh·meet·ur)—in the metric system, the tenth part of a meter.

Decoctions (dih·KOK·shuns)—product from steeping herbs in boiling water.

decolorization (dee·KUL·ur·ih·ZAY·shun)—the removal of color from the hair.

decolorize (dee·KUL·ur·yz)—a chemical process involving the lightening of natural pigment or artificial color from the hair.

decompose (dee·kum·POHZ)—to decay or rot; to separate into constituent parts; to bring to dissolution.

decomposition (dee·kahm·poh·ZIH·shun)—to separate or disintegrate into constituent parts or elements.

decreasing graduation (dee·KREES·ing GRAJ·oo·ay·shun)—graduation found within two nonparallel lines; in diminishes as it moves back from the face.

decrustation (dee·krus·TAY·shun)—the detachment or removal of a crust.

decurved (dee·KURVD)—curved or bent downward.

deep (DEEP)—extending below or far from the surface; a color of intense or dark hues; high saturation.

deep cervical artery (DEEP SUR·vih·kul ART·uh·ree)—the artery that supplies blood to the deep muscles of the neck.

deep fascia (DEEP FAYSH·uh)—fibrous tissue that penetrates deep in the body separating major muscle groups and anchoring them to bone.

deep kneading (DEEP NEED·ing)—a massage movement in which the flesh is lifted and squeezed with the hand.

deep temporal artery (DEEP TEM·puh·rul ART·uh·ree)—the artery that supplies blood to the temporal (temple) muscle and skull.

deep transverse massage (DEEP TRANZ·vurs muh·SAHZH)—massage that breaks down unwanted fibrous adhesions to restore mobility to the muscles.

defect (DEE·fekt)—an imperfection.

defective (dee·FEK·tiv)—imperfect; lacking in some physical quality.

deficiency (dih·FISH·en·see)—a lacking; something wanted.

deficiency disease (dih·FISH·en·see diz·EEZ)—a disease such as pellagra or scurvy, etc. caused by the lack of essential vitamins and other nourishment in the body.

define (dih·FYN)—to outline; to fix with precision an outline or boundary.

defluvium (duh·FLOO·vee·um)—to flow down; to lose something.

defluvium capilorum (duh·FLOO·vee·um kap·ih·LOH·rum)—complete loss of hair.

defluvium unguium (duh·FLOO·vee·um UN·gwee·um)—complete loss of nails.

deformed (dee·FORMD)— disfigured; misshaped; abnormal.

deformity (dee·FOR·mih·tee)—abnormal shape of a part of the body.

deft (DEFT)—skilled, dexterous.

degenerate (dee·JEN·ur·ayt)—to pass to a lower level of mental or physical qualities.

degenerative (dee·JEN·ur·uh·tiv)—a biochemical change caused by injury or disease and leading to loss of vitality, of function, etc; prone to deteriorate.

degrease (dee·GREES)—to remove grease or a greasy substance.

degree (duh·GREE)—to do in steps or stages; extent or amount; gradually. Term used to describe various units of measurement.

dehumidifier (dee·hyoo·MID·ih·fy·ur)—an apparatus designed to reduce moisture in the air.

dehydrate (dee·HY·drayt)—to deprive of water or to suffer loss of water; to dry out.

dehydrator (DEE·hy·drayt·ur)—an agent that removes or reduces water in the tissues of the body.

delicate (DEL·ih·kit)—exquisite and fine workmanship; fragile.

deltoid (DEL·toyd)—a triangular muscle covering the shoulder joint that allows the arm to be extended outward and to the side of the body.

demarcation (dee·mar·KAY·shun)—a line setting bounds or limits; in makeup, to blend colors to avoid a line of demarcation.

demi (DEM·ih)—less in size; partial.

demiwig (DEM·ih·wig)—a small hair piece; smaller than a full wig usually designed to be blended with a patron's own hair.

demonstration (dem·un·STRAY·shun)—to point out or prove; to describe by examples and experiments; a display; a teaching or performing technique.

denature (dee·NAY·chur)—to change the nature of something by chemical or physical means.

dendrites (DEN·dryts)—a treelike branching of nerve fibers extending from a nerve cell; short nerve fibers that carry impulses toward the cells.

dense (DENS)—close; thick; heavy; compact; crowded.

density (DEN·sih·tee)—the quality or condition of being close; thick; heavy.

dental (DEN·tul)—pertaining to the teeth.

dentifrice (DEN·tih·fris)—a powder, paste, or liquid used to clean the teeth.

denude (dee·NOOD)—to remove overlying matter or material; to expose to view; to clear the face of makeup.

deodorant (dee·OH·dur·unt)—a substance that conceals or removes offensive odors.

deodorize (dee·OH·dur·yz)—to free from odor.

depigment (dee·PIG·ment)—to cause the loss of pigment.

depilate (DEP·uh·layt)—to remove hair from the surface of the skin.

depilation (DEP·uh·lay·shun)—removal of superfluous hair.

depilatory (dih·PIL·uh·tohr·ee)—a substance, usually a caustic alkali preparation, used for the temporary removal of superfluous hair by dissolving it at the skin.

deplete (dee·PLEET)—to reduce; lessen; use up.

depleted (dee·PLEET·ud)—that which is exhausted; reduced.

depletion (dee·PLE·shun)—reduction or exhaustion in number or by draining away strength, power, or value.

deposit (dee·PAH·zit)—in hairdressing, describes a color product in terms of its ability to add color pigment to the hair. Color added equals deposit.

deposit-only color (dee·PAH·zit-OHN·lee KUL·ur)—a category of hair color products between permanent and semi-permanent colors. Formulated to deposit only color, not lift. They contain oxidation dyes and utilize low volume developer.

depot (DEEP·oh)—the site of an accumulation, as depot fat, which occurs in certain regions of the body as: hips, buttocks, abdominal walls, thighs, etc.

depress (dee·PRES)—to press down.

depression (dee·PRESH·un)—a hollow or sunken area; in psychiatry, a state of dejection, sadness, or melancholy.

depressor (dee·PRES·ur)—that which presses or draws down; a muscle that depresses.

depressor alae nasi (dee·PRES·ur AY·lee NAY·zye)—depressor septi; a muscle that contracts the nostril.

depressor anguli oris (dee·PRES·ur ANG·yoo·lye OH·ris)—a muscle that depresses the angle of the mouth.

depressor area (dee·PRES·ur AIR·ee·uh)—the vasomotor center that, when stimulated, can cause a drop in blood pressure and result in a slower heart rate.

depressor labii inferioris (dee·PRES·ur LAY·bee·eye in·FEER·ee·or·us)—quadratis labii inferioris; a muscle that depresses the lower lip.

depressor septi nasi (dee·PRES·ur SEP·tee NAY·zye)—a muscle that contracts the nostril.

depressor supercilii (dee·PRES·ur soo·pur·SIL·eye)—the portion of the orbicularis oculi muscle that draws the eyebrows downward.

depth (DEPTH)—distance from top to bottom; distance; in hairdressing, the degree of intensity and saturation of color. The lightness or darkness of a color. (*See* value, level.)

depth of side section (DEPTH UV SYD SEK·shun)—in hairstyling, the amount of hair in sectioning from the hairline to the back of the ear.

depth of top section (DEPTH UV TOP SEK·shun)—in hairstyling, the amount of hair sectioned from the hairline at the forehead to the crown of the head.

derivative (duh·RIV·uh·tiv)—that which is derived; anything obtained or deduced from another.

derm, derma, dermo (DURM, DURM·uh, DURM·oh)—pertaining to the skin.

derma (DUR·muh)—the true skin; the corium; the sensitive layer of the skin below the epidermis that extends to form the subcutaneous tissue.

dermabrasion (dur·muh·BRAY·zhun)—a technique to smooth scarred skin by sanding irregularities so scars blend better with the surrounding skin.

dermafat (DUR·muh·fat)—the adipose tissue of the skin.

dermal (DUR·mul)—pertaining to the skin.

dermal graft (DUR·mul GRAFT)—a skin graft using split or full thickness of skin for the grafting procedure.

dermal papilla (DUR·mul puh·PIL·uh)—an elevation of the projecting corium into the overlying epidermis.

dermal sense (DUR·mul SENS)—the perception of cold, heat, pain, pressure, or other sensations through the receptors of the skin.

dermatalgia (dur·muh·TAL·jee·uh)—pain accompanied by a burning sensation of the skin when no injury or other changes can be observed.

dermatherm (DUR·muh·thurm)—an apparatus designed to measure skin temperature.

dermatician (dur·muh·TISH·un)—one skilled in the treatment of the skin.

dermatitis (dur·muh·TY·tis)—an inflammatory condition of the skin; resulting either from the primary irritant effect of a substance or more frequently from the sensitization to a substance coming in contact with the skin.

dermatitis combustiones (dur·muh·TY·tis kum·bus·tih·OH·nees)—a type of dermatitis produced by extreme heat.

dermatitis, cosmetic (dur·muh·TY·tis kahz·MET·ik)—an inflammation of the skin caused by contact with some cosmetic product to which the individual may be allergic.

dermatitis, medicamentosa (dur·muh·TY·tis med·ih·kuh·men·TOH·suh)—a type of dermatitis caused by the internal use of medicines such as bromides.

dermatitis, occupational (dur·muh·TY·tis ahk·yoo·PAY·shun·ul)—an inflammation of the skin caused by the kind of employment in which the individual is engaged and by substances used on the job.

dermatitis seborrheica (dur·muh·TY·tis seb·or·EE·ih·kah)—a type of dermatitis found co-existing with seborrhea.

dermatitis venenata (dur·muh·TY·tis VEN·uh·nah·tuh)—an eruptive skin infection caused by contact with irritating substance such as chemicals or tints.

dermatodysplasia (dur·muh·toh·dis·PLAY·zeeuh)—a condition characterized by abnormal development of the skin.

dermatologist (dur·muh·TAHL·uh·jist)—a medical skin specialist; a physician who understands the science of treating the skin, its structures, functions, and diseases.

dermatology (dur·muh·TAHL·uh·jee)—the science that deals with the study of skin and its nature, structure, functions, diseases, and treatment.

dermatomycosis (dur·muh·toh·my·KOH·sis)—a superficial infection of the skin or its appendages caused by pathogenic fungus.

dermatoneurology (dur·muh·toh·noo·RAHL·uh·jee)—the study of the nerves of the skin in health and disease.

dermatopathic (dur·muh·toh·PATH·ik)—pertaining or attributable to disease of the skin.

dermatophyte (DUR·mah·toh·fyt)—a fungus parasitic on the skin.

dermatophytosis (dur·muh·toh·fy·TOH·sis)—commonly called athlete's foot.

dermatoplasty (DUR·muh·toh·plas·tee)—the science of skin grafting; an operation in which flaps of skin are used from another part of the body to replace lost or damaged skin.

dermatotherapy (dur·muh·toh·THAIR·uh·pee)—the treatment of the skin and its diseases.

dermatosis (dur·muh·TOH·sis)—any disease of the skin; usually a disease not characterized by inflammation.

dermatotrophic (dur·muh·toh·TROHF·ik)—affecting, infesting, or infecting the skin.

dermis, derma (DUR·mis, DUR·muh)—the layer below the epidermis; the corium or true skin.

dermoid (DUR·moyd)—resembling skin.

desensitize (dee·SEN·sih·tyz)—deprive of sensation; to cause the paralysis of a sensory nerve by blocking.

desiccate (DES·ih·kayt)—to deprive a substance of moisture; to dry.

desiccation (des·ih·KAY·shun)—the process of drying.

design (dee·ZYN)—arrangement of shapes, lines, and ornamental effects that create an artistic unit, as in hairstyling, makeup application, and the creation of fashions.

design component (dee·ZYN kahm·POH·nent)—one of four elements; texture, form, structure, and direction that make up a hair design.

design line (dee·ZYN·LYN)—the artistic concept of a finished hairstyle as expressed in its lines and shapes; a line used as a guide in creating the form of a design.

design, three dimensional (dee·ZYN THREE dih·MEN·shun·ul)—a sculpturing effect with hair, creating volume and/or indentation into a shape.

design, two dimensional (dee·ZYN TOO dih·MEN·shun·ul)—a pattern effect on a flat surface.

desmosine (DES·moh·sin)—one of two amino acids found in elastin; the other is isodesmosine.

desquamate (DES·kwuh·mayt)—to shed in scales; to shed the superficial layer of the skin.

desquamation (DES·kwuh·MAY·shun)—scaling of the cuticle.

destructive (dih·STRUK·tiv)—tending to destroy.

detergent (dee·TUR·jent)—a compound or solution used for cleansing; an agent that cleanses the skin and hair.

deteriorate (dee·TEER·ee·uh·rayt)—to grow worse; to become impaired in quality; to degenerate.

deterrent (dee·TUR·ent)—that which hinders or prevents.

detoxification (dee·tahk·sih·fih·KAY·shun)—reduction of toxic poisons; ridding the body of toxic substances.

detriment (DEH·trih·ment)—a cause of injury or damage.

detumescence (deh·too·MES·uns)—the subsiding of swelling; to go down.

develop (dee·VEL·up)—take effect; as during the process of a hair tint or lightener.

developer (dee·VEL·up·ur)—an oxidizing agent, such as 20-volume hydrogen peroxide solution; when mixed with an oxidation dye, it supplies the necessary oxygen gas to develop color molecules and create a change in hair color.

development time (dee·VEL·up·ment TYM)—the oxidation period required for the hair lightener or tint solution to act completely upon the hair.

device (dee·VYS)—an invention or contrivance of a simple nature for a particular use and purpose.

dewy (DOO·ee)—to appear moist; fresh; unblemished.

dexterity (deks·TAIR·ih·tee)—skill and ease in using the hands; expertness in manual acts.

dextral (DEKS·trul)—right-handed; right as opposed to left.

di (DYE)—a prefix denoting two-fold; double; twice; separation or reversal.

dia (DYE·uh)—a prefix denoting through; apart; asunder; between.

diabetic (dy·uh·BET·ik)—one who has diabetes, a disease associated with deficient insulin secretion.

diagnose (dy·ag·NOHS)—to determine the nature of a condition from the symptoms.

diagnosis (dy·ag·NOH·sis)—the determination of the nature of a disease from its symptoms.

diagonal (dy·AG·uh·nul)—a line with a slanting or sloping direction.

diagonal back design (dy·AG·uh·nul BAK dee·ZYN)—a design resulting in a backward flow of hair from the face.

diagonal forward design (dy·AG·uh·nul FOR·ward dee·ZYN)—a design resulting in a forward movement of hair onto the face.

diagonal left (dy·AG·uh·nul LEFT)—a diagonal line that travels to the left.

diagonal right (dy·AG·uh·nul RYT)—a diagonal line that travels to the right.

diagram (DY·uh·gram)—a figure for ascertaining or exhibiting certain relations between objects under discussion; an outline, figure, or scheme of lines, spaces, points; used in demonstrations, etc.

dialysis (dy·AL·uh·sus)—the process of separating different substances in solution by diffusion through a moist membrane or septum; separation.

diameter (dy·AM·ih·tur)—the length from one border to another of a straight line that passes through the center of an object.

diamond mesh (DY·uh·mund MESH)—a method of sewing up wefts into a diamond-shaped mesh.

diamond shape (DY·uh·mund SHAYP)—a figure bounded by four equal straight lines, having two angles acute and two obtuse.

diamond-shape face (DY·uh·mund SHAYP FAYS)—a face with a narrow forehead and chin, with the greater width across the cheekbones.

diaphoretic (dy·uh·fuh·RET·ik)—producing perspiration.

diaphragm (DY·uh·fram)—a muscular wall that separates the thorax from the abdominal region and helps to control breathing.

diaphysis (dy·AF·uh·sus)—the shaft of the bone between the enlarged end area of the bone.

diarthrotic joints (dy·ar·THRAH·tik JOYNTS)—freely movable joints.

diathermy (DY·uh·thur·mee)—the method of raising the temperature in the deep tissues by using high-frequency current; the application of oscillating electromagnetic fields to the tissues.

dichromatic (dy·kroh·MAT·ik)—having two colors.

dielectric (dy·ih·LEK·trik)—a nonconductor of direct electric current.

diet (DY·it)—a selection of foods in a regulated course of eating and drinking, especially for health reasons; to regulate kinds and amounts of food and drink for specific reasons.

dietetics (dy·uh·TET·iks)—the science of regulating the diet for hygenic or therapeutic purposes.

differentiation (dif·ur·en·chee·AY·shun)—division of the ovum into specialized cells that differ from one another and have specialized functions.

diffuse (dih·FYOOZ)—to pour out; to break down and spread in every way; scattered; not limited to one spot.

diffusion (dih·FYOO·zhun)—a spreading out; dialysis; the process by which substances move from areas of higher concentration to lower concentration.

digest (dy·JEST)—to prepare for absorption; to change food chemically in the alimentary canal for assimilation by the body.

digestion (dy·JES·chun)—the process of converting food into a form that can be readily absorbed; the breaking down of substances into simple forms, as food into simpler chemical compounds.

digestive enzymes (dy·JES·tiv EN·zymz)—chemicals that change certain kinds of food into a form capable of being used by the body.

digestive system (dy·JES·tiv SIS·tum)—the internal organs that change food into nutrients and wastes; the alimentary canal with its associated glands.

digit (DIJ·ut)—a finger or toe.

digital (DIJ·ut·ul)—pertaining to the fingers or toes.

digital artery (DIJ·ut·ul ART·uh·ree)—the artery that supplies blood to the fingers and toes.

digital function (DIJ·ut·ul FUNK·shun)—a massage technique using the fingertips in a rotating motion; pressing and rotating the fingers on the skin.

digitalis (dij·uh·TAL·us)—a drug used as a stimulant.

digital nerves (DIJ·ut·ul NURVZ)—sensory nerves of the fingers and toes; nerves that receive stimuli from the fingers or toes.

digital stroking (DIJ·ut·ul STROHK·ing)—a massage movement in which the fingertips are used to lightly glide over the face and neck.

digital tapotement (DIJ·ut·ul tah·POT·ment)—a massage movement to promote stimulation of blood to the skin surface; consists of light, tapping movements with the tips of the fingers.

digital vibration (DIJ·ut·ul vy·BRA·shun)—a massage movement using the tips of the fingers pressed on a pressure point, such as the temples, then using a rapid shaking movement for a few seconds.

digiti manus (DIJ·ih·ty MAN·us)—the digits of the hand.

digiti pedis (DIJ·ih·ty PED·us)—the digits of the foot.

digitus (DIJ·ih·tus)—finger.

digitus anularis (DIJ·ih·tus an·yuh·LAHR·is)—the ring finger, or second finger from the little finger, or third finger from the thumb side of the hand.

digitus demonstrativus (DIJ·ih·tus duh·MAHN·stray·tee·us)—the index finger.

digitus medius (DIJ·ih·tus MEE·dee·us)—the middle finger.

digitus minimus (DIJ·ih·tus MIN·ih·mus)—the last finger on the hand opposite the thumb.

dilate (DY·layt)—to enlarge; expand; distend.

dilator (dy·LAYT·ur)—that which expands or enlarges; an instrument for stretching or enlarging a cavity or opening.

dilute (dy·LOOT)—to make less concentrated, thinner, or more liquid by mixing with another substance, especially water.

dimension (dih·MEN·shun)—a measurement of width, height, thickness, or circumference.

dimensional coloring (dih·MEN·shun·ul KUL·ur·ing)—two or three different shades of the same color on the same head of hair.

dimensional design (dih·MEN·shun·ul dee·ZYN)—three-dimensional sculpturing effect with hair, creating volume or indentation into a shape and silhouette.

dimensional styling (dih·MEN·shun·ul STYL·ing)—hairstyling achieved by creating volume or indentation.

dimethylglyoxime (dy·meth·il·gly·AHR·seem)—compound used in ash testing; a compound used to detect nickel in a hair dye.

diminish (dih·MIN·ish)—to make smaller or less; to reduce.

dimple (DIM·pul)—a slight depression or indentation on the body, usually the cheeks or chin.

dioxide (dy·AHK·syd)—a chemical compound containing two atoms of oxygen to one of a metallic element.

diphtheria (dif·THEER·ee·uh)—an infectious disease in which the air passages, and especially the throat, become coated with a false membrane, caused by specific bacillus.

diplococcus (dip·loh·KOK·us)—a bacterium that occurs in groups of two; causes pneumonia.

diplomacy (dih·PLOH·muh·see)—the practice of negotiations; skill and tact when dealing with others.

direct current (dy·REKT KUR·ent)—an electric current constant in direction, as distinguished from an alternating current; the movement or flow of electricity in one direction.

direct dye (dy·REKT DYE)—a pre-formed color that dyes the fiber directly without the need for oxidation.

directional iron (dy·REK·shun·ul EYE·urn)—a curling iron with an oversized rod and groove used for the formation of straight, smooth lines.

directional roller (dy·REK·shun·ul ROHL·ur)—a roller used to direct the hair forward or backward to create a specific style.

direct point (dy·REKT POYNT)—in hairstyling, parting of curved or straight lines from a point to the outline of a circular shape.

dis (DIS)—a prefix denoting apart; away; asunder; between.

disarray (dis·uh·RAY)—lacking orderly arrangement; in a state of confusion.

disassemble (dis·uh·SEM·bul)—to take apart.

disc (DISK)—a circular plate or surface.

discard (DIS·kard)—to cast aside; to throw away.

discharge (dis·CHARJ)—to set free; to remove the contents or load; to relieve of responsibility; (DIS·charj)—the escape or flowing away of the contents of a cavity.

discharger (dis·CHARJ·ur)—an instrument for setting free electricity.

discolor (dis·KUL·ur)—to change or destroy the color.

discoloration (dis·kul·ur·AY·shun)—the development of an undesired color shade through chemical reaction.

discomfort (dis·KUM·fort)—to make uncomfortable or uneasy.

disconnect (dis·kuh·NEKT)—to sever or to terminate a connection.

discretion (dis·KRESH·un)—good judgment; the ability to make responsible decisions.

disease (dih·ZEEZ)—an abnormal state of all or part of the body making it incapable of carrying on its normal function.

disease carrier (dih·ZEEZ KAIR·ee·ur)—a healthy person who carries and may transmit disease germs to another person.

disentangle (dis·en·TANG·ul)—to free from clumping together; to straighten out snarls in hair.

disfigure (dis·FIG·yur)—to impair or destroy the beauty of a person or object.

disincrustation (dis·in·krus·TAY·shun)—a process used during a facial treatment to soften and emulsify grease deposits and blackheads in the follicles.

disinfect (dis·in·FEKT)—to free from infection.

disinfectant (dis·in·FEK·tent)—an agent used to destroy most bacteria and to sanitize implements.

disinfection (dis·in·FEK·shun)—the act of freeing one from infection.

disintegrate (dis·IN·tuh·GRAYT)—to separate or decompose a substance into its component parts; to reduce to fragments or powder.

dislocation (dis·loh·KAY·shun)—a bone displaced within a joint.

dispensary (dis·PEN·suh·ree)—a place where supplies are prepared and dispensed (given out).

dispersion (dis·PUR·zhun)—the act of scattering or separating; the incorporation of the particles of one substance into the body of another, comprising solutions, suspensions, and colloid solutions.

displacement (dis·PLAYS·ment)—volume or weight of fluid displaced by submerging something of equal weight into the fluid.

display (dis·PLAY)—to exhibit products to encourage sales.

disposable (dis·POH·zuh·bul)—designed to be discarded after use, as disposable products.

dissipate (DIS·ih·payt)—to dissolve.

dissociation (dih·soh·see·AY·shun)—the process by which combined chemicals are changed into simpler constituents.

dissoluble (dis·AHL·yuh·bul)—capable of being dissolved or decomposed.

dissolve (dih·ZAHLV)—to cause to become a solution; to break into parts; to disintegrate.

dissymmetry (dis·IM·uh·tree)—lack of symmetry.

distal (DIS·tul)—farthest from the center or median line.

distance (DIS·tans)—the degree or amount of separation between two objects or points.

distend (dis·TEND)—to expand; to swell.

distill (dis·TIL)—to extract the essence or active principle of a substance.

distillation (dis·tuh·LAY·shun)—the process of distilling.

distilled water (dis·TILD WAH·tur)—purified or refined water.

distribute (dis·TRIB·yoot)—to disperse through space or over an area; to arrange; in hairdressing and design, distribution refers to the direction hair is combed in relation to its base parting.

disulfide (dy·SUL·fyd)—a chemical compound in which two sulphur atoms are united with a single atom of an element, i.e., carbon; an amino acid found in hair.

disulfide links (dy·SUL·fyd LINKS)—bonds or cross linkages between the polypeptide chains of the hair cortex.

Dr. Vodder's Manual Lymph Drainage (DAHK·tur VAHD·urz MAN·yoo·ul LIMF DRAYN·ij)—a method of gentle massage along the surface lymphatics to accelerate functioning of the lymphatic system.

dominant (DAHM·ih·nent)—the prominent part or position; large or more impressive, as a dominant facial feature.

dorsal (DOR·sul)—pertaining to the back of a part.

dorsal nasal artery (DOR·sul NAY·zul ART·uh·ree)—artery that supplies blood to the dorsum of the nose.

dorsal vertebrae (DOR·sul VURT·uh·bray)—the bones of the vertebral or spinal column located in the midsection of the back.

dorso, dorsi (DOR·soh, DOR·sy)—pertaining to the back of the body; denoting relationship to a dorsum or to the posterior aspect of the body.

double (DUB·ul)—combined with another; repeated; having two parts.

double adhesive plaster (DUB·ul ad·HEE·siv PLAS·tur)—plaster that is adhesive on both sides, used on the adhesive patch to hold a hair piece in position.

double application tint (DUB·ul ap·lih·KAY·shun TINT)—a product requiring two separate applications to the hair, a softener or lightener followed by a penetrating tint; also called a two-process tint.

double bond (DUB·ul BAHND)—a chemical bond consisting of two bonds between two atoms of a molecule, each bond formed by shared electrons.

double chin (DUB·ul CHIN)—a fleshy fold under the chin giving the appearance of two chins.

double flat wrap (DUB·ul FLAT RAP)—a hair wrap in which one end paper is placed under, and one paper over, the strand of hair that is being wrapped for permanent waving.

double halo (DUB·ul HAY·loh)—in permanent waving, a technique using two rows of rods around the face area.

double knotting (DUB·ul NAHT·ing)—the method employed to attach the hair to the netting in the formation of hair pieces.

double process (DUB·ul PRAH·ses)—A technique requiring two separate procedures in which the hair is decolorized or pre-lightened with a lightener (bleach) before the depositing color is applied; two-step coloring.

double-prong clips (DUB·ul-PRAWNG KLIPS)—small clips with short prongs used to hold pin curls flat; also used in other shaping, rolling, and setting of hair.

dove tail (DUV TAYL)—a connecting line in a style between two or more shapes.

downblending (DOWN·BLEND·ing)—blending the hair down from the crown.

down elevation (DOWN el·uh·VAY·shun)—downward angle cutting of hair.

down stroke (DOWN STROHK)—a stroke made with a razor while shaving; in facials, stroking lightly upward and downward with the tips of fingers.

downward (DOWN·ward)—in hairdressing, toward the shoulder down from a part in the hair; in facials, strokes and movements from top to bottom as from cheeks to chin.

downward angle cutting (DOWN·ward ANG·ul KUT·ing)—a technique in haircutting; hair cut in graduating lengths from short to long.

downy hair (DOWN·ee HAYR)—soft, lightweight hair growth; fine hair.

drab (DRAB)—a shade that has no red or gold tones; usually a dull brown or gray color. See ash, dull.

drabber (DRAB·ur)—a concentrated coloring agent designed to reduce the presence of red or gold tones.

drabbing agent (DRAB·ing AY·jent)—a chemical used to eliminate red or gold tones from the hair color.

drab color (DRAB KUL·ur)—a hair color lacking red and gold tones; colors such as ash, gray, silver, white, platinum, smoky, or steel gray.

drag (DRAG)—a term to describe a feeling of resistance when a product is applied; the opposite of slip or ease of application.

drape (DRAYP)—a cape or covering placed on a customer to protect clothing while receiving salon services; a coverlet placed over a customer during a facial treatment.

draped hair (DRAYPT HAYR)—to arrange a section of hair in a curved or draped effect; to allow a portion of hair to fall into a curved design.

draw (DRAW)—in haircutting, to bring the section of hair through the fingers to hold it taut while cutting and shaping.

drawing cards (DRAW·ing KARDS)—in the manufacture of wigs, two identical pieces of leather with steel prongs, used to disentangle and properly arrange hair.

drawn through parting (DRAWN THROO PART·ing)—in the manufacture of wigs, a specially prepared portion of a wig in which the hair, after being knotted, is drawn through a fine silk material, which gives the appearance of the natural scalp.

drench (DRENCH)—to saturate; to soak; to wet thoroughly.

dressing (DRES·ing)—arranging hair in a style; a substance applied to the hair; a salve or pomade.

droop (DROOP)—to hand downward; be limp; lifeless; lacking bounce or elasticity.

drop crown (DRAHP CROWN)—permanent waving technique for long hair using crown rods on extended stems to achieve a smooth crown effect.

dropping a wave (DRAHP·ing uh WAYV)—the act of discontinuing a wave rather than carrying it around the entire head.

drug (DRUG)—chemical used in dyeing; a substance other than food intended to affect the structure or function of the body; a chemical compound or substance used in some medications.

dry cell (DRY SEL)—a battery; a direct current (DC) source.

dry clean (DRY KLEEN)—to clean with a substance or with a solvent, other than water, such as tetrachloride.

dry cleaner (DRY KLEEN·ur)—one who cleans clothing; a solution for cleaning fabric or wigs.

dry cut (DRY KUT)—a technique for cutting the hair while it is dry; to cut hair before it is shampooed, or after it has been shampooed and dried.

dryer (DRY·ur)—an apparatus for drying the hair; hair dryer; a device to absorb moisture.

dryer chair (DRY·ur CHAYR)—a chair to which a hair dryer is attached.

dry hair (DRY HAYR)—hair lacking sufficient or normal oils; a condition that may be temporary or chronic in nature; hair that is free from moisture.

dry hair shampoo (DRY HAYR sham·POO)—a shampoo formulated for dry hair.

dry heat (DRY HEET)—heat produced in a dry airtight cabinet containing an active fumigant; used to sanitize implements and keep them clean until ready for use.

drying lamp (DRY·ing LAMP)—an infrared lamp used to dry wet hair during a haircutting procedure.

dry sanitizer (DRY SAN·ih·tyz·ur)—an airtight, specially constructed cabinet containing a disinfectant or active fumigant such as formalin; used to keep implements sanitary.

dry shampoo (DRY sham·POO)—a substance used to cleanse the hair without the use of soap and water.

dry skin (DRY SKIN)—skin that is deficient in oil and/or moisture.

ducktail (DUK·tayl)—in hairstyling, a style popular during the 1950s and revived in the 1980s; the hair is cut short and brushed to a center point at the back of head and napeline.

duct (DUKT)—a passage or canal for fluids.

duct gland (DUKT GLAND)—gland that produces a substance that travels through small tubelike ducts; examples are the sudoriferous (sweat) glands and sebaceous (oil) glands.

ductless gland (DUKT·lis GLAND)—a gland that has no excretory duct but releases secretions directly into the blood or lymph.

dull (DUL)—used to describe hair or hair color without sheen. (*See* drab.)

duodenum (doo·uh·DEE·num)—the part of the small intestines just below the stomach.

duplicated movements (DOOP·lih·kayt·ud MOOV·ments)—movements performed by a patient with a therapist and are considered resistive or assistive exercises.

durability (door·uh·BIL·ih·tee)—the quality of being able to last for a long time without significant wear or deterioration.

dusky (DUS·KEE)—somewhat dark in shade or coloring, especially dark skin.

dye (DYE)—to stain or color; a chemical compound or mixture formulated to penetrate the hair and effect a change in hair color; made from plants, metals, or synthetic compounds; artificial pigment.

dye brush (DYE BRUSH)—a small, flat, long-handled brush designed for the application of hair coloring or hair treatment products.

dye intermediate (DYE in·tur·MEE·dee·it)—a material that develops into color only after reaction with developer (hydrogen peroxide); also known as oxidation dyes.

dye remover (DYE ree·MOOV·ur)—a prepared commercial product that removes tint from the hair; also called color remover.

dye solvent (DYE SAHL·vunt)—a chemical solution that is employed to remove artificial color from the hair.

dye stain remover (DYE STAYN ree·MOOV·ur)—a chemical substance used to remove tint stains from the skin following the hair tinting procedure.

dye stuff (DYE STUF)—a raw color ingredient.

dynel (DY·nel)—a synthetic fiber, resembling wool, which is employed in the manufacture of machine-made wigs and hair pieces.

dyschromia (dis·KROH·mee·uh)—abnormal pigmentation of the skin.

dyskeratoma (dis·kair·uh·TOH·muh)—a skin tumor; warty growth; a brownish, red nodule with a soft, yellowish keratotic plug appearing on the face or scalp.

dyskeratosis (dis·kair·uh·TOH·sis)—imperfect keratinization of individual epidermal cells.

dysvitaminosis (dis·vih·tah·min·OH·sis)—a disorder due to an excess of or a deficiency of a particular vitamin or vitamins.

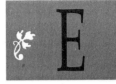

ear (EER)—the organ of hearing and equilibrium.

earlap (EER·lap)—the external ear, especially the ear lobes.

ear lobe (EER lohb)—the soft, fleshy lower part of the external ear.

earphone (EER·fohn)—a listening device held near or inserted into the ear as a hearing aid.

ear protector (EER proh·TEK·tur)—a plastic ear-shaped shell used over the ears as a protection during the hair drying procedure.

earth color (URTH KUL·ur)—any of several pigments or paints prepared from materials found in the earth; examples are: umber, chalk, clay, ocher, and charcoal.

earwax (EER·waks)—a yellowish-brown substance secreted by the glands lining the passages of the external ear; also called cerumen.

eau de cologne (OH duh kah·LOHN)—a fragrant toilet water.

ebony (EB·un·ee)—a hard, dark, almost black wood used for fine furnishings; a term used to describe a deep, dark skin tone.

eccentric contraction (ek·SEN·trik kun·TRAK·shun)—a type of isotonic muscle contraction, when the distance between the ends of a contracting muscle increases.

ecchymosis (ek·ih·MOH·sus)—a discoloration such as a bluish spot caused by the rupture of a small blood vessel beneath the surface of the skin; a bruise.

eccrine (EK·run)—pertaining to the eccrine glands and their secretions.

eccrine glands (EK·run GLANZ)—small sweat glands distributed over the surface of the skin of the human body; the glands that produce secretions important for heat regulation and hydrating the skin.

ecderon (EK·dur·ahn)—the epithelial, outermost layer of the skin and mucous membrane.

eclectic (ek·LEK·tik)—selecting from various sources; composed of elements or methods drawn from various sources.

ecology (ee·KAHL·uh·jee)—the study of the environmental relations of organisms.

ectal (EK·tul)—external; outer.

ecthyma (ek·THY·muh)—a virus disease that forms ulcerating pustules on the skin.

ecto (EK·toh)—a prefix denoting without; outside; external.

ectoderm (EK·tuh·durm)—the outermost layer of the three primary germ layers in an embryo that develops into skin, the nervous system, and sense organs.

ectodermic (ek·tuh·DUR·mik)—pertaining to the outer layer of cells formed from the inner cell mass in the embryonic cell.

ectomorph (EK·tuh·morf)—a person who is characterized by a lean, lanky body structure.

ectothrix (EK·toh·thriks)—a fungal parasite that affects the hair shaft.

ectylotic (ek·tih·LAHT·ik)—describing an agent that removes warts.

eczema (EG·zuh·muh)—an inflammatory, itching disease of the skin.

eczematization (ek·zee·muh·tih·ZAY·shun)—the presence or formation of eczema or like irritation by allergic reaction or physical or chemical irritants.

eczematoid reaction (ek·ZEE·muh·toyd ree·AK·shun)—a dermal and epidermal inflammatory condition characterized by edema and scaling.

eczematosis (ek·zee·muh·TOH·sus)—any eczematous skin disease.

eczematous (ek·ZEE·muh·tus)—having the characteristics of eczema.

edema, oedema (ih·DEE·muh)—an abnormal accumulation of clear watery fluid in the lymph spaces of the tissues.

edge (EJ)—the cutting side of a blade.

edging (EJ·ing)—the process of cutting the sideburn and nape area; feathering.

effect (uh·FEKT)—consequence; result.

effector (uh·FEK·tur)—a gland or muscle that responds to stimulation.

efferent (EF·uh·rent)—conveying outward, as efferent nerves conveying impulses away from the central nervous system, from brain to muscles.

efferent lymphatic (EF·uh·rent lim·FAT·ik)—a vessel conveying lymph away from a lymph node.

efferent neuron (EF·uh·rent NOO·rahn)—a neuron conducting impulses away from a nerve center.

effete (eh·FEET)—worn out; incapable of further vital use; exhausted of energy.

efficacious (eh·ih·KAY·shus)—possessing the quality of being effective.

efficiency (ih·FISH·un·see)—usefulness; quality or degree of being able to produce results; economic productivity.

efficient (ih·FISH·unt)—characterized by energetic and useful activity.

effilate (EF·ih·layt)—to cut the hair strand by a sliding movement of the scissors.

effilating (EF·ih·layt·ing)—a method of cutting and tapering hair in the same operation by a sliding movement of the scissor.

effleurage (EF·loo·rahzh)—a light, continuous stroking movement in massage.

efflorescence (ef·luh·RES·uns)—a rash or eruption of the skin.

effluvium (eh·FLOO·vee·um)—an ill-smelling emanation or exhalation.

effusion (eh·FYOO·zhun)—the act of pouring out; the escape of fluid from the blood vessels or lymphatics into a tissue or cavity.

egg (EG)—ovum; a round or oval reproductive body produced by female birds, fish, etc.; used primarily as a food and in some products such as shampoos and facial masks.

egg oil (EG OYL)—fatty oil extracted from the yolk of eggs; used in some types of cosmetic creams and ointments.

egg powder (EG POW·dur)—pulverized egg shell; used in many cosmetics including bath preparations, shampoos, facial masks, and creams.

eggshell nails (EG·shell NAYLZ)—nails that are abnormally thin, translucent, and blue-white and more flexible than normal; onychotrophic condition.

Egyptian henna (ih·JIP·shun HEN·uh)—a cosmetic used for dyeing the hair; a color varying from reddish-orange to coppery brown.

elastic (ih·LAS·tik)—capable of returning to the original form after being stretched; having the ability to stretch and return to the original form.

elastic band (ih·LAS·tik BAND)—a flexible band used in wigs to make them adjustable; a band of elasticized material used to hold hair off the face during a facial treatment or makeup; a fastening band on a perm wave rod.

elastic cartilage (ih·LAS·tik KART·ul·ij)—a resistant cartilage found in the external ear and larynx.

elasticity of hair (ih·las·TIS·ut·ee UV HAYR)—the ability of the hair to stretch and return to normal; important in the ability of hair to retain curl or withstand chemical treatments.

elasticity of muscles (ih·las·TIS·ut·ee UV MUS·ulz)—ability of muscles to return to their original shape after being stretched.

elastin (ih·LAS·tun)—a protein base similar to collagen, which forms elastic tissue.

elastoma (ih·las·TOH·muh)—a tumor formed by an excess of elastic tissue fibers or abnormal collagen fibers of the skin.

elastosis senilis (ih·las·TOH·sis seh·NIL·is)—degeneration of the elastic connective tissues in advanced age.

elbow (EL·boh)—the joint of the arm between the upper arm and the forearm.

elder (sambucus) (EL·dur)—a shrub of the honeysuckle family, the oil from which is used to soften the skin; provides mineral salts and amino acids that help reduce hardening effects of keratinization and aging of skin cells.

electrical (ih·LEK·trih·kul)—consisting of, containing, producing, or operated by electricity.

electrical sterilizer (ih·LEK·trih·kul STAIR·uh·lyz·ur)—a cabinet electrically heated and used to keep implements sanitized.

electric clippers (ih·LEK·trik KLIP·urz)—an electrically powered implement used to cut and trim hair, especially on the neck area.

electric comb (ih·LEK·trik KOHM)—a comb heated electrically and used in blow-dry styling of the hair.

electric current (ih·LEK·trik KUR·unt)—the flow of electric charge.

electric facial mask (ih·LEK·trik FAY·shul MASK)—a contoured pad heated electrically and placed over the fact to soften grease deposits and to induce deep penetration of beneficial products into the skin.

electric hair roller (ih·LEK·trik HAYR ROHL·ur)—a cylindrical roller designed to retain heat and used to style hair while it is dry.

electric heater (ih·LEK·trik HEET·ur)—as used in permanent waving, a heating device connected to a permanent wave machine.

electricity (ih·lek·TRIS·ih·tee)—a form of energy, that when in motion, exhibits magnetic, chemical, or thermal effects.

electricity, animal (ih·lek·TRIS·ih·tee, AN·uh·mul)—the free electricity in the body.

electricity, chemical (ih·lek·TRIS·ih·tee, KEM·ih·kul)—electricity generated by chemical action in a galvanic cell.

electricity, franklinic (ih·lek·TRIS·ih·tee, frank·LIN·ik)—a friction or static electricity.

electricity, frictional (ih·lek·TRIS·ih·tee, FRIK·shun·ul)—electricity produced by friction.

electricity, galvanic (ih·lek·TRIS·ih·tee, gal·VAN·ik)—electricity generated by chemical action in a galvanic cell.

electricity, induced or inductive (ih·lek·TRIS·ih·tee, in·DOOST OR in·DUK·tiv)—electricity produced by proximity to an electrified body.

electricity, magnetic (ih·lek·TRIS·ih·tee, mag·NET·ik)—electricity developed by bringing a conductor near the poles of a magnet.

electricity, static (ih·lek·TRIS·ih·tee, STAT·ik)—frictional electricity.

electricity, voltaic (ih·lek·TRIS·ih·tee, vohl·TAY·ik)—galvanic or chemical electricity.

electric pressing iron (ih·LEK·trik PRES·ing EYE·urn)—a curling iron designed with a larger barrel for straightening curly hair.

electric sanitizer (ih·LEK·trik SAN·ih·tyz·ur)—a dry sanitizer unit containing an ultra-violet lamp that keeps implements sanitary.

electric shaver (ih·LEK·trik SHAYV·ur)—an electrically powered device used to remove facial and body hair.

electric straightening comb (ih·LEK·trik STRAYT·un·ing KOHM)— a comb with a wooden handle and metal teeth designed with a heating element and used to straighten curly hair.

electric styling brush (ih·LEK·trik STYL·ing BRUSH)—an implement that combines a hand-held dryer with a brush; used to style hair.

electrification (ih·lek·trih·fih·KAY·shun)—the process of applying electricity to the body by holding an electrode in the hand and charging the body with electricity.

electrocoagulation (ih·lek·troh·koh·ag·yoo·LAY·shun)—the single-needle shortwave method of electrolysis; the use of high-frequency current to remove superfluous hair.

electrode (ih·LEK·trohd)—a pole of an electric cell; an applicator for directing the electric current from the machine to the client's skin.

electrode jel (ih·LEK·trohd JEL)—a jel used to improve contact between the electrode and the skin when the electrode is used in a specific treatment.

electrologist (ih·lek·TRAHL·uh·just)—one who removes hair and various skin imperfections by means of an electric current applied to the body with a needle-shaped electrode.

electrology (ih·lek·TRAHL·uh·jee)—the science of electricity.

electrolysis (ih·lek·TRAHL·ih·sis)—decomposition of a chemical compound or body tissues, particularly hair roots, by means of electricity.

electrolyte (ih·LEK·troh·lyt)—any compound that, in solution, conducts a current of electricity.

electrolytic (ih·lek·troh·LIT·ik)—pertaining to electrolysis.

electrolytic cup (ih·lek·troh·LIT·ik KUP)—an appliance used to cleanse the skin before giving a facial or body massage.

electrolytic rebonding (ih·lek·troh·LIT·ik ree·BAHND·ing)—chemical process involving reformation of electromagnetic or ionic bonds.

electromagnet (ih·lek·troh·MAG·net)—a mass of soft iron surrounded by a coil of wire; a current passing through the wire will make the iron core magnetic.

electromotive force (ih·lek·troh·MOH·tive FORS)—something that moves or tends to move electricity.

electron (ih·LEK·trahn)—a basic negatively charged particle found outside the nucleus of an atom, arranged in orbits or shells.

electronic tweezing (ih·lek·TRAHN·ik TWEEZ·ing)—the use of high-frequency current in removal of superfluous hair.

electrophobia (ih·lek·troh·FOH·bee·uh)—a morbid fear of electricity.

electropositive (ih·lek·troh·PAHZ·ih·tiv)—relating to or charged with positive electricity.

electrostatic (ih·lek·troh·STAT·ik)—pertaining to static electricity.

electrotherapeutics (ih·lek·troh·thair·uh·PYOO·tiks)—the application of electricity for therapeutic purposes.

element (EL·uh·ment)—the simplest form of basic matter; a substance that cannot be broken down into a simpler substance without loss of identity; of the more than 100 elements, examples are: iron, sulfur, hydrogen, mercury, carbon.

elementary (el·uh·MEN·tuh·ree)—basic introductory; relating to the simplest elements or principles of something.

elements in hair (EL·uh·ments IN HAYR)—elements commonly found in hair are: nitrogen, oxygen, carbon, sulfur, hydrogen, and phosphorus.

elevate (EL·uh·vayt)—to raise; to make higher.

elevation (el·uh·VAY·shun)—a term employed in hair shaping (cutting) and styling to indicate the angle or degree hair is held from the head.

elevation, high (el·uh·VAY·shun, HYE)—when hair is approximately the same length when extended at right angels from the scalp; in high elevation hair is held 90 degrees from the headform.

elevation, low (el·uh·VAY·shun, LOH)—hair is held 15 degrees from the headform creating a slight amount of layering.

elevation, medium (el·uh·VAY·shun, MEE·dee·um)—the hair is held 45 degrees from the headform.

eleventh cranial nerve (ee·LEV·unth CRAY·nee·ul NURV)—nerve that affects the muscles of the neck and back.

eliminate (ih·LIM·ih·nayt)—to rid the body of; to excrete; to set aside.

elimination (ih·lim·ih·NAY·shun)—act of expelling or excreting.

eliminative (ih·LIM·ih·nuh·tiv)—relating to or tending to eliminate.

ellipse (ih·LIPS)—a wide oval curve.

elutriate (ee·LOO·tree·ayt)—purify by washing, separating, and straining.

emaciation (ih·may·shee·AY·shun)—the state of being wasted away physically; loss of fat of the body; extreme leanness.

embed (em·BED)—to fix firmly in surrounding matter.

embellish (em·BEL·ish)—to decorate; to add something; to adorn.

embolus (EM·boh·lus)—a blood clot that breaks loose and floats in the blood, causing possible death if it becomes lodged in the lungs, heart, or brain.

embryo (EM·bree·oh)—an organism in the early stages of development; a developing human from the moment of conception to the end of the eighth week after fertilization.

embryology (em·bree·AHL·uh·jee)—science dealing with the development of the embryo.

embryonic extract (em·bree·AHN·ik EKS·trakt)—substances taken from any living thing in the earliest stages of life and used in some types of medicinal and cosmetic preparations.

emerald (EM·uh·ruld)—a bright green precious stone; a deep, rich green color.

emery board (EM·ur·ee BORD)—a disposable manicuring instrument having rough cutting ridges; used to file or remove the free edge of the nail.

emit (ee·MIT)—to send out; to give off light, heat, sound.

emollient (ih·MAHL·yunt)—an agent that softens or smooths the surface of the skin.

emollient cream (ih·MAHL·yunt KREEM)—a specially prepared cream used in facial and body massage.

emphasize (EM·fuh·syz)—to give importance or prominence to; to enhance facial features by use of cosmetics.

emphysema (em·fuh·ZEE·muh)—abnormal presence of air or gas in body tissues; a disease of the lungs marked by swelling of air spaces and destructive changes in the alveolar walls.

emulsified (ih·MUL·suh·fyd)—made into an emulsion.

emulsifier (ih·MUL·suh·fy·ur)—a substance, as gelatin, gum, etc., that helps keep oils and liquids in suspension to prevent separation of ingredients.

emulsion (ih·MUL·shun)—substantially permanent mixture of two or more liquids that are normally nonsoluble, and are held in suspension by emulsifiers.

enamel (in·AM·ul)—gloss; polish.

encephalic (en·suh·FAL·ik)—pertaining to the brain.

encephalitis (en·SEF·uh·ly·tus)—a viral disease causing inflammation of the brain or meninges.

enclose (en·KLOHZ)—to close in; confine.

end (END)—termination.

end bonds, peptide bonds (END BAHNDZ, PEP·tyd BAHNDZ)—the chemical bonds that join amino acids to form the long chains characteristic of all proteins.

endepidermis (end·ep·ih·DUR·mus)—the inner layer of the epidermis.

endermic (en·DUR·mik)—acting through the skin by absorption, as a product applied to the skin.

endermosis (en·dur·MOH·sus)—the application of a product to the skin by rubbing.

enderon (EN·dur·ahn)—the deeper part of the skin or mucous membrane; as distinguished from the epidermis or epithelium.

endo (EN·doh)—a prefix denoting inner; within.

endocardium (EN·doh·kar·dee·um)—innermost layer of the heart.

endocrine (EN·duh·krin)—secreting directly into the bloodstream as a ductless gland; secreting internally.

endocrine gland (EN·duh·krin GLAND)—one of several ductless glands, as the thyroid and pituitary and suprarenal glands, whose hormonal secretions are released directly into the blood stream.

endocrine obesity (EN·duh·krin oh·BEE·sut·ee)—a condition causing weight gain due to dysfunction of the endocrine glands.

endocrine system (EN·duh·krin SIS·tum)—a group of specialized organs that manufacture hormones.

endocrinology (EN·duh·krin·ahl·uh·jee)—the study of the endocrine glands and their function.

endoderm (EN·duh·derm)—a layer of cells developing in human fetus to produce tissue for specialized function.

endomorph (EN·duh·morf)—an individual having a body build characterized by roundness, large viscera, and fat accumulation; large of trunk and thighs.

end organ (END OR·gun)—the termination of nerve fiber in the skin, muscle, mucous membranes, etc.

endosteum (en·DAHS·tee·um)—the membrane covering the inner surface of bone in the medullary cavity.

endothelial (en·duh·THEE·lee·ul)—a thin lining of the interior of the heart, blood vessels, lymphatics, etc.

endotoxin (en·doh·TAHK·sun)—a toxic substance found in some forms of bacteria.

end papers (END PAY·purz)—absorbent papers used to control the ends of hair in wrapping and winding hair on rods or rollers.

end permanent (END PUR·muh·nent)—a permanent wave applied only to the ends of the hair.

ends, hair (ENDZ, HAYR)—the last inch of the hair furthest away from the scalp.

energy (EN·ur·jee)—internal or inherent power or capacity for performing work.

enfleurage (ahn·flur·AHZH)—a process of extracting perfume by placing blossoms in glass trays lined with odorless fat: the fat takes up the fragrance and when mixed with alcohol then distilled, provides the essential oils used in fine perfumes.

enhance (en·HANS)—to increase beauty or attractiveness; to add value and desirability.

enlarged pores (en·LARJD PORZ)—follicles (pores) that have been stretched due to accumulation of sebum and dead surface cells.

insure (in·SHUR)—to make sure or secure.

entangle (en·TANG·gul)—to intertwine the hair in a confused manner.

environment (en·VY·run·ment)—the surrounding conditions; influences or forces that influence or modify.

enzyme (EN·zym)—an organic compound, frequently a protein, capable of accelerating or producing high catalytic action that will promote a chemical change or initiate a chemical process.

eosin (EE·oh·sin)—a synthetic, organic red dye used in cosmetics, especially in lip and cheek coloring.

epi (EP·ih)—a prefix denoting upon, beside.

epicardium (ep·ih·KARD·ee·um)—the protective outer layer of the heart.

epicranium (ep·ih·KRAY·nee·um)—a broad band of muscles covering the cranium.

epicranius (ep·ih·KRAY·nee·us)—the occipito frontailis; the scalp muscle.

epidemic (ep·uh·DEM·ik)—common to many people; excessively prevalent, as a disease.

epidermabrasion (ep·ih·DURM·uh·bray·zhun)—cosmetic skin peeling achieved with chemicals or special machines; sloughing off the outermost layer of the skin.

epidermal (ep·ih·DUR·mul)—pertaining to or arising from the outer layer of the skin.

epidermin (ep·ih·DUR·min)—a regenerating substance; an extract of animal tissues that has been used in the renewal of destroyed skin, such as in wounds and burns.

epidermis (ep·uh·DUR·mis)—the outer epithelial layer of the skin.

epilate (EP·ih·layt)—to remove hair from below the skin surface; to uproot hair.

epilation (ep·uh·LAY·shun)—the removal of hair by the roots.

epilatory (uh·PIL·uh·toh·ree)—a substance used to remove hair by pulling it out of the follicle.

epilepsy (EP·ih·lep·see)—a chronic nervous disease caused by abnormal electrical activity in the CNS, characterized by sudden loss of consciousness and seizures.

epileptic (ep·ih·LEP·tik)—one affected by epilepsy.

epinephrine (ep·ih·NEF·run)—a hormone secreted by the medulla of the adrenal glands in response to emergency; used as an injection for the relief of some allergic reactions.

epiphysis (ih·PIF·uh·sus)—the enlarged area on the end of the long bones.

epithelial (ep·ih·THEE·lee·ul)—having the nature of epithelium.

epithelial cell (ep·ih·THEE·lee·ul SEL)—one of various kinds of cells that form the epidermis and lines hollow organs, such as the stomach and all passages.

epithelial tissue (ep·ih·THEE·lee·ul TISH·oo)—pertaining to cells that form the epidermis; a protective layer that functions in the process of absorption, excretion, secretion, and protection.

epithelioma (ep·ih·thee·lee·OH·muh)—a malignant growth consisting of epithelial cells.

epithelium (ep·ih·THEE·lee·um)—a cellular tissue or membrane, with little intercellular substance, covering a free surface or lining of a cavity.

eponychium (ep·oh·NIK·ee·um)—the extension of cuticle at base of nail; the quick of the nail.

equal (EE·kwal)—uniform; even; exactly the same in measurement or amount.

equal blending (EE·kwal BLEND·ing)—in hair styling, the blending of hair that is one length at an equal distance from the scalp.

equation (ee·KWAY·zhun)—a method of expressing a chemical reaction by using chemical formulas and symbols.

equilibrium (ee·kwoh·LIB·ree·um)—the state of balance between two or more forces acting within or upon a body in such a way that stability is maintained.

equipment (ee·KWIP·ment)—supplies and instruments required to perform a particular service.

equivalent (ee·KWIV·uh·lent)—a state of being or having equal values; equal in volume, area, force, etc.

eradicate (ih·RAD·ih·kayt)—to destroy thoroughly.

eradication (ih·rad·ih·KAY·shun)—act of plucking by the roots; destroying utterly.

erecter pilae (ih·REK·tur PEE·lye)—minute muscles located at the base of each hair that contract when the skin becomes cold, causing the hair to stand erect; compression of skin glands; gooseflesh.

erector (ih·REK·tur)—an elevating muscle.

erector muscle (ih·REK·tur MUS·ul)—a muscle that produces erection; for example, the arrector pili, fanlike muscles attached to hair follicles, which contract, especially when cold, causing the hair to stand up in a "gooseflesh" manner.

erosion (ih·ROH·zhun)—the eating away of tissue.

eructation (ee·ruk·TAY·shun)—belching; that which is forced out.

eruption (ih·RUP·shun)—a visible lesion of the skin due to disease; marked by redness or papular condition or both.

erysipelas (er·uh·SIP·uh·lus)—an acute infectious disease accompanied by a diffused inflammation of the skin and mucous membrane.

erythema (er·uh·THEE·muh)—a superficial blush or redness of the skin.

erythematous (er·uh·THEM·ut·us)—pertaining to or characterized by abnormal redness of the skin caused by a congestion of capillaries.

erythrasma (er·ih·THRAZ·muh)—eruption of reddish brown patches in the axillae and groin, especially due to the presence of a fungus.

erythrism (ER·uh·thrizm)—exceptional redness of the hair, beard, and skin.

erythrocyte (ih·RITH·ruh·syt)—a red blood cell; red corpuscle, and carries oxygen from lungs to body cells and carbon dioxide from cells to lungs.

erythrosis (er·ih·THROH·sis)—a reddish or purple discoloration of the skin and mucous membranes.

eschar (ES·kur)—a dry crust of dead tissue or a scab caused by heat or a corrosive substance.

esophagus (eh·SOF·uh·gus)—the canal leading from the pharynx to the stomach.

essence (ES·unz)—the extract of a plant or food containing the distinctive properties of the plant or food such as might be used in perfumes.

essential (ih·SEN·shul)—important in the highest degree; necessary; indispensable.

essential fatty acid (ih·SEN·shul FAT·ee AS·ud)—any of the polyunsaturated fatty acids that are required in the diet, including linoleic, linolenic, and arachidonic acids.

essential oils (ih·SEN·shul OYLZ)—any class of volatile oils that impart the characteristic odors to plants; in perfumes and flavorings.

ester (ES·tur)—an organic compound formed by the reaction of an acid and an alcohol.

esthetic, aesthetic (es·THET·ik)—of or relating to beauty; describing beauty in art and nature; appreciation of beauty.

esthetician, aesthetician (es·thuh·TISH·un)—a specialist in or devotee of esthetics; one whose occupation is in the cleansing, preservation of health, and beautification of the skin and body; one who gives therapeutic facial treatments.

esthetics, aesthetics (es·THET·iks)—the branch of cosmetology that deals with the health and beautification of the skin and the entire body.

estrogen (ES·truh·jin)—any of various substances that influence estrus or produce changes in the sexual characteristics of female mammals.

ether (EE·thur)—a substance obtained from distilling alcohol with sulphuric acid, used as an anesthetic.

etheric oils (ih·THAIR·ik OYLZ)—oils from the leaves of certain plants (rosemary, sage, thyme); used in herbal essence therapy.

ethics (ETH·iks)—principles of good character and proper conduct.

ethmoid (ETH·moyd)—resembling a sieve; a bone forming part of the walls of the nasal cavity.

ethmoid bone (ETH·moyd BOHN)—a light, spongy bone between the eye sockets; forms part of the nasal cavity.

ethmonasal (eth·moh·NAY·zul)—pertaining to the ethmoid and nasal bones.

ethnic (ETH·nik)—belonging to or distinctive of a particular racial or cultural division.

ethyl acetate (ETH·ul AS·uh·tayt)—a colorless liquid with a fruity odor that occurs in fruits and some berries; used as a solvent in nail polish and polish remover.

ethyl alcohol (ETH·ul AL·kuh·hawl)—the basis of some alcoholic beverages; used in cosmetic products, such as astringents, antiseptics, and fragrances.

ethyl methacrylate (ETH·ul meth·AK·ruh·layt)—a compound of ethyl alcohol and methacrylic acid used in the chemical formulation of many sculptured nails.

etiology (eet·ee·AHL·uh·jee)—the science of the causes of disease and their mode of operation.

eucalyptus (yoo·kuh·LIP·tus)—an oil from the eucalyptus plant; used for its stimulating properties and often called "blue gum."

eukeratin (yoo·KAIR·uh·tin)—a true keratin found in hair, nails, feathers, hoofs, horns, etc.

eumelanin (yoo·MEL·uh·nin)—one of two types of melanin that gives color to hair.

European hair (yoor·uh·PEE·un HAYR)—fine quality human hair, usually from European countries, used in constructing wigs and hair pieces.

evaporate (ih·VAP·uh·rayt)—to disburse in the form of vapor.

evaporation (ih·vap·uh·RAY·shun)—the product of changing from liquid to vapor form.

evascularization (eh·vas·kyoo·lar·ih·ZAY·shun)—the destruction of a vessel or a duct that conveys blood to a part of the body.

ex (EKS)—a prefix denoting out of; from; away from.

exaggerate (eg·ZAJ·ur·ayt)—to delineate extravagantly; to enlarge or increase beyond the normal.

excess (EK·ses)—more than a normal amount.

excitation (ek·sy·TAY·shun)—the act of stimulating or irritating.

excoriate (ek·SKOR·ee·ayt)—to wear away, scrape, or strip off the skin.

excoriation (ek·skor·ee·AY·shun)—act of stripping or wearing off the skin; an abrasion.

excrement (EKS·kruh·ment)—waste material expelled from the body; also called feces.

excrescence (ik·SKRES·uns)—a disfiguring outgrowth.

excrete (eks·KREET)—to eliminate from the blood or tissue from the body as through the kidneys or sweat glands.

excretion (eks·KREE·shun)—that which is thrown off or eliminated from the body; a substance that is produced by some cells, but in itself is of no further use to the body; the act or process of excreting.

excretory (EKS·kruh·toh·ree)—pertaining to or serving for excretion; organs of elimination.

exercise (EK·sur·syz)—a putting into action, use, or practice; exertion for the sake of improvement.

exfoliation (eks·foh·lee·AY·shun)—peeling and shredding of the horny layer of the skin; a process that normally follows inflammation or occurs in some skin diseases.

exfoliative dermatitis (eks·FOH·lee·ay·tiv dur·muh·TY·tus)—any dermatitis where there is excessive hair loss and denudation of the skin.

exhalation (eks·huh·LAY·shun)—the act of breathing outward, expelling carbon dioxide from the lungs.

exhaustion (ek·ZAWS·chun)—loss of vital and nervous power from fatigue or protracted disease.

exocrine gland (EK·suh·krin GLAND)—a gland that secretes to an epithelial surface directly or through ducts.

exothermic (ek·soh·THUR·mik)—characterized by or formed with the giving off of heat.

exotic (eg·ZAHT·ik)—unusual, striking, or different.

expansion (eks·PAN·shun)—distention, dilation, or swelling; the distance a completed sculptured form extends into space.

expel (eks·PEL)—to force out; to eject or dislodge; to remove a blackhead from a follicle.

experiment (ek·SPIHR·ih·ment)—to test; discover or illustrate a truth, principle, or effect; to try.

expert (EKS·purt)—an experienced person; one who has special knowledge in a particular subject.

expertise (ek·spur·TEES)—knowledge or skill in a particular field.

expiration (ek·spih·RAY·shun)—the act of breathing out; expelling air from the lungs.

expire (ek·SPYR)—to breathe out air from the lungs; to exhale; to die.

exposure (eks·POH·zhoor)—state of being open to view or unprotected, as from the weather.

exquisite (ek·SKWIH·zit)—rare; delicate; showing a high degree of excellence of craftsmanship.

extend (ek·STEND)—to open or stretch more or to full length.

extensibility (eks·ten·sih·BIL·ih·tee)—capable of being extended or stretched.

extension (eks·TEN·shun)—a type of fantasy hair piece in which the hair is sewn to a wire covered with tubular ribbon; the extension is used to add space but not density to a coiffure.

extensor (ik·STEN·sur)—a muscle that serves to extend or straighten out a limb or part.

extensor carpiradialis (ik·STEN·sur KAR·pih·ray·dee·ay·lis)—a strong muscle in the wrist that operates with other muscles to bend the hand backward.

extensor digitorum longus (ik·STEN·sur dij·ih·TOR·um LONG·us)—a muscle that bends the foot upward and enables the toes to be extended.

exterior (eks·TEE·ree·ur)—outside.

external (eks·TUR·nul)—pertaining to the outside.

external carotid artery (eks·TUR·nul kuh·RAHT·ud ART·uh·ree)—artery that supplies blood to the anterior parts of the scalp, ear, face, neck, and side of the head.

external jugular vein (eks·TUR·nul JUG·yuh·lur VAYN)—the vein located on the side of the neck.

external maxillary artery (eks·TUR·nul MAK·sah·lair·ee ART·uh·ree)—the artery that supplies blood to the mouth and the lower region of the face.

external respiration (eks·TUR·nul res·pih·RAY·shun)—the exchange of gases between the air in the atmosphere and air in the lungs: then the exchange of air in the lungs and the pulmonary capillaries.

external vertebral plexuses (eks·TUR·nul VURT·uh·brul PLEK·sus·sis)—veins located anterior and posterior to the vertebral column.

externus (eks·TUR·nus)—external; pertaining to the outside.

extracellular (eks·truh·SEL·yuh·lur)—outside of a cell or cells.

extract (EKS·trakt)—a solid obtained by evaporating a solution of a drug; to draw out; to extract a blackhead.

extracurricular (ek·struh·kuh·RIK·yuh·lur)—pertaining to activities or studies that are in addition to a regular course of study; supplementary.

extraocular muscle (ek·struh·AHK·yah·lur MUS·ul)—the six small voluntary muscles that control the movement of the eyeball within its orbit.

extravagant (ek·STRAV·uh·gant)—overly lavish; excessive.

extreme (eks·TREEM)—to a very great or to the greatest degree; to the farthest point.

extremity (ek·STREM·ih·tee)—the distant end or part of any organ; a hand or foot.

extricate (EKS·trih·kayt)—to disentangle.

extrusion (ek·STROO·zhun)—a forcing out or expulsion as the expelling of a blackhead.

exudation (ek·suh·DAY·shun)—act of discharging sweat, moisture, or other liquid from a body through pores or incisions; oozing out.

exudative eczema (EK·suh·day·tiv EG·zuh·muh)—an acute form of dermatitis in which serum is exuded; also called "weeping eczema."

exude (EKS·ood, eks·OOD)—to discharge slowly from a body through pores or incisions, as sweat.

exuviate (ig·ZOO·vee·ayt)—to cast off; to shed; as to shed skin.

exuviation (ig·ZOO·vee·AY·shun)—the shedding of epidermal structures; the act of shedding.

eye (EYE)—the organ of vision.

eyeball (EYE·bawl)—the ball-shaped part of the eye; the globe of the eye.

eyebrow (EYE·brow)—the bony ridge upon which hair grows in an arch above the eye.

eyebrow arching (EYE·brow ARCH·ing)—the plucking, trimming, or waxing of the brow hair to create a neat arched effect.

eyebrow brush (EYE·brow BRUSH)—a small, short handled brush used to groom the eyebrows.

eyebrow comb (EYE·brow KOHM)—a small comb with a short handle used for grooming the eyebrows.

eyebrow pencil (EYE·brow PEN·sul)—a pencil used to add color and shape to the eyebrows.

eyebrow remover (EYE·brow ree·MOOV·ur)—the product, such as wax, or implement, such as tweezers or a shaver, used to remove superfluous hair from the eyebrows.

eyebrow tint (EYE·brow TINT)—a metallic salt dye formulated to be used in tinting eyebrows and eyelashes.

eye color (EYE KUL·ur)—the color of the iris of the eye; color in eye makeup products.

eye cream (EYE KREEM)—a cream or emollient formulated for the delicate skin around the eyes; some of the ingredients used in eye creams are: beeswax, cholesterol, lanolin, sodium benzoate, boric acid, mineral oil, almond oil, ascorbyle palmitate, and lecithin.

eye cup (EYE KUP)—a small cup with a curved rim to fit the eye; used when washing or applying lotion or liquid to the eye.

eyedrops (EYE·drahps)—a specially formulated cleansing wash for the eyes that is dispensed with an eyedropper.

eyehole (EYE·hohl)—an opening for the eyes, as in a gauze mask.

eyelash adhesive (EYE·lash ad·HEE·siv)—a product that is used to make artificial eyelashes adhere to the natural lash line; surgical adhesive.

eyelash brush (EYE·lash BRUSH)—a small, long-handled brush with short bristles used to groom the eyelashes and to apply mascara to the lashes.

eyelash comb (EYE·lash KOHM)—a small comb with a long-handle designed to comb and curl the eyelashes.

eyelash curler (EYE·lash KUR·lur)—an implement designed to fit the curve of the eyelid so when lashes are pressed between two parts, they will be curled upward.

eyelashes (EYE·lash·iz)—the hair of the eyelids.

eyelashes, artificial (EYE·lash·iz, ar·tih·FISH·ul)—individual lash hair on a strip, applied with adhesive to the natural lash line.

eyelash remover (EYE·lash ree·MOOV·ur)—a liquid used to remove artificial eyelashes by dissolving the adhesive that fastens the lashes to the natural lash line.

eyelash tint (EYE·lash TINT)—a metallic salt dye formulated to be used in dyeing eyelashes and eyebrows.

eyelid (EYE·lid)—the movable fold of skin over the eye; the protective covering of the eyeball.

eyeliner (EYE·lyn·ur)—a pencil or liquid makeup used to outline the eyes.

eye makeup (EYE MAYK·up)—cosmetics created especially for the enhancement of brows, lashes, and eyelids.

eye pads (EYE PADZ)—cotton pads shaped to fit over the eyelids during a facial treatment.

eye shadow (EYE SHAD·oh)—a cosmetic applied on the eyelids to accentuate or contour them.

eye tabbing (EYE TAB·ing)—the application of individual artificial eyelashes.

eyewash (EYE·wash)—a soothing lotion to alleviate fatigue and to cleanse the eyes.

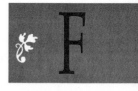

face (FAYS)—the front portion of the head comprising the area from forehead to chin and ear to ear; the forehead, eyes, nose, mouth, cheeks, and chin.

face framing (FAYS FRAYM·ing)—a frame formed by lightening (one or two shades) a narrow section of hair around the face.

face lift (FAYS LIFT)—in cosmetic surgery, rhytidectomy, the removal of excess skin to correct sagging areas of the face.

face powder (FAYS POW·dur)—a fine cosmetic powder sometimes tinted and scented that is used to add a matte or dull finish to the face.

facial (FAY·shul)—pertaining to the face; also, the seventh cranial nerve.

facial arteries (FAY·shul ART·uh·reez)—the arteries that supply blood to the face.

facial bowl (FAY·shul BOHL)—a specially designed bowl used during the spraying procedure of a facial treatment; also called a couvette.

facial chair (FAY·shul CHAYR)—a reclining chair with a headrest.

facial cream (FAY·shul KREEM)—a product in cream form used during a facial treatment for specific purposes, such as cleansing and hydrating.

facial feature (FAY·shul FEE·chur)—a distinctive part of the face, such as the eyes, nose, mouth, cheeks, or chin.

facial hair (FAY·shul HAYR)—any hair on the face; whiskers, beard, mustache, eyebrows; superfluous facial hair, usually found on upper lip and between the eyebrows.

facial index (FAY·shul IN·deks)—a number that expresses the ratio of the breadth of the face to the length multiplied by 100.

facial machines (FAY·shul muh·SHEENZ)—specially constructed apparatus, appliances, and equipment used to give facial treatments.

facial mask (FAY·shul MASK)—a mask of gauze or wax with openings for eyes and nose, used with products to benefit specific skin conditions; types include oil mask and wax mask.

facial massage (FAY·shul muh·SAHZH)—a series of movements designed to benefit the facial muscles, skin, and tissues; a procedure given by a trained esthetician to stimulate, tone, cleanse, and beautify the skin.

facial movements (FAY·shul MOOV·ments)—a massage procedure where certain manipulation and movements are used in facial treatment to benefit the skin.

facial muscles (FAY·shul MUS·ulz)—pertaining to the muscles of the face. (*See* muscles.)

facial nerve (FAY·shul NURV)—the seventh cranial nerve, one of a pair that serves to activate the muscles that control facial expressions.

facial pack (FAY·shul PAK)—a product placed on the face for beneficial purposes, such as tightening the skin, cleansing the follicles, and removing impurities from the skin.

facial proportions (FAY·shul proh·POR·shunz)—the dimensional relationship of one facial feature to another, to be considered in makeup artistry and hairstyling.

facial salon (FAY·shul sul·LAHN; SAL·ahn)—a salon or shop where clients receive facial treatments.

facial steamer (FAY·shul STEEM·ur)—an apparatus used to apply steam at a comfortable temperature to the face during a facial treatment.

facial towel (FAY·shul TOW·ul)—a small towel, usually of white cotton terry cloth about 16 × 24 inches (40.64 cm × 60.96 cm) used to apply warm, moist steam to the face during a facial treatment or a shaving procedure.

facial treatment (FAY·shul TREET·munt)—a cosmetic treatment applied to the face and neck generally for preventive or corrective purposes and for the general enhancement of skin and muscle tone.

facial veins (FAY·shul VAYNZ)—veins located on the anterior side of the head. (*See* veins.)

facioplasty (FAH·shee·oh·plas·tee)—plastic surgery of the face.

fad (FAD)—a style that is accepted for a short period of time and then disappears.

fade (FAYD)—to become indistinct; to gradually disappear; to lose color through exposure to the elements or other factors.

Fahrenheit (FAYR·un·hyt)—pertaining to the Fahrenheit thermometer or scale; water freezes at 32°F and boils at 212°F.

fair (FAYR)—light in color; pleasing to the eye.

fake (FAYK)—artificial; false, such as hair or eyelashes.

fall (FAWL)—an artificial section of hair placed across the back of the head.

fall point (FAWL POYNT)—point at crown of head from which hair grows in a circular direction.

false (FAWLS)—artificial, such as hair or eyelashes; to deceive or pretend.

fancy (FAN·see)—extravagant; elaborate; not ordinary.

fantail comb (FAN·tayl KOHM)—a comb with a tapering tail used for sectioning and parting hair, and for use in wrapping and smoothing; also called a rattail comb.

fantasy (FAN·tuh·see)—a type of hair piece that is intended only as a form of art and not for practical usage.

faradic (fuh·RAD·ik)—relating to an alternating and interrupted current that produces a mechanical reaction without a chemical effect.

faradic current (fuh·RAD·ik KUR·unt)—an induced interrupted current.

faradism (FAR·uh·diz·um)—a form of electrical treatment used for stimulating activity of the tissues.

fascia (FAYSH·uh)—a sheet of connective tissue covering, support-ing, or binding together internal parts of the body.

fascial (FAY·shul)—relating to a fascia.

fascicle (FAS·ih·kul)—a small band or a bundle of muscle or nerve fibers; fasciculus.

fashion (FASH·un)—the prevailing style during a particular period of time.

fashionable (FASH·un·uh·bul)—conforming to the mode of dress; behavior or lifestyle prevailing in a society at a given time.

fat (FAT)—adipose tissue; a greasy, soft solid material found in animal tissues; plump; obese.

fatigue (fuh·TEEG)—physical or mental exhaustion.

fatty acid (FAT·ee AS·ud)—an acid derived from the saturated series of open chain hydrocarbons.

fatty alcohols (FAT·ee AL·kuh·hawlz)—cetyl, lauryl, myristye, stearyl; these are solid alcohols used in creams and lotions.

favus (FAY·vus)—a contagious parasitic disease of the scalp, characterized by yellowish crusts.

feather cut (FEH·thur KUT)—a basic hair shaping consisting of a smooth crown surrounded by tapered ends.

feather edge (FEH·thur EJ)—a very thin fringe of hair resembling the edge of a feather.

feathering (FEH·thur·ing)—shortening the hair in a graduated effect. (*See* tapering.)

feature (FEE·chur)—distinctive parts of the face (nose, mouth, chin, lips, cheeks, etc.).

fecal (FEE·kul)—relating to the discharge from the bowel during defecation.

feel (FEEL)—to examine with the hands; to explore to determine or get an impression through the sense of touch; as to examine the texture of the hair.

felon (FEL·un)—paronychia of the nail; a painful inflammation of a fingernail or toenail.

felt (FELT)—an unwoven, matted type of fabric.

feminine (FEM·uh·nin)—pertaining to the female sex; womanly.

femur (FEE·mur)—the thigh bone; the long bone extending from the pelvis to the knee; also called the femoral bone.

fennel (FEN·ul)—an herb used in cookery and in medical and aromatic preparations.

ferment (fur·MENT)—to cause or undergo fermentation.

fermentation (fur·mun·TAY·shun)—a chemical decomposition of organic compounds into more simple compounds, brought about by the action of an enzyme.

ferrous sulfate (FAIR·us SUL·fayt)—a salt of sulfuric acid derived from iron.

fertilization (fur·tih·lih·ZAY·shun)—the union of the male and female reproductive cells.

fester (FES·tur)—to develop inflammation and pus.

fetid (FET·ud)—having a foul odor.

fever (FEE·vur)—rise of body temperature above normal, which is 98.6°F or about 37°C.

fever blister (FEE·vur BLIS·tur)—an acute skin disease characterized by the presence of vesicles over an inflammatory base; herpes simplex.

fiber (FY·bur)—a slender, threadlike structure that combines with others to form animal or vegetable tissue.

fiber rod (FY·bur RAHD)—a rod composed of fibrous material, not metal.

fiber tape (FY·bur TAYP)—a type of self-sticking tape made with nonwoven fibers; it is well suited for protection from wire endings.

fibrillar (FY·brih·lur)—having a fibrous form or structure.

fibrin (FY·brun)—the active agent in coagulation of the blood.

fibrinogen (fy·BRIN·uh·jun)—a substance capable of producing fibrin.

fibrocartilage (fy·broh·KART·ul·ij)—cartilage found between the vertebrae and the pubic symphysis.

fibroma (fy·BROH·muh)—a tumor composed mainly of fibrous or fully developed connective tissue.

fibrosis (fy·BROH·sus)—the formation of fibrous tissue.

fibrous (FY·brus)—containing, consisting of, or like fibers.

fibrous connective tissue (FY·brus kuh·NEK·tiv TISH·oo)—closely arranged fibers that form tendons and ligaments.

fibula (FIB·yuh·luh)—the outer and smaller of two bones forming the lower part of the human leg from the knee to the ankle.

fifth cranial nerve (FIFTH KRAY·nee·ul NURV)—a large sensory nerve of the face; controls chewing.

filament (FIL·uh·munt)—a threadlike structure.

file (FYL)—a hardened steel instrument having cutting ridges, for the removal of portions of anything; nail file; used to remove portion of the free edge of the nail.

filler (FIL·ur)—a preparation used to recondition and/or add color to lightened, tinted, or damaged hair; a commercial product used to provide fill for porous spots in the hair during tinting, lightening, and permanent waving. (*See* color refresher.)

fill-in curl (FIL·in KURL)—a pin curl used between roller shapings for continuous style.

film (FILM)—a membranous covering causing opacity; thin skin.

filter (FIL·tur)—anything porous through which liquid is passed to cleanse or strain it.

filterable virus (FIL·tuh·ruh·bal VY·rus)—living organisms so small they can pass through the pores of a porcelain filter; causes common cold.

fine (FYN)—being of small diameter, not coarse or thick.

fine hair (FYN HAYR)—a hair fiber that is relatively small in diameter or circumference.

finesse (fih·NES)—delicate skill.

finger (FING·gur)—one of the digits of the hand; little or fourth finger, ring finger, middle finger, forefinger or index finger; the thumb is sometimes called the first finger.

finger air waving (FING·gur AYR WAYV·ing)—a technique of rolling the hair over the fingers while air waving, as opposed to using a brush.

finger bowl (FING·gur BOHL)—a small bowl used to hold water for soaking the fingers during a manicure procedure; a small bowl used to cleanse the fingers following the serving of food.

finger breadth (FING·gur BREDTH)—the width of a finger, about 3/4 to one inch.

finger curls (FING·gur KURLZ)—elongated, spiral wound curls resembling the fingers; long curls.

finger dexterity (FING·gur deks·TAIR·ih·tee)—skill and ease in using the fingers.

fingernail (FING·gur·nayl)—the horny protective substance (hard keratin) on the upper surface of the fingers and thumb; the nail.

fingernail brush (FING·gur·nayl BRUSH)—a small brush with semihard bristles, used to cleanse the fingers and nails during the manicure procedure.

fingernail buffer (FING·gur·nayl BUF·ur)—a padded implement used for polishing the nails without nail enamel; used to stimulate blood to the nail bed.

fingernail composition (FING·gur·nayl kahm·poh·ZIH·shun)—the material that composes the nail, mainly keratin, a protein substance that forms the base of all horny tissue.

fingernail file (FING·gur·nayl FYL)—a steel instrument with fine filing edges designed for filing and shaping the fingernails; an emery board with sandpaper surfaces is also used to smooth and shape the nails.

fingernail mender (FING·gur·nayl MEN·dur)—an adhesive product used to mend split or broken nails.

fingernail polish (FING·gur·nayl PAHL·ish)—a clear or colored enamel used to beautify and protect the nails.

fingernail polish remover (FING·gur·nayl PAHL·ish ree·MOOV·ur) —a product containing acetone, usually formulated with some water, lanolin fragrance, and coloring agents; used to remove nail enamel.

fingernail reconstruction (FING·ur·nayl ree·kahn·STRUK·shun)—a process in which a substance is applied to the natural nail, then shaped to form an artificial nail to replace the damaged natural nail or to add length to the nail.

fingernail repair (FING·gur·nayl ree·PAYR)—the art of restoring and mending damaged nails by replacing the natural nail with an artificial nail or by sculpturing technique.

fingernail sculpturing (FING·gur·nayl SKULP·chur·ing)—a technique using a product to build and form realistic artificial nails.

fingernail shapes (FING·gur·nayl SHAYPS)—the general classification of nail shapes, as square, rounded, oval, and pointed.

finger shield (FING·gur SHEELD)—a small metal cap worn to protect the finger.

finger stall (FING·ur STAWL)—a finger-shaped covering of plastic or rubber; used as a protector for sensitive or injured fingers.

finger test (FING·gur TEST)—a test given to determine the degree of porosity in the hair.

fingertip (FING·gur·tip)—the extreme end of a finger.

finger wave (FING·gur WAYV)—the process of setting the hair in a pattern of waves through the use of the fingers, a comb, and a setting solution.

finger wave comb (FING·gur WAYV KOHM)—a small tapered comb used to sculpture finger waves in the hair.

finish (FIN·ish)—the final phase of a combout; the final touches to achieve a desired effect or to correct imperfections.

finishing cream (FIN·ish·ing KREEM)—an emulsion composed of stearic acid in water, utilized before makeup is applied.

finishing knot (FIN·ish·ing NAHT)—the technique used in securing the final strand of hair, on a wig or hair piece, to make certain that the hair does not become loose.

finishing rinse (FIN·ish·ing RINS)—a conditioning rinse used as the final step of a shampoo or chemical service to close the cuticle and normalize the pH of the hair.

firelighting (FYR·lyt·ing)—a coloring technique of tone on tone, red on red by single- or doubl-tinting process, depending on the desired results.

first-degree burn (FIRST-duh·GREE BURN)—a mild burn characterized by some pain and reddening of the skin, and less severe than a second- or third-degree burn.

first-quality hair (FIRST-KWAHL·ih·tee HAYR)—human hair in good condition used in wigs and hair pieces.

fishhook (FISH·hook)—a flaw in the curling of hair that results in the tip of the hair bending in a direction opposite to that of the rest of the curl.

fish oil (FISH OYL)—a fatty oil from fish used in the manufacture of soaps; hydrogenated fish oil.

fish skin (FISH SKIN)—a special material, used in wiggery, to cover the tips of springs or in some cases the entire spring, to prevent rust and discoloration.

fission (FISH·un)—reproduction of bacteria by cellular division; the splitting of an atomic nucleus.

fissure (FISH·ur)—a narrow opening made by separation of parts; a furrow; a slit.

fitting (FIT·ing)—pertaining to the adjusting of a wig or hair piece to the proper size.

fixative (FIK·suh·tiv)—a hairdressing used to keep hair in place; in cold waving, an agent that stops the chemical action of the cold waving solution and sets or hardens the hair; a chemical agent capable of stopping the processing of the chemical hair relaxer and hardening the hair in its new form; neutralizer; stabilizer.

flabby (FLAB·ee)—wanting firmness; flaccid.

flaccid (FLAS·id)—flabby; relaxed; being without bone.

flagella (fluh·JEL·uh)—slender whiplike processes that permit locomotion in certain bacteria.

flair (FLAYR)—a sense of artistry; natural talent or ability.

flake (FLAYK)—a small particle of a substance; to scale or chip as shedding of the skin in a dandruff condition; sloughing off of the epidermis due to dryness.

flammable (FLAM·uh·bul)—capable of being easily ignited and burning with great rapidity.

flare (FLAYR)—to spread outward; to add width.

flare curl (FLAYR KURL)—a pin curl that is rolled and placed so that it stands slightly away from the scalp; semi-standup curl.

flat (FLAT)—having a horizontal surface with no hollows or projections.

flatter (FLAT·ur)—to display to advantage; to enhance the individual's facial features through hairstyle or makeup.

flattop hairstyle (FLAT·top HAYR·styl)—a hairstyle for men in which the hair is cut short on top so that the ends create a horizontal line.

flat weft (FLAT WEFT)—the most common type of weaving hair on silks; woven on three silks.

flat winding (FLAT WYND·ing)—winding the hair on a rod without twisting.

flaxen (FLAK·sun)—a pale, straw color; a term used to describe light blonde hair.

fleshy (FLESH·ee)—pertaining to fullness, plumpness; as fleshy cheeks.

flex (FLEKS)—to bend, especially repeatedly; as to exercise a muscle.

flexible (FLEK·sih·bul)—capable of being bent; pliable; not stiff.

flexor (FLEK·sur)—a muscle that bends or flexes a part or a joint.

flexor carpiulnaris (FLEK·sur KAR·pih·ul·nair·us)—the extensor muscles of the wrist, which are involved in bending the hand backward.

flick (FLIK)—a quick, sharp movement.

flip (FLIP)—to turn over or up; a hairstyle with the ends of the hair turned upward.

floral fragrance (FLOR·ul FRAY·grentz)—a fragrance characterized by the scent of one flower.

floral bouquet (FLOR·ul boo·KAY)—a combination of flower fragrances.

floral perfume (FLOR·ul pur·FYOOM)—perfume made from flowers.

florid (FLOR·ud)—flushed; tinged with red; ruddy.

flow (FLOH)—smooth movement; free and graceful movement.

fluctuate (FLUK·choo·ayt)—to shift back and forth; to move like a wave.

fluff (FLUF)—hair that is combed so that it has a soft, airy effect.

fluid (FLOO·id)—a nonsolid substance; liquid or gas.

fluid dram (FLOO·id DRAM)—a measure equal to one eighth of a fluid ounce, 60 minims, or 3.70 cubic centimeters.

fluid movement (FLOO·id MOOV·ment)—the appearance of a finished coiffure achieved from a predetermined change of direction in the setting pattern.

fluid ounce (FLOO·id OWNS)—one sixteenth of a pint (29.5737 cubic centimeters).

fluorescent (flur·ES·ent)—an ability to emit light after exposure to light; the wave length of the emitted light being longer than that of the light absorbed.

flush (FLUSH)—to become red in the face due to emotion, fever, or a skin condition that causes blood to rush to the under surface of the skin; to blush.

flyaway (FLY·uh·way)—of or pertaining to an excessive electrostatic condition of hair that causes individual hair strands to repel one another and stand away from the head.

fly weft (FLY WEFT)—fine weaving used for the top row of postiche made of weft.

foam (FOHM)—a bubbly or frothy mass produced by products such as soap, detergents, or bath beads.

foamer (FOH·mur)—a substance that creates an excessive amount of foam.

foil (FOYL)—a very thin sheet of metal once used in the construction of permanent wave pads; presently used in color technique of slicing or weaving out small strands of hair and placing in color, covered foil for processing.

fold (FOHLD)—to turn or bend back so that one part covers or lies alongside another; to close or wrap; wind; the space between two folded parts.

folic acid (FOH·lik AS·ud)—vitamin B complex, found in green, leafy vegetables and some animal products.

follicle (FAWL·ih·kul)—a small secretary cavity or sac; the depression in the skin containing the hair root.

follicular (fah·LIK·yuh·lar)—affecting or arising from the follicles.

folliculitis (fah·lik·yuh·LY·tis)—an inflammation of any follicle.

folliculose (fah·LIK·yuh·lohs)—full of follicles.

folliculosis (fah·lik·yuh·LOH·sis)—a disease in which there is excessive development of the follicles.

fomentation (foh·men·TAY·shun)—made by soaking a towel in the liquid and wrapping it around the part of the body to be treated.

Food and Drug Administration (FDA) (FOOD AND DRUG ad·min·ih·STRAY·shun)—an agency of the United States Federal Government responsible for ensuring that cosmetics, drugs, and foods are safe, correctly packaged, and truthfully labeled.

foot (FOOT)—the terminal section of the limb of a vertebrate animal upon which it stands, rests, or moves.

footrest (FOOT·rest)—a small stool or platform upon which to place the feet; the extension of the service chair used in a salon upon which the client may place his or her feet.

foramen (fuh·RAY·mun)—a passage or opening through a bone or membrance.

forces (FOR·sez)—the causes that produce change or stop the motion of a body; representation of curvature motion; clockwise or counterclockwise.

forearm (FOR·arm)—the part of the arm between the elbow and the wrist.

forehead (FOR·hed)—the part of the face from the eyebrows to the hairline.

foreign matter (FOR·un MAT·ur)—undesirable substance or particles from outside the body, found on or in the skin, hair, nails, or body, occurring where they are not normally found.

forelock (FOR·lok)—a small section of hair growing over the forehead.

foreside (FOR·syd)—the front part or front side.

form (FORM)—the outline of the overall hairstyle as seen from all angles.

formaldehyde (for·MAL·duh·hyd)—a pungent gas possessing powerful disinfectant and preservative.

formalin (FOR·muh·lin)—a 37% to 40% disinfectant solution of formaldehyde in water.

formation (for·MAY·shun)—the manner in which a thing is formed or shaped.

formula (FOR·myuh·luh)—a prescribed method or rule; a recipe or prescription mixture of two or more ingredients.

formulate (FOR·myoo·layt)—the art of mixing to create a blend or balance of two or more ingredients.

forward curls (FOR·word KURLZ)—curls directed toward the face; curls wound in a clockwise direction on the left side of the head; on the right side of the head such curls would be in a counterclockwise direction.

forward wave (FOR·word WAYV)—a wave shaped toward the face.

fossa (FAHS·uh); pl., **fossae** (FAHS·ee)—a depression, furrow, or sinus below the level of the surface of a part.

foul (FOWL)—offensive to the senses; disagreeable or unpleasant.

foundation base (fown·DAY·shun BAYS)—in wig making, the supporting base upon which the hair is fastened and secured; a cosmetic, usually tinted, in liquid, cream, or powdered form, used as a base for makeup applications.

foundation cream (fown·DAY·shun KREEM)—a cream sometimes used in place of a colored makeup base or as a protective film applied before the makeup base and/or powder.

foundation, net (fown·DAY·shun, NET)—a fine, stiffened net used for most foundational hair pieces.

fraction (FRAK·shun)—a quantity less than a unit; a part of something.

fracture (FRAK·chur)—the breaking or cracking of a bone or cartilage.

fragile hair (FRAJ·il HAYR)—hair that is lacking in normal flexibility, tensile strength, and resilience and is usually brittle an easily broken.

fragilitas (fruh·JIL·ih·tus)—brittleness.

fragilitas crinium (fruh·JIL·ih·tus KRY·nee·um)—brittleness of the hair.

fragment (FRAG·ment)—a small detached portion.

fragrance (FRAY·grentz)—a pleasant, agreeable odor; a product ingredient used to enhance cosmetic and other products; products used on the person, such as perfume, toilet water, cologne, etc.

fragrant (FRAY·grent)—having an agreeable odor.

frail (FRAYL)—easily broken or damaged; delicate.

frame (FRAYM)—in hairstyling, hair arranged to create a pleasing outline for the face.

franchise (FRAN·chyz)—authorization given by owner, corporation, group, or founder to do business under their regulations.

fraudulent claim (FRAWD·yuh·lunt CLAYM)—a claim characterized by, founded on, or obtained by fraud.

frayed (FRAYD)—worn away, especially an edge of cloth, by friction or use.

freckle (FREK·ul)—a yellow or brown spot on the skin; lentigo.

free edge (FREE EJ)—part of the nail body extending over the fingertip.

free hand (FREE HAND)—a hand position and kind of stroke used when shaving the face.

free styling (FREE STYL·ing)—a technique using the fingers of one hand with a hand-held dryer in the other; to direct and style the hair.

French braiding (FRENCH BRAYD·ing)—a technique of hair braiding using four strands of hair interlaced close to the head to form a pattern.

French flow technique (FRENCH FLOH tek·NEEK)—a styling technique that employs double rollers or pin curls in an oblong design.

French fluff (FRENCH FLUF)—a combination of prepared tint and shampoo that is applied to the hair like a regular shampoo; adds some color and brightness to faded hair. (*See* soap cap.)

French knot (FRENCH NAHT)—in hairstyling, a hairstyle where the hair is smoothed off the face and gathered into a twisted roll at the nape of the neck; also called classic knot or chignon.

French lacing (FRENCH LAYS·ing)—the technique of combing small sections of hair from the ends toward the scalp causing it to form a cushion upon which the hair is combed into the desired style; also called teasing.

French seam (FRENCH SEEM)—a hairstyle created by combing the hair at the back of the head into a smooth, vertical, flat roll with the ends of the hair folded under.

French twist (FRENCH TWIST)—a vertical seamlike arrangement at the back of the head.

frequency (FREE·kwen·see)—the number of complete cycles per second of current produced by an alternating current generator; standard frequencies are 25 and 60 cycles per second.

freshener (FRESH·un·ur)—a mild liquid cosmetic usually used on the skin following the removal of cleansing cream; skin freshening lotion.

friction (FRIK·shun)—the resistance encountered in rubbing one body against another; a deep rubbing movement requiring pressure on the skin while moving it over the underlying structure.

fringe (FRINJ)—hair that partially or completely covers the facial area near the hairline; a small hair piece.

frizzy (FRIZ·ee)—hair formed into small, tight curls or narrow waves.

frontal (FRUNT·ul)—in front; relating to the forehead; the bone of the forehead.

frontal artery (FRUNT·ul ART·uh·ree)—the supraorbital artery, which supplies blood to the forehead and upper eyelids.

frontal bone (FRUNT·ul BOHN)—the bone forming the forehead; the anterior part of the skull forming the forehead.

frontalis (frun·TAY·lus)—anterior or front portion of the epicranium; muscle of the scalp.

frontal nerve (FRUNT·ul NURV)—a somatic sensory nerve that innervates the skin of the upper eyelids, the forehead, and the scalp.

frontal vein (FRUNT·ul VAYN)—the diploic vein of the frontal bones.

frostbite (FRAWST·byt)—injury to the skin and subcutaneous tissues caused by exposure to extreme cold.

frosting (FRAWST·ing)—to lighten or darken (reverse frosting) small, selected strands of hair over the entire head to blend with the rest of the hair.

frosting cap (FRAWST·ing KAP)—a plastic caplike head covering with small holes through which strands of hair are pulled to the surface to be tinted, lightened, or darkened as desired.

fruity blend (FROO·tee BLEND)—pertaining to fragrances based on the aromas of various fruits and combinations of fruits, as lemon, lime, peach, etc.; used in grooming products.

fuchsia (FYOO·shuh)—a bright bluish-red color.

full base (FUL BAYS)—placement of a roller or a curl directly and completely on its base.

full complement (FUL KAHM·pluh·ment)—complete; containing all of the essential or required substances.

fuller's earth (FUL·urz URTH)—a soapy clay often used as a foundation for packs and masks.

fulling (FUL·ing)—a massage movement in which the limb is rolled back and forth between the hands.

full stem (FUL STEM)—a curl or curling device, such as a roller, that is rolled up to the base part.

full stem curl (FUL STEM KURL)—a curl that is fastened completely off its base to give mobility to the curl; also called long stem curl.

full twist (FUL TWIST)—a ropelike winding of the hair on the rod in spiral permanent waving.

fume (FYOOM)—a smoke, vapor, or gas, especially one that is irritating.

fumigant (FYOO·mih·gant)—a gaseous substance capable of destroying pathogenic bacteria, used to keep clean objects sanitary.

fumigate (FYOO·mih·gayt)—disinfect by the action of smoke or fumes.

function (FUNK·shun)—the normal or special action for which a part is especially suited or used.

fundamental (fun·duh·MEN·tul)—basic; essential; basic rule or principle.

fundus (FUN·dus)—coiled base of the sweat gland.

fungicide (FUN·jih·syd)—a substance formulated to destroy fungi.

fungus (FUN·gus)—a vegetable parasite; a spongy growth of diseased tissue on or in the body.

furfurol (FUR·fuh·rahl)—a colorless aromatic fluid obtained in the distillation of bran with sulphuric acid.

furrow (FUR·oh)—a groove; wrinkle.

furuncle (FYOO·rung·kul)—a small skin abscess (boil).

fuscin (FUS·in)—the black pigment of the retina.

fuscous (FUS·kus)—grayish brown; dusky.

fuse (FYOOZ)—to liquify by heat; a special device that prevents excessive current from passing through a circuit.

fusion (FYOO·zhun)—the act of uniting, blending, or melting together; something formed by fusing.

fuzz (FUZ)—fine, lightweight hair.

galea aponeurotica (GAY·lee·uh ap·uh·noo·RAHT·ih·kuh)—the flat tendon joining the frontalis and occipitalis muscles in the scalp.

gallon (GAL·un)—a liquid measure equal to 4 quarts or 8 pints; in metric 3.78 liters.

galvanic current (gal·VAN·ik KUR·unt)—a direct, continued current having a positive and a negative pole; named for Galvani (1737-1798).

galvanic machine (gal·VAN·ik muh·SHEEN)—an apparatus with attachments designed to produce galvanic current; used in the treatment of facial and scalp conditions.

galvanic multiple needle technique (gal·VAN·ik MUL·tih·pul NEE·dul tek·NEEK)—a technique used to remove superfluous hair permanently by use of galvanic current and several needles.

galvanic skin response (GSR) (gal·VAN·ik SKIN ree·SPAHNS)—the electrical reaction of the skin to stimulus by the galvanometer; used to measure the skin's responses to electrical current.

galvanism (GAL·vuh·niz·um)—a constant current of electricity, the action of which is chemical.

galvanothermy (gal·vuh·noh·THUR·mee)—the production of heat by galvanism; used in therapeutic treatments.

gamma globulin (GAM·uh GLAHB·yuh·lin)—a globulin in the blood plasma that contains antibodies effective against pathogenic microorganisms.

gamma rays (GAM·uh RAYZ)—a kind of powerful electromagnetic radiation having a frequency greater than X rays.

ganglion (GANG·glee·un); pl., **ganglia** (GANG·glee·uh)—subcutaneous tumors; bundles of nerve cells in the brain, in organs of special sense of forming units of the sympathetic nervous system.

gangrene (gang·GREEN)—the dying of tissue due to interference with local nutrition.

gardenia (gar·DEE·nee·uh)—a tropical flower of yellow or white whose essence is used in perfumery.

garlic (GAR·lik)—a member of the onion family of vegetables; used in cookery, some cosmetics, and medicines; nutritionally, it provides sulphur to hair follicles and skin, regulates oil glands, and speeds removal of toxins from the system.

gastric (GAS·trik)—pertaining to the stomach.

gastric juice (GAS·trik JOOS)—the digestive fluid secreted by the glands of the stomach.

gastrointestinal (gas·troh·in·TES·tun·ul)—pertaining to both the stomach and intestines.

gaudy (GAW·dee)—showy; garish; flashy.

gauge (GAYJ)—to estimate; appraise; judge.

gauze (GAWZ)—a thin open-meshed cloth used for dressings and for facial masks in some types of facial treatments.

gauze grit (GAWZ GRIT)—a wide meshed gauze generally used as the underneath layer of a hair piece.

gauze mask (GAWZ MASK)—a mask made by cutting a piece of thin open mesh cloth (cheesecloth) to fit over the client's face and neck; the material is moistened with warm water, applied to the face, then the mask ingredients such as fresh crushed fruit or other thin substance is applied over the cloth. The purpose of the gauze is to keep the mask from running or crumbling.

gauze, silk (GAWZ, SILK)—a fine gauze silk material, having a flesh look, and used in the construction of wigs and hair pieces.

gel (JEL)—a substance comprised of a solid and a liquid that exists as a solid or semi-solid mass.

gelatine (JEL·ut·un)—the tasteless, odorless, brittle substance extracted by boiling bones, hoofs, and animal tissues; used in various foods, medicines, etc.

gene (JEEN)—the ultimate unit in the transmission of hereditary characteristics.

general circulation (JEN·ur·ul sir·kyoo·LAY·shun)—the blood circulation from the heart throughout the body and back again to the heart.

general infection (JEN·ur·ul in·FEK·shun)—an infection affecting large areas of the body.

generator (JEN·ur·ay·tur)—one who, or that which, generates, causes, or produces.

generic (juh·NAIR·ik)—pertaining to a genus or class of related things.

generic product (juh·NAIR·ik PRAHD·ukt)—a product, especially a drug, not protected by a trademark and not registered.

genetics (juh·NET·iks)—the science that deals with the heredity and variation of organisms.

gentian (JEN·chun)—an American herb used in astringents and cleansing products.

genuine (JEN·yoo·in)—authentic; real.

geriatrics (jeer·ee·AH·triks)—the branch of medicine that deals with the physical and psychological changes that affect humans during the aging process.

germ (JURM)—a microorganism that causes disease; a microbe; a bacillus.

germicidal (jer·muh·SYD·ul)—destructive to germs.

germicide (JER·muh·syd)—any chemical that will destroy germs.

germination (jer·muh·NAY·shun)—the formation of an embryo from an impregnated ovum; the first act of growth in a germ, seed, or bud.

germinative (JER·muh·nayt·iv)—having power to grow or develop.

germinative layer (JER·muh·nayt·iv LAY·ur)—stratum germinativum; the deepest layer of the epidermis resting on the carium.

germ layer (JURM LAY·ur)—any of three primary layers of cells from which the various organs of most embryos develop by further differentiation.

gerontology (jair·un·TAHL·uh·jee)—the scientific study of the processes and problems of aging.

gift spots (GIFT SPAHTS)—leukonychia; spots of whiteness on the nails, often caused by a blow to the nail or by nutritional deficiency.

ginger (JIN·jur)—a product of a tropical plant used in medicinal preparations and in cookery.

ginseng (JIN·sang)—an herb native to China and North America; used as a stimulant and in some hair and skin preparations.

glabrous (GLAY·brus)—smooth; without hair.

glamor, glamour (GLAM·ur)—fascinating, alluring, and often illusory glorification.

gland (GLAND)—a secretory organ of the body; glands vary in size and function.

glandular (GLAN·juh·lur)—pertaining to a gland.

glimmer (GLIM·ur)—a rouge that imparts a glossy appearance.

glint (GLINT)—brightness; luster; shine.

globule (GLAHB·yool)—a small, spherical droplet of fluid or semi-fluid material.

glomus tumor (GLOH·mus TOO·mur)—a tumor affecting the digits; usually painful, bluish, and benign.

glossal (GLAWS·ul)—pertaining to the tongue.

glossing (GLAWS·ing)—a technique in hair tinting and conditioning that creates a highlight effect on the hair.

glossopharyngeal (glahs·oh·far·eh·JEE·ul)—the ninth cranial nerve; pertaining to the pharynx and tongue.

glossy (GLAWS·ee)—smooth and shining; highly polished.

glucose (GLOO·kohs)—a monosaccharide (dextrose) found in fruit and other foods and in the blood; the chief source of energy for living organisms; used in the treatment of dehydration.

glued wig (GLOOD WIG)—a type of wig in which glue is placed on the base or netting, and the hair is attached to the glued surface.

glutamate (GLOOT·uh·mayt)—a salt or ester of glutamic acid used to enhance the flavor of foods; used as an antioxidant in cosmetics to prevent spoilage.

glutamic acid (gloo·TAM·ik AS·ud)—an amino acid from vegetable or grain protein, used in cosmetics as an antioxidant and as a softener in permanent wave solutions.

gluteus muscle (GLOOT·ee·us MUS·ul)—any of three muscles of the buttocks.

glutin (GLOO·tin)—a protein obtained from gelatin.

glycerin (GLIS·ur·in)—a colorless, oily substance obtained by hydrolysis of fats and by synthesis; manufactured from the natural substance, glycerol; used as a solvent, emollient, and humectant.

glycerol monostearate (GLIS·ur·awl mahn·oh·STEE·rayt)—pure white or cream-colored, waxlike solid with faint odor; used as an emulsifying agent for oils, waxes, and solvents; acts as a protective coating for various cosmetics.

glycine (GLY·seen)—aminoacetic acid.

glycogelatin (gly·koh·JEL·uh·tin)—an ointment base containing gelatin and glycerin.

glycogen (GLY·kuh·jen)—animal starch.

glycol (GLY·kawl)—any dihydric aliphatic alcohol; ethylene alcohol; useful as a solvent.

glycolic acid (gly·KAHL·ik AS·ud)—a possible intermediate in the metabolism of carbohydrates and proteins, found in cane sugar and some fruit.

goiter (GOYT·ur)—enlargement of the thyroid gland.

gold (GOHLD)—in hairdressing, a term used to indicate the presence of yellow tones; not ashy.

gold bands (GOHLD BANDZ)—uneven effect and brassy areas, occurring in some hair lightening procedures.

golden (GOHL·dun)—bright, like the color of gold; golden blond; the color of gold tones.

golden seal (GOHL·dun SEEL)—an herb having a yellow rootstock; a source of hydrosline (a crystalline alkaloid); used in astringents as a mild antiseptic; used for acne, dandruff, and like conditions.

gonads (GOH·nadz)—primary sex glands; ovaries and testes.

gonorrhea (gahn·uh·REE·uh)—a contagious venereal disease caused by the presence of the gonococci bacteria in the genital tract, characterized by discharge and burning sensation when urinating.

gooseflesh (GOOS·flesh)—skin marked by a raised appearance around the hair follicles caused by the contraction of the arrectore pilorum muscles; a condition caused by cold or emotional changes affecting the body; goose bumps.

gouty arthritis (GOW·tee ar·THRY·tis)—arthritis caused by high levels of uric acid in blood that results in pain and inflammation of joints.

grab (GRAB)—to react very rapidly to some stimulus; in haircoloring, pertaining to color that takes quickly.

graceful (GRAYS·ful)—pleasing in form, line, or movement.

graduate (GRAJ·oo·ayt)—in hairstyling, to layer the hair.

graduated haircut (GRAJ·oo·ayt·ud HAYR·kut)—a haircut in which subsections of hair are cut in layers longer from the inner layer to the outer layer; a haircut displaying up-angle cutting.

gram (GRAM)—the basic unit of mass or weight in the metric system.

granular layer (GRAN·yuh·lur LAY·ur)—the stratum granulosum of the skin.

granules (GRAN·yoo·ulz)—small grains or particles. In haircoloring, granules contain melanin pigment.

granulosum (gran·yoo·LOH·sum)—grandular layer of the epidermis.

grapefruit oil (GRAYP·froot OYL)—an oil obtained from the fresh peel of the grapefruit; used in fragrances and fruit flavorings.

grape-seed oil (GRAYP-seed OYL)—an oil expressed from grape seeds; used in hypoallergenic lubricating creams and lotions.

graphite (GRAF·yt)—a soft, black form of carbon used in pencils and as a pigment in some cosmetics.

GRAS. (generally recognized as safe)—a list established by Congress in 1958 to designate food additives that are not harmful when used as intended.

grattage (grah·TAHZH)—the scrubbing, scrapping, or brushing of a part during treatment.

gravity (GRAV·ih·tee)—the effect of the attraction of the earth upon matter; the quality of having weight.

gray (GRAY)—any achromatic color mixture of black and white; gradation of black and white.

grayed (GRAYD)—in coloring, dulled or diluted by the addition of gray.

gray hair (GRAY HAYR)—hair with decreasing amounts of natural pigment; hair with no natural pigment is actually white; white hair looks gray when mingled with the still pigmented hair.

grease (GREES)—oil; fat; oily matter.

great auricular (GRAYT aw·RIK·yuh·lur)—a nerve at sides of neck affecting the face, ears, neck, and parotid gland.

greater multangular (GRAY·tur mul·TANG·yuh·lur)—trapezium; bone of the wrist.

greater occipital (GRAY·tur ahk·SIP·ut·ul)—sensory and motor nerve affecting the splenius complexus and scalp, located in back of head.

great saphenous vein (GRAYT sah·FEE·nus VAYN)—a large superficial vein in the leg.

great toe (GRAYT TOH)—the first inner digit of the foot.

green (GREEN)—the color between blue and yellow in the spectrum; the result of mixing equal parts of yellow and blue (primary colors) to achieve the secondary color, green.

green algae (GREEN AL·jee)—a class of algae in which the cells containing chlorophyll are dominant; source of chlorophyll used in some grooming products.

green soap (GREEN SOHP)—a soft soap made from hydroxides of potassium and sodium, and containing linseed oil; used as a cleanser for certain skin problems; also called tincture of green soap.

greige (GRAYZH)—a color between gray and beige as seen in some unfinished, unprocessed, or raw fibers.

grip (GRIP)—to hold firmly; to grasp.

gristle (GRIS·ul)—cartilage, the tough, elastic connective tissue in the body.

grit gauze (GRIT GAWZ)—a very firm, wide-meshed gauze; used in the manufacture of wigs underneath the silk gauze top layer; the grit gauze is the material into which the hair is knotted and anchored.

grizzled (GRIZ·uld)—streaked or flecked with gray; graying.

groom (GROOM)—to make neat or tidy.

groove (GROOV)—the hollow part of a curling iron into which the rod fits; a long, narrow depression.

gross (GROHS)—in mathematics, a unit of quantity comprising 12 dozen.

ground (GROWND)—in electricity, the connection of an electrical current with the earth through some form of conductor, such as a ground wire that connects an electrical apparatus with the ground object.

ground wire (GROWND WYR)—a wire that connects an electric current to a ground.

growth (GROHTH)—lengthening of hair, nails, etc.; the process of growing larger, longer; increase in size or maturity; abnormal formation of tissue, such as a tumor.

growth direction (GROHTH dih·REK·shun)—the direction in which the hair grows from the scalp.

growth pattern (GROHTH PAT·urn)—the direction in which the hair grows.

guarantee (gair·un·TEE)—a contract, pledge, promise to pay or act according to agreement.

guide (GYD)—something that serves as a model to follow or provides information; a rule to follow.

guideline (GYD·lyn)—in hairdressing, a hair strand used for a general shaping pattern; hair usually at the hairline cut to a specific length to serve as a guide for determining the length of the rest of the section.

gum (GUM)—a water soluble viscous vegetable secretion.

gum arabic (GUM AIR·uh·bik)—acacia gum; a gum obtained from African acacia trees; used in facial masks, hair sprays, setting lotions, and powders; a stabilizer, emulsifier, and gelling substance.

gummy (GUM·ee)—a gumlike substance; sticky.

gum tragacanth (GUM TRAJ·uh·kanth)—a gum that binds substances together in a compact form.

guttate (GUT·ayt)—droplike form, characterizing certain cutaneous lesions.

gynecology (gy·nuh·KAHL·uh·jee)—the science and branch of medicine dealing with the diseases of women, particularly those affecting the sexual organs.

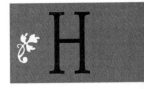

H (AYCH)— in chemistry, the symbol for hydrogen.

hack (HAK)—in haircutting, to cut the hair in an irregular or unskilled fashion; in massage, to use short chopping movements with the side of the hand.

hacking (HAK·ing)—a chopping stroke made with the edge of the hand in massage.

hackle (HAK·ul)—an oblong board designed with metal upright teeth through which hair or other fiber is pulled to remove tangles; a disentangling device used in wig making.

hair (HAYR)—a slender threadlike filament of protein keratin; an appendage or outgrowth of the skin of the head and body.

hair analysis (HAYR uh·NAL·ih·sis)—the examination of the hair to determine its condition, such as strength, elasticity, porosity, moisture content, etc.; the study of the mineral and chemical content of hair.

hair analyzer (HAYR AN·ul·y·zur)—an instrument designed to test the hair for chemical content and/or to determine its condition.

hairband (HAYR·band)—an elasticized band used to hold the hair in place during a facial treatment; a decorative ribbon or material worn to hold the hair back from the face.

hair bleaching (HAYR BLEECH·ing)—diffusing the natural pigment of the hair so it appears almost colorless. (*See* hair lightening.)

hair bobbing (HAYR BAHB·ing)—the term once used to describe the cutting of women's and children's hair.

hairbrush (HAYR·brush)—an implement designed with bristles on one end and a handle on the other; used for grooming and styling the hair.

hair buld (HAYR BULB)—the part of the hair that holds the root; the part that enclosed the hair papilla; the lower extremity of the hair.

hair canal (HAYR kuh·NAL)—the space in the hair follicle occupied by the hair root.

hair care products (HAYR KAYR PRAHD·ukts)—products formulated especially for the hair to condition, cleanse, and beautify the hair.

hair cell (HAYR SEL)—an epithelial cell with hairlike out growths, especially those in the organ of Corti in the inner ear.

hair clip (HAYR KLIP)—a metal or plastic device with prongs that open and close to secure a curl or curler, or subsection of hair in place.

hair clipper (HAYR KLIP·ur)—an implement designed to cut and trim the hair.

hair clipping (HAYR KLIP·ing)—removing the hair by the use of hair clippers; removing split hair ends of the hair with scissors.

hair cloth (HAYR KLAWTH)—a protective covering placed around the client's shoulders to protect clothing during haircutting or other hair care procedures.

hair, coarse (HAYR, KORS)—hair that is extremely large in circumference.

haircolor (HAYR·kul·ur)—an industry-coined term referring to artificial haircolor products.

hair color (HAYR KUL·ur)—the color of hair created by nature.

hair color filler (HAYR KUL·ur FIL·ur)—a product used to fill porous spots in the hair and deposit base color during the lightening, tinting, or perming process.

hair coloring (HAYR KUL·ur·ing)—the science and art of changing the color of the hair.

hair coloring brush (HAYR KUL·ur·ing BRUSH)—a flat, short-bristled brush with a long, pointed handle, designed to be used in applying a coloring product to the hair.

hair coloring classification (HAYR KUL·ur·ing klas·ih·fih·KAY·shun)—the four main categories of hair coloring; temporary, semipermanent, deposit only, and permanent.

hair coloring tint (HAYR KUL·ur·ing TINT)—oxidative color; also called penetrating tint, synthetic tint, para tint, and amino tint; used in permanent hair coloring.

hair color processing machine (HAYR KUL·ur PRAH·ses·ing muh·SHEEN)—a machine designed to increase the developing action of tints.

hair color remover (HAYR KUL·ur ree·MOOV·ur)—a product formulated to remove tint from the hair.

hair color rinse (HAYR KUL·ur RINS)—a temporary rinse used to color and highlight the hair.

hair color spray (HAYR KUL·ur SPRAY)—a spray, usually gold or silver, applied from an aerosol container, generally used for shows and special effects.

hair composition (HAYR kahm·poh·ZIH·shun)—hair is chiefly composed of protein keratin; the primary elements in average hair are: carbon, 50.65%; hydrogen, 6.36%; nitrogen, 17.14%; sulfur, 5.0%; and oxygen, 20.85%; hair also contains phosphorus in measurable amounts; the exact composition varies with the type of hair, depending to a large extent on age, race, sex, and color.

hair condition (HAYR kun·DIH·shun)—average condition; the state of health of a generally healthy, normal head of hair.

hair conditioner (HAYR kun·DIH·shun·ur)—a product formulated to be used in the hair to improve its health and appearance.

hair cortex (HAYR KOR·teks)—the layer of hair between the cuticle and the medulla.

hair cowlick (HAYR KOW·lik)—a tuft of hair standing up.

hair crayons (HAYR KRAY·uns)—sticks of coloring material compounded with soaps or synthetic waxes; used to retouch the hair growth between tintings.

haircut (HAYR·kut)—the act of cutting the hair; the result of cutting the hair.

haircut, blunt (HAYR·kut, BLUNT)—refers to a haircut in which there is no elevation; hair is cut off squarely, without taper, so all hairs are the same length.

haircut circular (HAYR·kut SIR·kyuh·lur)—a haircut with medium to high elevation that blends when combed in any direction.

haircut, geometric (HAYR·kut jee·uh·MET·rik)—haircut using straight lines, zig-zag, and unusual designs; the front perimeter and sides are cut into flattering designs.

hair cuticle (HAYR KYOO·tih·kul)—the outside, horny layer of the hair composed of transparent, overlapping cells pointing away from the scalp toward the hair ends.

haircut, reverse elevation (HAYR·kut ree·VURS el·uh·VAY·shun)—the longest length of hair is at the lower hairline with the hair cut progressively shorter toward the crown and toward the front hairline.

haircut, shag (HAYR·kut, SHAG)—a haircut combining high and low elevation with fringed effect around the hairline.

haircut, tailored neckline (HAYR·kut TAYL·urd NEK·lyn)—a hairline length with low elevation in the nape section; haircut with fitted napeline.

haircut tapering (HAYR·kut TAY·pur·ing)—cutting the hair at various lengths within the strands.

haircut thinning (HAYR·kut THIN·ing)—cutting off small strands of hair at the scalp to reduce bulk.

haircutting (HAYR·kut·ing)—shortening and thinning of the hair, and molding the hair into a becoming style; hair shaping.

haircutting comb (HAYR·kut·ing KOHM)—a comb specifically designed to be used in haircutting; usually it is narrow with short, fine teeth.

haircutting implements (HAYR·kut·ing IM·pluh·ments)—the tools used to cut, trim, and shape the hair: scissors, thinning shears, straight razor, combs, hair clippers, razors, and safety guards.

haircutting kit (HAYR·kut·ing KIT)—a case designed to hold the implements used in haircutting.

haircutting lotion (HAYR·kut·ing LOH·shun)—a liquid applied to wet hair before cutting to aid the cutting process.

haircutting shears (HAYR·kut·ing SHEERZ)—scissors designed to cut and shape the hair; special thinning shears are used to remove excess bulk.

haircut under elevation (HAYR·kut UN·dur el·uh·VAY·shun)—the shortest length of the hair is at the lower hairline; hair is cut progressively longer toward the top of the head, causing each layer to overlap to cover hair underneath; used in "page boy" styles.

hair density (HAYR DEN·sih·tee)—the amount of hair strands per square inch on the scalp, generally broken into categories according to color; approximate number of hairs: blond hair, 140,000; brown hair, 110,000; black hair, 108,000; red hair, 90,000.

hair design (HAYR dee·ZYN)—the art of styling the hair; a specific style or trend.

hair, direction (HAYR dih·REK·shun)—the direction in which the hair flows in the final combout.

hair disease (HAYR dih·ZEEZ)—disease affecting the hair or scalp. (*See* trichology.)

hairdresser (HAYR·dres·ur)—a term for cosmetologist.

hairdresser's dermatitis (HAYR·dres·urz der·mah·TYT·us)—an inflammation of the skin caused by coming in contact with irritating substances used in hairdressing procedures.

hairdressing (HAYR·dres·ing)—art of arranging the hair into various becoming shapes or styles.

hairdressing adhesive (HAYR·dres·ing ad·HEE·siv)—a substance used to hold small curls in place.

hair dryer (HAYR DRY·ur)—a machine used to dry the hair; chair with drying hood; hand-held hair dryer.

hair drying lamp (HAYR DRY·ing LAMP)—an infrared lamp with a reflector designed to dry wet hair.

hair dyeing (HAYR DY·ing)—giving the hair new and permanent color by impregnating it with a coloring agent.

hair elasticity (HAYR ee·las·TIS·ut·ee)—the ability of hair to stretch and return to its original form without breaking.

hair ends (HAYR ENDZ)—the last one to on- half inch of hair growth furthest from the scalp.

hair filler (HAYR FIL·ur)—a commercial product used to provide fill for porous spots in the hair during tinting, lightening, and permanent waving.

hair, fine (HAYR, FYN)—hair that is extremely small in circumference.

hair follicle (HAYR FAHL·ih·kul)—the depression in the skin containing the hair root.

hair glands (HAYR GLANZ)—the sebaceous glands (oil glands) of the hair follicles.

hair goods (HAYR GOODS)—wigs, hair pieces, and decorative items for the hair.

hair lace (HAYR LAYS)—a net foundation made or stiffened human hair that is used in wig making.

hair lacquer (HAYR LAK·ur)—a product used to hold a hairstyle in place; usually used in spray form.

hairless (HAYR·les)—without hair; bald.

hairlift (HAYR·lift)—an instrument employed to raise hair into proper balanced position while combing.

hair lightening (HAYR LY·ten·ing)—a chemical process involving the diffusion of the natural color pigment or artificial color from the hair.

hairline (HAYR·lyn)—the line around the top of the head at which the hair ends, the edge of the growth of the hair around the face.

hairline tip (HAYR·lyn TIP)—the thin line at the tip of the nail where excess nail polish is removed during the manicure.

hair loss (HAYR LAWS)—alopecia; unnatural loss of hair or premature baldness.

hair net (HAYR NET)—a cap-shaped, open mesh head covering made of nylon or rayon, used to hold the hair in place while drying; also made in a three-cornered scarf style, which is tied over the head.

hair oil (HAYR OYL)—an oil used to lubricate dry hair and scalp.

hair ornament (HAYR OR·nuh·ment)—a decorative object added to the finished hairstyle; comb, ribbon, feathers, bow, clasp, etc.

hair papilla (HAYR puh·PIL·uh)—a small cone-shaped elevation at the bottom of the hair follicle.

hair parting (HAYR PART·ing)—separating the hair by a line to comb or create a set, or as an aid in styling the hair; the sectioning of hair to apply tint or bleach to the scalp.

hair piece (HAYR PEES)—toupee; a small wig used to cover top or crown of the head; added piece of hair used in some women's hairstyles.

hairpin (HAYR·pin)—a slender, elongated "U"-shaped pin of plastic or metal, used to secure the hair in place; a pin shaped like a clasp with ridges or plain sides.

hair porosity (HAYR puh·RAHS·ut·ee)—the ability of hair to absorb moisture.

hair pressing (HAYR PRES·ing)—a method of temporarily straightening overcurly hair by means of a heated iron or comb.

hair pressing cream (HAYR PRES·ing KREEM)—a cream used in hair pressing as a protective lubricant for the hair.

hair pressing oil (HAYR PRES·ing OYL)—an oily or waxy mixture used in hair pressing.

hair relaxer (HAYR ree·LAKS·ur)—a chemical product used to soften or remove natural curl from the hair.

hair relaxing (HAYR ree·LAKS·ing)—a method used to chemically straighten overcurly hair so that it can be styled in less curly arrangements.

hair restorer (HAYR ree·STOR·ur)—a haircoloring preparation containing metallic dye; not used professionally.

hair roll (HAYR ROHL)—a sausagelike shape, in various lengths; used to fill under hair to create special effects.

hair roller (HAYR ROHL·ur)—a tube-shaped device made of metal, plastic, or other material of various lengths and diameters; used to set hair following a shampoo.

hair roller pick (HAYR ROHL·ur PIK)—a toothpick-shaped plastic pick used to hold a hair roller in place.

hair roller pin (HAYR ROHL·ur PIN)—a flat, long, closed "U"-shaped pin, used to secure hair rollers.

hair root (HAYR ROOT)—that part of the hair contained within the follicle, below the surface of the scalp.

hair sample (HAYR SAM·pul)—a swatch of hair taken from a client's hair for purposes of testing or matching.

hair set (HAYR SET)—the technique of placing the hair into roller or pin curl patterns, finger waving, or other manipulations, then combing and brushing into a finished style.

hair set tape (HAYR SET TAYP)—a type of tape that is used to assist in the foundation of hairlines and curves when the hair is too short to set on rollers or in pin curls.

hair setting product (HAYR SET·ing PRAHD·ukt)—a lotion, spray, or gel used to make the hair easier to set and to hold the finished style in place.

hair shaft (HAYR SHAFT)—the portion of hair that projects beyond the skin, consisting of an outer layer, the cuticle; an innermost layer, the medulla; and an in-between layer called the cortex.

hair shapers (HAYR SHAYP·urz)—an implement for haircutting shaped like a straight razor with a safety guard.

hair shaping (HAYR SHAYP·ing)—the art of haircutting; molding the hair into a style.

hair shingling (HAYR SHING·gling)—the technique of cutting the hair close to the nape with the hair becoming gradually longer toward the crown.

hair slithering (HAYR SLITH·ur·ing)—the process used in thinning and tapering the hair at the same time, using scissors.

hair softener (HAYR SAW·fen·ur)—a hair pomade, hair cream, cream rinse, or similar substances that tend to remain on the hair for better texture and control.

hair spray (HAYR SPRAY)—a hair cosmetic applied in the form of a mist.

hair straightener (HAYR STRAYT·en·ur)—a chemical agent or an iron used to straighten overcurly hair.

hair straightening (HAYR STRAYT·en·ing)—straightening over-curly hair by use of chemical agents or a heated mechanical device.

hair stream (HAYR STREEM)—the natural direction in which the hair grows after leaving the follicle.

hairstyle (HAYR·styl)—a way of wearing the hair; a coiffure.

hairstyling (HAYR·styl·ing)—the art of dressing the hair.

hairstylist (HAYR·styl·ist)—a specialist in the creation and design of hair fashions.

hair, superfluous (HAYR, soo·PUR·floo·us)—unwanted or excess hair on the face or body.

hair test (HAYR TEST)—a sampling of how the hair will react to a particular treatment.

hair texture (HAYR TEKS·chur)—the general quality of hair as to coarse, medium, or fine; the feel of the hair.

hair thinning (HAYR THIN·ing)—a procedure to reduce the bulk and density of hair.

hair tint (HAYR TINT)—a permanent hair coloring.

hair tinting (HAYR TINT·ing)—the act of chemically adding pig-ment to either virgin or tinted hair.

hair tint test (HAYR TINT TEST)—the testing of a product on the client's skin to determine predisposition to the ingredients in the product to be used; a test to determine the reaction of a tint on a sample strand of hair.

hair tonic (HAYR TAHN·ik)—a liquid product for cleansing the hair and toning the scalp.

hair transplant (HAYR TRANZ·plant)—a surgical procedure for transferring tufts of hair from one area of the scalp to a bald area.

hair treatment (HAYR TREET·munt)—a procedure using appropriate products to improve the condition of the hair and scalp.

hair trim (HAYR TRIM)—trimming; cutting the hair slightly; following the existing lines.

hair weaving (HAYR WEEV·ing)—the practice of sewing wefts of hair into a foundation, attached to the remaining hair on the head, in an effort to eliminate the appearance of baldness.

hair weft (HAYR WEFT)—a section of woven hair.

hairy (HAYR·ee)—having excessive hair growth; hirsute.

hairy nevus (HAYR·ee NEE·vus)—a mole; a pigmented, brownish growth covered with hair.

half base (HAF BAYS)—the placement of a roller or a curl one-half off the base.

half moon (HAF MOON)—in manicuring, a term pertaining to the light, crescent shape at the base of each nail, which may be polished or left unpolished; lunula.

half stem (HAF STEM)—a technique by which a curl is rolled and placed one-half off its base; pertains to rollers, pin curls, and perm wave rods.

half tone (HAF TOHN)—a semitone, halfway between a highlight and a shadow.

half twist (HAF TWIST)—a term used in permanent waving to designate a type of winding, flat on one side of the rod and twisted on the other side in each revolution.

half wig (HAF WIG)—a hair piece formed on one-half of a wig base to blend with the natural hair on the head.

halitosis (hal·uh·TOH·sus)—offensive odor from the mouth; foul breath.

hallux (HAL·uks)—the first and innermost digit of the foot; the great toe.

halo (HAY·loh)—lengths of layered hair, on a ventilated or wefted foundation band, which is used over the top of the head or to encircle the head.

halo lightening (HAY·loh LYT·un·ing)—lightening the hairline area to create a halo effect.

halo wrap (HAY·loh RAP)—a permanent wave created by wrapping vertical rods at the perimeter.

halve (HAV)—to divide into two equal parts; to take half.

hamamelis (ham·uh·MEE·lus)—a shrub of eastern North America having hazel-like leaves and small yellow flowers appearing after the leaves have fallen; witch hazel is an extract of this plant, and is used as an astringent.

hamate (HAY·mayt)—hooked, unciform; a bone of the wrist.

hamstring (HAM·string)—in human anatomy, one of the tendons at the back of the knee; tendon of the biceps, flexor femoris.

hand (HAND)—in human and primate anatomy, the part of the upper limb distal to the forearm and comprising the corpus, metacarpul, and fingers (digits); the part attached to the wrist, top, or back of the hand, palm, fingers, and thumb.

hand care (HAND KAYR)—pertaining to beneficial exercises and grooming of the hands and nails.

hand care products (HAND KAYR PRAHD·ukts)—any cream, lotion, or other preparation used to soften and smooth the skin of the hands and to aid in care of the nails.

hand clippers (HAND KLIP·urz)—an implement used in haircutting. (*See* clippers.)

hand-held implement (HAND-HELD IM·pluh·ment)—an item, such as a blow-dryer, clippers, scissors, and facial apparatus, held in the hand and used to perform a service.

handmade (HAND·mayd)—made by hand, as differentiated from machine made.

hand massage (HAND muh·SAHZH)—a series of massage movements for the hands, included with a manicure.

hand mirror (HAND MEER·ur)—a small mirror with a handle used in the salon to enable the client to view the back and sides of the finished hairstyle.

handtied (HAND·tyd)—a process in wig making whereby individual hairs are inserted in the mesh foundation and knotted individually with the aid of a needle; this type of wig is also referred to as a ventilated hair piece.

hanging curls (HANG·ing KURLZ)—curls hanging downward from the head.

hangnail (HANG·nayl)—a tear in a strip of epidermis at the side of the nail; agnail.

hard (HARD)—firm; solid; difficult.

hardener (HARD·un·ur)—a substance used to strengthen the fingernails.

hard goods (HARD GOODZ)—pertaining to apparatus, machines, implements; also hardware.

hard press (HARD PRES)—a technique in thermal hair straightening of repeating the procedure to remove all the curl.

hard rubber (HARD RUB·ur)—a substance used in the manufacture of combs for the cosmetology and barbering industry.

hard soap (HARD SOHP)—a soap made with sodium hydroxide; a white solid, bar-shaped soap, or a yellowish or white powdered soap.

hard sore (HARD SOR)—also called a chancre sore; a primary lesion that forms a hard crust.

hard water (HARD WAW·tur)—water containing certain minerals and metallic salts as impurities; does not lather with soap.

harmony (HAR·muh·nee)—an orderly or pleasing arrangement of shapes and lines.

haversian canals (huh·VUR·zhun kuh·NALZ)—small channels through which the blood vessels divide in the bone.

hay fever (HAY FEE·vur)—allergy caused by plant pollens in the air.

hazel (HAY·zul)—a medium yellowish-brown color.

H-bond (AYCH-BAHND)—a hydrogen bond.

head (HED)—the part of a vertebrate animal at the top or front of a spinal column containing the sense organs: eyes, ears, nose, and the mouth.

headband (HED·band)—a band, usually of material, worn to hold the hair back from the face.

headdress (HED·dres)—an ornamental addition to the hair; the style in which the hair has been arranged; a coiffure.

head lice (HED LYS)—small, flat insects that may infect humans; an external parasite (pediculus capitis) found on the head.

heal (HEEL)—to cure.

health (HELTH)—state of being whole or sound in body and mind.

heart (HART)—a hollow muscular organ that by contracting rhythmically, keeps up the circulation of the blood.

heat (HEET)—high temperature; to be or become warm or hot.

heat, electric (HEET ee·LEK·trik)—the heat produced in a conductor by the passage of an electric current through it.

heater (HEET·ur)—an apparatus used to warm products used in some grooming services; an example is the electric heater for warming wax used in facials and to remove superfluous hair.

heating cap (HEET·ing KAP)—an insulated cap, containing interwoven electric wires, which is used for heating the hair and scalp in some corrective treatment.

heating coil (HEET·ing KOYL)—electric coil that heats the air in a hair dryer.

heat lamp (HEET LAMP)—a reddish-brown, coated glass bulb that produces infrared light; used as an aid in heat treatments.

heat rash (HEET RASH)—also called miliaria; an acute, inflammatory disease of the sweat glands characterized by lesions and itching papules; prickly heat.

heat regulation (HEET reg·yuh·LAY·shun)—a system of permanent waving employing either machines or chemicals to generate heat; a means of controlling the amount of heat generated by chemical or mechanical means.

heat rollers (HEET ROHL·urz)—electric or steam preheated rollers for setting the hair.

heat treatment (HEET TREET·munt)—a treatment given with the aid of a heat lamp, which produces infrared light.

heat wave (HEET WAYV)—a permanent wave accomplished by changing the hair structure from an ordinary and natural straightness to one of curliness or waviness by using heat and mild chemicals.

heat waving (HEET WAYV·ing)—a method of permanent waving using machines or chemicals to produce heat.

heavy hair (HEV·ee HAYR)—dense, thick hair having more than average weight and mass.

heavy side of the head (HEV·ee SYD UV THE HED)—the side of the head to which most of the hair is directed.

Heberden's disease (HEE·bur·denz dih·ZEEZ)—arthritis; a degenerative joint disease affecting the fingers and hand; often deforming the bone structure.

heel (HEEL)—in human anatomy, the round, posterior part of the foot behind the arch and back of the ankle; also the heel of the hand, the part of the hand near the wrist and adjoining the thumb.

height (HYT)—the distance from the base to the top.

helcoma (hel·KOH·muh)—an ulcer.

helical (HEEL·ih·kul)—shaped like a spiral.

helical winding (HEEL·ih·kul WYND·ing)—winding the hair from the scalp to the ends;. (*See* spiral waving.)

heliotherapy (hee·lee·oh·THAIR·uh·pee)—the therapeutic use of solar energy; use of the sun's rays as a beneficial treatment.

helix (HEE·liks)—spiral formation; the structural arrangement of polypeptide chains in the hair.

hem (HEM)—the bent-over edge of a piece of material that has been turned under to avoid fraying; in wig work, the netting and the binding.

hemal, haemel (HEE·mul)—relating to the blood or blood vessels.

hematidrosis, hemidrosis (hem·uh·tih·DROH·sus, hem·uh·DROH·sus)—the excretion of sweat stained with blood or blood pigment.

hematocyst (heh·MAT·uh·sist)—a cyst containing blood.

hematocyte (heh·MAT·uh·syt)—a blood corpuscle.

hematology (hee·muh·TAHL·oh·jee)—the science of the blood, its functions, composition, and diseases.

hematoma (hee·muh·TOH·muh)—mass of blood trapped in tissue or cavity as a result of internal bleeding.

hemi (HEM·ih)—a prefix signifying half.

hemifacial (hee·ih·FAY·shul)—pertaining to one side of the face.

hemoglobin; haemoglobin (HEE·muh·gloh·bun)—the coloring matter of the blood; the oxygen-carrying pigment in the blood and iron-containing protein in red blood cells.

hemophilia (hee·moh·FEE·lee·uh)—disease characterized by slow blood clotting and excessive bleeding.

hemopoietic tissue (hee·muh·poy·ET·ik TISH·oo)—tissue found in bone marrow and the vascular system.

hemorrage (HEM·uh·rij)—heavy or uncontrollable bleeding.

hemostatic (hee·muh·STAT·ik)—a substance used to control bleeding; also referred to as a styptic.

henna (HEN·uh)—the leaves of an Asiatic plant, lawsone, used as a dye, imparting a reddish tint; also used as a cosmetic.

henna, compound (HEN·uh KAHM·pownd)—Egyptian henna to which has been added one or more metallic preparations to alter color and adhere like a coating to the hair. (*See* progressive dye.)

henna intensifier (HEN·uh in·TEN·sih·fy·ur)—an additive for henna that increases its color value.

henna leaves (HEN·uh LEEVZ)—leaves of the henna plant from which a red dye is extracted; the dye may be used on hair but is not used on eyebrows or eyelashes.

henna shampoo (HEN·uh sham·POO)—a shampoo to which henna has been added to add color and luster to the hair.

henna, white (HEN·uh, WHYT)—magnesia plus peroxide and ammonia.

herb (URB, HURB)—a plant with leaves, stems, or parts used in cookery and in medicinal and cosmetic preparations.

herbal (URB·ul)—pertaining to herbs.

herbal extracts (URB·ul EKS·trakts)—substances from herbs used in various products.

herbal shampoo (URB·ul sham·POO)—shampoo containing substances extracted from bark, roots, and herbs known to aid in cleansing the hair and scalp; shampoo to which saponin products have been added.

herbal therapy (URB·ul THAIR·uh·pee)—the use of etheric oils of plants and natural oils, applied to the skin as a stimulant and to impart a sense of physical well being.

hereditary (huh·RED·ih·teh·ree)—descending from ancestor to heir; genetically transmitted from parent to offspring.

heredity (huh·RED·ih·tee)—the genetic capacity of the organism to develop ancestral characteristics; the transfer of qualities or disease from parent to offspring.

herpes (HER·peez)—an inflammatory disease of the skin caused by a viral infection and characterized by small vesicles in clusters.

herpes facialis (HER·peez fah·she·AY·lis)—a type of herpes simplex affecting the face, usually the lips and mouth; coldsore.

herpes simplex (HER·peez SIM·pleks)—fever blister; cold sore; viral infection.

hexachlorophenol (heks·uh·kloh·roh·FEE·nohl)—white, free-flowing powder, essentially odorless; used as a bactericidal agent in antiseptic soaps, deodorant products, including soaps and various cosmetics.

hidroa (hy·DROH·uh)—a skin lesion associated with or caused by profuse sweating.

hidrosis (hid·ROH·sus)—abnormally profuse sweating.

high caloric diet (HY kal·OR·ik DY·ut)—a diet containing 3,000 or more calories per day.

high colored (HY KUL·urd)—deep or brilliant rosy color; exaggerated color.

high elevation (HY el·uh·VAY·shun)—haircutting term indicating that hair is held 90 degrees or more from the head form and then cut, causing it to fall in a layered effect.

high fashion (HY FASH·un)—a current fashion trend in clothing, hairstyling, or hair coloring.

high fashion blonding (HY FASH·un BLAHND·ing)—the special process of coloring in which the hair is lightened and then toned.

high-frequency current (HY-FREE·kwen·see KUR·ent)—current with a high vibration.

high-frequency machine (HY-FREE·kwen·see muh·SHEEN)—a machine that produces violet rays, used for facial and scalp treatments.

high frequency, tesla (HY FREE·kwen·see TES·luh)—violet ray; an electric current of medium voltage and medium amperage.

high lift tinting (HY LIFT TINT·ing)—a single-process color with a higher degree of lightening action and a minimum amount of color deposit.

highlight (HY·lyt)—brightness or luster added to hair by some artificial means; a lighter cosmetic applied to a facial feature to improve its contours.

highlighting (HY·lyt·ing)—coloring some of the hair strands lighter than the natural color to add the illusion of sheen; generally not strongly contrasting from the natural color; applying a lighter cosmetic to a facial feature to improve its contours.

highlighting shampoo tint (HY·lyt·ing sham·POO TINT)—a permanent hair tint mixed with peroxide and shampoo; used when a very slight change in hair shade is desired.

high molecular weight (HY muh·LEK·yuh·lur WAYT)—large size and density of a specific molecular construction.

high style (HY STYL)—the newest hair fashion; an up-to-the minute design.

hip (HIP)—in human anatomy, the part of the body below the waist on either side of the pelvis.

hip bone (HIP BOHN)—the innominate bone.

hirsute (HUR·soot, hur·SOOT)—hairy; having coarse, long hair; shaggy.

hirsuties (hur·SOO·shee·eez)—hypertrichosis; growth of an unusual amount of hair in unusual locations, as on the faces of women or the backs of men; hairy; superfluous hair.

hirsutism (HUR·suh·tiz·um)—pertaining to an excessive growth or cover of hair, especially in areas not normally covered with excessive hair.

histologists (his·TAHL·uh·jists)—those who apply themselves to the science of histology.

histology (his·TAHL·uh·jee)—the science of the minute structure of organic tissues; microscopic anatomy.

hives (HYVZ)—urticaria; a skin eruption.

hoary (HOR·ee)—gray or white with age.

Hodgkin's disease (HAHJ·kinz dih·ZEEZ)—a disease characterized by enlargement of the lymph nodes, lymphoid tissue, and the spleen; a progressive and sometimes fatal condition, named after Dr. Thomas Hodgkin (1798-1866).

hold (HOLD)—pertaining to the ability of a hair spray to keep a hairstyle in place.

holding angle (HOLD·ing ANG·gul)—angle at which the hand is held while cutting hair from the headform.

homeostasis (hoh·mee·oh·STAY·sus)—the maintenance of normal, internal stability in the organism.

homogenizer (huh·MAHJ·uh·nyz·ur)—a substance that produces a uniform suspension of emulsions from two or more normally immiscible substances.

homogenous (huh·MAHJ·uh·nus)—having the same nature or quality; a uniform character in all parts.

hone (HOHN)—a fine grit stone used to sharpen a cutting tool, such as a razor; used for haircutting or for shaving the beard.

honey (HUN·ee)—mel; the product of the honey bee; considered to be a health-giving food and sometimes used in facial and other cosmetic products.

honeycomb base (HUN·ee·kohm BAYS)—a lightweight, openly woven base on a wig through which a person's own hair can be pulled through the openings and blended with the artificial wig hair.

honeysuckle (HUN·ee·suk·ul)—a large climbing shrub with white or crimson flowers, valued for its pleasing fragrance; used in perfumery.

hops (HAHPS)—a climbing herb with scaly fruit; produces an astringent and moisturizing substance; provides amino acids for cell renewal.

horizontal (hor·ih·ZAHN·tul)—parallel to the horizon; level; opposed to vertical.

hormone (HOR·mohn)—a secretion produced in and by one of the endocrine glands, such as the pituitary, thyroid, adrenals, etc., and carried by the blood stream or body fluid to another part of the body or body organ to stimulate functional activity.

hormone cream (HOR·mohn KREEM)—a cosmetic containing hormones.

horny (HOR·nee)—composed of or resembling horns; a keratoid substance; having the hard texture of horns.

horse chestnut (HORS CHES·nut)—a tree bearing chestnutlike fruit, digitate leaves, and clusters of flowers; used in preparations for facial treatments; said to tighten pores, stimulate, and speed healing of the skin.

horsetail (HORS·tayl)—an herb with hollow, jointed stems used in products for the skin and hair; contains vitamin C and acts as an astringent and healing substance.

hot brush (HAHT BRUSH)—an electric curling iron with metal body and firm bristles, shaped like a round brush; used to style the hair when it is dry.

hot comb (HAHT KOHM)—a thermal iron used in hair pressing; also an electric appliance designed to dry the hair as it is being styled.

hot iron (HAHT EYE·urn)—another term for curling iron.

hot oil (HAHT OYL)—a warmed oil used in facial and manicure treatments.

hot rollers (HAHT ROHL·urz)—rollers that are preheated before being placed in the hair.

hue (HYOO)—pertaining to a particular color, tint, or shade; gradation of color.

human hair (HYOO·mun HAYR)—hair that grows on a human being; the facial, head, or body hair of a person.

human hair wig (HYOO·mun HAYR WIG)—a wig made with Asiatic or European hair, considered to be of excellent quality.

humectant (hyoo·MEK·tent)—a substance that absorbs moisture or promotes retention of moisture; a substance having affinity for water, with the stabilizing action on water content of a material.

humeral (HYOO·mur·ul)—pertaining to the humerus; the shoulder or shoulders.

humerus (HYOO·muh·rus)—the bone of the upper part of the arm.

humid (HYOO·mid)—containing moisture, vapor, or water; damp.

humidity (hyoo·MID·ih·tee)—dampness; a moderate amount of wetness especially of the atmosphere.

hyacinth (HY·uh·sinth)—a fragrant bell-shaped flower cultivated for use in perfumery; the color purple-blue.

hyaline (HY·uh·lin)—cartilage found in the nose, trachea, and on the ends of bones and in movable joints.

hydrate (HY·drayt)—a compound formed by the union of water with some other substance; to combine a substance with water; to add moisture to the skin.

hydrating agent (HY·drayt·ing AY·jent)—a substance used in facial treatments to restore moisture to a dry (dehydrated) skin.

hydration (hy·DRAY·shun)—the chemical union of a substance with water.

hydro (HY·droh)—a prefix denoting water; hydrogen.

hydrocarbon (hy·droh·KAR·bun)—charcoal; any compound consisting only of hydrogen and carbon.

hydrochloric acid (hy·droh·KLOR·ik AS·ud)—a compound of hydrogen and chlorine.

hydrocyst (HY·droh·sist)—a cyst containing a watery fluid.

hydrocystoma (hid·roh·sis·TOH·muh)—a variety of sudamina appearing on the face, especially of women in middle and advanced life.

hydrogen (HY·druh·jun)—in chemistry, the symbol H; the lightest element; it is an odorless, tasteless, colorless gas found in water and all organic compounds.

hydrogenate (hy·DRAHJ·uh·nayt)—to combine or treat with hydrogen.

hydrogenated lanolin (HY·druh·jen·ayt·ud LAN·ul·un)—lanolin treated with hydrogen so that it retains its emollient qualities while losing unwanted odor, color, and tackiness; used in cosmetic preparations such as creams, lotions, powders, sprays, suntan products, hair, and nail preparations and perfumes.

hydrogen bond (physical bond) (HY·druh·jun BAHND)—in chemistry, the bond formed between two molecules when the nucleus of a hydrogen atom, originally attached to a fluorine, nitrogen, or oxygen atom of a second molecule of the same or different substance.

hydrogen bond in hair (HY·druh·jun BAHND IN HAYR)—in hair chemistry; the molecular association between an atom of hydrogen and an atom of oxygen in the hair forming an electromagnetic bond; gives strength and elasticity to hair and form to the hair when it is dry.

hydrogen ion concentration (HY·druh·jun EYE·ahn kahn·sen·TRAY·shun)—also called pH, a measure of the degree of acidity or alkalinity of an aqueous solution and expressed on a scale of 0-14, where 7 is neutral, 0.0-6.9 indicates decreasing acidity, and 7.1-14.0 indicates increasing alkalinity.

hydrogen peroxide (HY·druh·jun puh·RAHK·syd)—a powerful oxidizing agent; in liquid form it is used as an antiseptic, as a neutralizer, and for the activation of lighteners and hair tints; the most common strength for cosmetology use is 6% (20 volume). Also referred to as a developer, available in liquid and cream.

hydrolysis (hy·DRAHL·uh·sus)—chemical process of decomposition involving splitting of a bond with the addition of the elements of water (hydrogen and oxygen).

hydrolyze (HY·droh·lyz)—to decompose as a result of the incorporation and splitting of water; the two resulting products divide the water: the hydroxyl group being attached to one and the hydrogen atom to the other.

hydrolyzed elastin (HY·druh·lyzd ih·LAS·tun)—the product (hydrolysate) of animal ligaments and other connective tissue used in creams formulated to help retain the skin's elasticity.

hydromassage (hy·druh·muh·SAHZH)—massage by means of moving water.

hydrometer (hy·DRAHM·ut·ur)—an instrument used to measure the strength (volume) of peroxide and other liquids.

hydrophilic (hy·drah·FIL·ik)—capable of combining with or attracting water.

hydrophobia (hy·druh·FOH·bee·uh)—rabies in humans; morbid fear of water.

hydroquinone (hy·droh·kwin·OHN)—a chemical compound used as an antioxidant and bleaching agent in some cosmetic preparations.

hydrosis (hy·DROH·sis)—excretion of perspiration.

hydrosoluble (hy·droh·SAHL·yoo·bul)—soluble in water.

hydrotherapy (hy·druh·THAIR·uh·pee)—the scientific use of water in the treatment of injuries, diseases, or for mental well-being; physical therapy using water.

hydroxic cellulose (hy·DRAHK·sik SEL·yuh·lohs)—a chemical employed as a thickening agent; a chemical used to make a watery liquid thick.

hydroxide (hy·DRAHKS·yd)—any compound formed by the union of OH (one oxygen atom joined with one hydrogen atom) with a group of atoms known as a radical.

hygiene (HY·jeen)—the science of preserving health.

hygienic (hy·JIEN·ik)—having to do with preserving health.

hygroscopic (hy·gruh·SKAHP·ik)—readily absorbing and retaining moisture.

hyoid (HY·oyd)—pertaining to the "U"-shaped bone situated at the base of the tongue that supports the tongue and its muscles; also called "Adam's Apple."

hyper (HY·pur)—a prefix denoting excessive; above normal; above; beyond.

hyperacidity (hy·pur·uh·SID·ih·tee)—an excess of acidity.

hyperemia (hy·puh·REE·mee·uh)—the presence of an excessive quantity of blood in a part of the body.

hyperhidrosis, hyperidrosis (hy·per·hy·DROH·sus, hy·pur·ih·DROH·sis)—excessive sweating.

hyperkeratinization (HY·pur·kair·uh·tin·ih·zay·shun) —*see* hyperkeratosis.

hyperkeratosis (hy·pur·kair·uh·TOH·sis)—hypertrophy (excessive growth) of the corneous (horny) layer of the skin and associated with hypertrophy of the prickle cell layer, and the granular layer of the skin.

hyperkeratosis subungualis (hy·pur·kair·uh·TOH·sis sub·un·GWAY·lis)—hypertrophy affecting the nail bed.

hyperostosis (hy·puh·rahs·TOH·sus)—excessive growth or thickening of bone tissue.

hyperpigmentation (hy·pur·pig·men·TAY·shun)—a condition characterized by the production of more melanin in some areas of the skin than in others.

hyperplasia (hy·pur·PLAY·zhuh)—excessive formation of tissue; an increase in the size of a tissue or organ because of an increase in the number of cells.

hypersecretion (hy·pur·suh·KREE·shun)—excessive secretion.

hypersensitivity (hy·pur·sen·sih·TIV·ih·tee)—unusually affected by external agencies or influences to which a normal individual does not react.

hypertrichosis, hypertricosis (hy·pur·trih·KOH·sis)—a condition of excessive development or abnormal growth of the hair; superfluous hair.

hypertrophica, acne (hy·pur·TRAHF·ih·kuh, AK·nee)—vulgaris in which the lesions leave conspicuous pits and scars upon healing.

hypertrophy (hy·PUR·truh·fee)—abnormal increase in the size of a part or an organ; overgrowth; abnormal growth.

hypertrophy (hy·PUR·truh·fee)—enlargement of muscle due to repeated forceful muscle activity.

hypo (HY·poh)—a prefix denoting under;, beneath; lower state of oxidation.

hypoallergenic (hy·poh·al·ur·JEN·ik)—having a lower than usual tendency to cause allergic reactions.

hypodermal (hy·poh·DUR·mul)—lying beneath the epidermis.

hypodermic (hy·poh·DUR·mik)—of or relating to parts beneath the skin; placed or introduced beneath the skin.

hypodermis (hy·poh·DUR·mis)—in human anatomy, the subcutaneous tissue.

hypoglossal (hy·poh·GLAHS·ul)—under the tongue; the twelfth cranial nerve.

hyponychium (hy·poh·NIK·eeum)—the thickened stratum corneum of the epidermis that lies underneath the free edge of the nail.

hypothalamus (hy·poh·THAL·uh·mus)—the part of the brain that regulates many metabolic body processes.

hypothenar (hy·PAHTH·uh·nahr, hy·poh·THEEN·ur)—the fleshy eminence on the palm of the hand over the metacarpal bone of the little finger; also the prominences of the palm at the base of the fingers.

hypothermia (hy·poh·THER·mee·uh)—a condition of abnormally low body temperature.

hypothesis (hy·PAHTH·uh·sis)—an assumption or theory proposed to account for facts.

hypoxia (hip·AHK·see·uh)—inadequate supply of oxygen in the tissues.

hyssop (HIS·up)—an herb of the mint family; used in medicine and cosmetic preparations; valued as an astringent and for its healing properties.

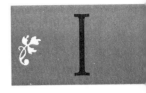

ice (YS)—frozen water.

ice bag (YS BAG)—also called ice pack; a flexible, waterproof container used to hold ice; it is wrapped in a towel and applied to the part of the face or body to be treated.

ice cube (YS KYOOB)—frozen water in the shape of a small block; used in ice bags and in some facial procedures to contract the pores.

ice pick scars (YS PIK SKARZ)—large visible open pores that look as if the skin has been punctured with an ice pick or similar object; this scar is caused by a deep pimple or cyst that has destroyed the follicle as infection worked its way to the surface of the skin.

ichthyosis (ik·thee·OH·sis)—a skin disease in which the skin becomes rough with diminished sweat and sebaceous secretion; fishskin disease.

ichthyotic (ik·thee·AHT·ik)—characterized by a skin disease accompanied by scaling.

icing (YS·ing)—in haircoloring, a term for frosting only half of the head, either the front or back of the head.

ide (YD)—a word termination denoting certain types of compounds.

identical (y·DEN·tih·kul)—exactly alike or equal.

illumination (ih·loo·mih·NAY·shun)—the action or state of making light, luminous or shining; in hair coloring, a process whereby one area of the head is lightened two or three shades.

imagery (IM·ij·ree)—the forming of a mental image; creative thinking.

imbalance (im·BAL·ens)—the state of being out of balance.

imbibition (im·buh·BISH·un)—the act of sucking up moisture.

imbricated (IM·brih·kayt·ud)—overlapped, as scales in skin disease.

imbrications (im·bruh·KAY·shunz)—cells arranged in layers overlapping one another; tiny overlapping of scales found in the hair cuticle; overlapping of layers of tissue in the closure of wounds or repair of defects.

immerse (ih·MURS)—to plunge into; dip; submerge in a liquid.

immersion (ih·MUR·shun)—plunging or dipping into a liquid especially so as to cover completely.

immiscible (im·IS·uh·bul)—not capable of being mixed, as oil and water.

immobile (ih·MOH·bul)—incapable of being moved; motionless.

immune (ih·MYOON)—safe from attack; protected from disease by vaccination or natural defenses.

immunity (im·YOO·net·ee)—freedom from or resistance to disease; the body's ability to destroy bacteria that have gained entrance, and thus resist infection.

immunodermatology (im·yoo·noh·dur·muh·TAHL·uh·jee)—the study of the immune system as related to skin disorders and their treatment.

immunology (im·yoo·NAHL·uh·jee)—the branch of medical science that deals with immunity to diseases.

impair (im·PAYR)—to make worse; to render less than perfect; to cause to lose quality.

impearl (im·PURL)—to make pearly; to pearlize a cosmetic product to give a sheen.

impedance (im·PEED·ens)—the resistance in an electric current to an alternating current.

impenetrable (im·PEN·uh·troh·bul)—incapable of being penetrated.

imperfect (im·PUR·fikt)—falling short of perfection; defective; unfinished.

impermeable (im·PUR·mee·uh·bul)—impenetrable; not capable of being penetrated; impervious to moisture.

impervious (im·PUR·vee·us)—impenetrable; incapable of being passed through.

impetigo (im·puh·TEE·goh)—an eruption of pustules, caused by staphylococci or streptococci, which rupture or become crusted; occurring chiefly on the face around the mouth and nostrils.

implant (im·PLANT)—to imbed; to insert and fix firmly.

implement (IM·pluh·ment)—an instrument or tool.

impregnated (im·PREG·nayt·ud)—fertilized; saturated.

impure (im·PYOOR)—containing some form of contamination; lacking purity; adulterated.

in (IN)—a prefix denoting not; negative; within; inside.

inactive electrode (in·AK·tiv ih·LEK·trohd)—the opposite pole from the active electrode.

inappropriate (in·uh·PROH·pree·ut)—unsuitable, not fitting; as a hairstyle unsuitable for facial structure.

incandescent (in·kan·DES·ent)—giving forth light and heat.

inch (INCH)—a measure of length equal to the twelfth part of a foot; 2.54 centimeters.

incision (in·SIZH·un)—a cut; a cut of soft body tissue made with a knife or similar instrument.

inclined (in·KLYND)—forming an angle with a line or plane; bent or bowed.

include (in·KLOOD)—to make a part of something; add to a category; comprise.

incombustible (in·kahm·BUS·tih·bul)—fireproof; not flammable.

increase layering (in·KREES LAY·ur·ing)—cutting to produce a layered effect with progressively longer lengths.

increasing graduation (in·KRESS·ing graj·oo·WAY·shun)—graduation within two nonparallel lines; it increases as it moves back from the face.

incretion (in·KREE·shun)—the secreting of a substance, such as oil, from the sebaceous glands.

incrust (in·KRUST)—also encrust; to form a crust or a coating.

incrustation (in·krus·TAY·shun)—the state of having crusts or scales; the formation of a crust or hard coating.

incubation (in·kyoo·BAY·shun)—the act or process of hatching or developing; the period of time between infection of an individual with an infectious disease and the appearance of symptoms.

incurable (in·KYOOR·uh·bul)—not capable of being cured.

incurvate (IN·kur·vayt)—to cause to curve inward.

indelible (in·DEL·ih·bul)—cannot be removed, erased, blotted out, or eliminated; permanent; lasting.

indemnity (in·DEM·nih·tee)—compensation for loss.

indent (IN·dent)—an inward depression or hollow.

indentation (in·den·TAY·shun)—the curved depth, valley, or hollowness created by the formation of curls or waves in the hair.

indentation curl (in·den·TAY·shun KURL)—pin curl technique in which the stem is combed flat against the scalp and the curl is rolled up to stand up away from the head; used to create a hollow or valley in the finished style.

indentation roller (in·den·TAY·shun ROHL·ur)—setting technique in which the stem is combed flat against the scalp and the roller is rolled upward, away from the head; used to create a hollow or valley in the finished style.

index (IN·deks)—an alphabetical list of items from a printed work; the first finger next to the thumb.

Indian cress (IN·dee·an KRES)—an herb used in some skin care products and as a dandruff control agent; contains amino acids, sulphur, and antibiotics.

indicator (IN·dih·kay·tur)—an apparatus or instrument used to show changes in conditions, such as color or the degree of acidity or alkalinity.

indigo (IN·dih·goh)—a blue dye.

indirect point (IN·dih·rekt POYNT)—partings of an oval shape using curved or straight lines; the first parting is out of the circumference, then intersections all form one point.

indispensable (in·dis·PEN·suh·bul)—absolutely necessary.

individual (in·dih·VIJ·oo·ul)—separate; distinguished from others of the same kind.

individual eyelashes (in·dih·VIJ·oo·ul EYE·lash·ez)—separate, artificial eyelashes that are applied to the eyelids one at a time.

individualize (in·dih·VIJ·oo·uh·lyz)—to distinguish from others; to give a client a particular hairstyle or hair cut.

induction (in·DUK·shun)—the process by which an electrified or magnetic state is produced through nearness with a charged body or presence in a magnetic field.

inductor (in·DUK·tur)—an electrical apparatus or part that acts inductively upon another.

indurata, acne (in·dyoo·RAH·tuh AK·nee)—deeply seated papular eruptions with hard tubercular lesions.

indurate (IN·dyuh·rut)—to make hard or firm.

induration (in·dyuh·RAY·shun)—the process or act of hardening; a spot or area of hardened tissue.

inefficiency (in·ih·FISH·un·see)—quality, state, or fact of being wasteful of time or energy or not producing the effect intended or desired within a given expenditure of time or energy.

inelasticity (in·ih·las·TIS·ih·tee)—in cosmetology, the ability to stretch but not return to its former shape, as overbleached or limp hair; aging skin or muscles.

inert (in·URT)—inactive; lacking the power to move.

infect (in·FEKT)—to cause infection; to contaminate.

infection (in·FEK·shun)—the invasion of body tissues by disease germs.

infection, general (in·FEK·shun, JEN·ur·ul)—the result of disease germs gaining entrance into the bloodstream and circulating throughout the entire body.

infection, local (in·FEK·shun, LOH·kul)—infection confined to only certain portions of the body such as an abscess.

infectious (in·FEK·shus)—capable of spreading infection.

infectious allergy (in·FEK·shus AL·ur·jee)—delayed hypersensitivity induced by an infectious agent.

infectious dermatitis (in·FEK·shus dur·muh·TY·tis)—an inflamed irritation of the skin resulting from the irritating effect of a substance.

infectious mononucleosis (in·FEK·shus mahn·uh·noo·klee·OH·sis)— a contagious disease characterized by a swelling of the lymph nodes, fever, and sore throat; also called glandular fever.

inferior (in·FEER·ee·ur)—situated lower down or nearer the bottom or base; of lesser quality.

inferioris (in·FEER·ee·or·us)—below; lower.

inferior labial artery (in·FEER·ee·ur LAY·bee·ul ART·ur·ee)—artery that supplies blood to the lower lip.

inferior labial nerve (in·FEER·ee·ur LAY·bee·ul NURV)—in the skin of the lower lip.

inferior labial vein (in·FEER·ee·ur LAY·bee·ul VAYN)—a vein that drains the region of the lower lip into the facial vein.

inferior maxilla (in·FEER·ee·ur mak·SIL·uh)—the lower jawbone or mandible.

inferior ophthalmic vein (in·FEER·ee·ur ahf·THAL·mik VAYN)— a vein that supplies blood to the eye, orbit, and adjacent facial structures.

inferior palpebral nerve (in·FEER·ee·ur PAL·puh·brul NURV)— a nerve that receives stimuli for the lower eyelid.

inferior palpebral vein (in·FEER·ee·ur PAL·puh·brul VAYN)— a vein that drains blood from the lower eyelids to the facial veins.

inferior terbinate (in·FEER·ee·ur TUR·bih·nayt)—the nasal concha; an irregular scroll-shaped bone situated on the lateral wall of the nasal cavity.

inferior vena cava (in·FEER·ee·ur VEE·nuh KAYV·uh)—the large vein that carries blood to the heart from the abdomen, feet, and legs; located in front of the vertebral column to the right of the aorta.

infiltrate (in·FIL·trayt)—to pass through; to filter or permeate.

infiltration (in·fil·TRAY·shun)—the process or act of passing through or into another substance, such as cells or fluid passing into tissues or other cells.

inflammable (in·FLAM·uh·bul)—tending to be easily ignited.

inflammation (in·fluh·MAY·shun)—a condition of some part of the body as a protective response reaction to injury, irritation, or infection characterized by redness, heat, pain, and swelling.

inflate (in·FLAYT)—to swell or distend by filling with air or gas.

influenza (in·floo·EN·zuh)—an acute, highly contagious viral disease characterized by sudden onset, fever, prostration, and severe aches and pains; grippe.

informal (in·FORM·ul)—not in the usual or prescribed form; relaxed; casual.

infra (IN·fruh)—a prefix denoting below; lower.

inframandibular (in·fruh·man·DIB·yuh·lur)—below the lower jaw.

infraorbital (in·fruh·OR·bih·tul)—below the orbit, in the floor of the orbit; a sensory and motor nerve affecting the cheek muscles, nose, and upper lip.

infrared (in·fruh·RED)—pertaining to that part of the spectrum lying outside the visible spectrum and below the red rays.

infratrochlear (in·fruh·TRAHK·lee·ur)—sensory nerve affecting the lacrimal sac, the skin of the nose, and the inner muscle of the eye.

ingestion (in·JES·chun)—the act of taking substances, especially food, into the body.

ingredient (in·GREE·dee·unt)—any part of a compound; that which enters into the composition of a mixture.

ingrown (IN·grohn)—growing inward; an ingrown hair or nail.

ingrown hair (IN·grohn HAYR)—a hair that has grown so that the normally free end is embedded in or underneath the skin, sometimes causing an infection.

ingrown nail (IN·grohn NAYL)—a nail that has grown into the flesh instead of toward the tip of the finger or toe, sometimes causing an infection.

inhalation (in·huh·LAY·shun)—the breathing in of air or other vapors.

inhale (in·HAYL)—to draw in the breath; to inspire.

inhibit (in·HIB·it)—to check or restrain; prohibit.

inhibition (in·hih·BISH·un)—the diminution or arrest of the function in an organ.

inject (in·JEKT)—to force into; to force fluid through a syringe or needle; to force fluid into an injector rod.

injectable fillers (in·JEK·tuh·bul FIL·urz)—injections of collagen used to raise depressions, deep scars, and deep aging lines.

injector rod (in·JEK·tur RAHD)—a permanent wave rod designed with openings into which wave lotion and neutralizer may be injected after the hair is wound on the rod.

injury (IN·joor·ee)—damage or hurt.

inner (IN·ur)—interior; internal; inward.

inner and outer circle (IN·ur AND OUT·ar SUR·kul)—terms employed in hair sectioning to indicate an inner section with a preshaped base and an outer section with a slanted or oblique base.

inner and outer technique (IN·ur AND OWT·ur tek·NEEK)— in hairdressing, the technique of expanding a circle.

inner circle (IN·ur SUR·kul)—in hair sectioning, a pieshaped base; the outer circle is on a slanted base.

innermost (IN·ur·mohst)—the inmost part; the farthest inward from the outermost part.

inner perimeter (IN·ur puh·RIM·ih·tur)—in hairstyling, the hair length and density in the inner area excluding the hairline.

innervation (in·ur·VAY·shun)—distribution of nerves in a part of the body.

innominate (in·AHM·uh·nut)—having no specific name or names; anonymous; generally applied to certain anatomical structures.

innominate artery (in·AHM·uh·nut ART·uh·ree)—an artery that distributes blood to the right side of the head and to the right arm.

innominate bone (in·AHM·uh·nut BOHN)—one of two large irregular bones that form the pelvis; hipbone.

innominate veins (in·AHM·uh·nut VAYNZ)—veins of the neck.

innovate (IN·uh·vayt)—to create or introduce something new and original, such as a new hairstyle.

innovation (in·uh·VAY·shun)—to introduce new methods or ideas.

inoculation (in·ahk·yuh·LAY·shun)—the injection of a disease agent to cause a mild form of the disease to build immunity to that disease.

inorganic (in·or·GAN·ik)—composed of matter not arising from natural growth or living organisms; without carbon.

inorganic chemistry (in·or·GAN·ik KEM·is·tree)—the branch of chemistry dealing with compounds lacking carbon, or containing carbon only in the form of cyanides, carbides, or carbonates.

inorganic hair dye (in·or·GAN·ik HAYR DYE)—a nonvegetable, nonanimal hair-coloring material.

inorganic nutrients (in·or·GAN·ik NOO·tree·ents)—minerals needed in the daily diet.

insanitary, unsanitary (in·SAN·ih·teh·ree, un·SAN·ih·teh·ree)—not sanitary or healthful; unclean enough to be injurious to health.

inseparable (in·SEP·ar·uh·bul)—incapable of being separated.

insert (in·SURT)—to put or thrust in; to set, so as to be within.

insertion (in·SUR·shun)—act of inserting; that which is set in; portion of muscle at more movable attachment.

inside (IN·syd)—an inner side or surface.

inside curve (IN·syd KURV)—a concave (inward) curve cut in the hair.

inside movement (IN·syd MOOV·ment)—pertaining to an indentation, a curve, or movement keeping the hair close to the head.

insolation (in·suh·LAY·shun)—exposure to the rays of the sun; sunstroke.

insoluble (in·SAHL·yuh·bul)—incapable of being dissolved or very difficult to dissolve.

inspiration (in·spur·AY·shun)—the feeling or impulse leading to a creative idea; the act of inhaling.

inspire (in·SPYR)—to influence or motivate a person; to inhale.

instantaneous (in·stan·TAY·nee·us)—done, occurring, or acting immediately.

instant hair roller (IN·stant HAYR ROHL·ur)—an electronically heated hair roller used to style the hair while it is dry.

instep (IN·step)—the dorsal part of the human foot on the medial side; the arched upper part of the foot.

instructor (in·STRUK·tur)—one who instructs; a teacher; a licensed cosmetologist with teaching credentials; a person with the required licenses and experience to teach a subject or subjects.

instrument (IN·struh·ment)—device or tool for performing cosmetology work.

insulate (IN·suh·layt)—to separate by nonconductors to prevent transfer of electricity of heat.

insulation (in·suh·LAY·shun)—nonconducting substance.

insulator (IN·suh·layt·ur)—a nonconducting material or substance used to cover electric wires.

insulin (IN·suh·lin)—a hormone secreted by the pancreas that regulates carbohydrate and fat metabolism.

insurance (in·SHUR·ens)—protection against loss or injury.

integument (in·TEG·yuh·ment)—a covering, especially the skin.

integumentary system (in·TEG·yuh·ment·uh·ree SIS·tum)—pertaining to the skin and its functions.

intensify (in·TEN·sih·fy)—to increase; to make stronger or more intense.

intensity (in·TEN·sih·tee)—the amount of force per unit area, as of heat, light, or current; the quality of being intense; used in haircoloring to describe the "strength" of the color's toxidity, whether mild, medium, or strong.

inter- (IN·tur)—a prefix denoting amid; between; among.

intercellular (in·tur·SEL·yuh·lur)—between or among cells.

intercostal (in·tur·KAHS·tul)—between the ribs.

intercostal muscles (in·tur·KAHS·tul MUS·ulz)—muscles lying between adjacent ribs.

intercostal nerves (in·tur·KAHS·tul NURVZ)—the branches of the thoracic nerves in the intercostal spaces (spaces between the ribs).

interior (in·TEER·ee·ur)—inner or internal part of anything; situated within; occurring or functioning on the inside.

interlace (in·tur·LAYS)—to weave strands of hair.

interlocking (in·tur·LAHK·ing)—a type of back combing that does not pack or mat the hair at the scalp; this technique causes the strands of hair to cling to each other and gives better control.

intermediate (in·tur·MEE·dee·ut)—between two extremes; being or occurring at the middle place or degree.

intermediate supraclavicular nerve (in·tur·MEE·dee·ut soo·pruh·kluh·VIK·yuh·lur NURV)—nerve that receives stimuli from the skin of the anterior part of the neck and chest wall.

intermittent heat (in·tur·MIT·ent HEET)—interrupted heating period; electric current turned on and off during a steaming procedure.

intermuscular (in·tur·MUS·kyuh·lur)—situated between the muscles.

internal (in·TUR·nul)—pertaining to the inside; inner part.

internal absorption (in·TUR·nul ab·SORP·shun)—the normal digestive assimilation of foods and liquids.

internal carotid artery (in·TUR·nul kuh·RAHT·ud ART·uh·ree)—the artery that distributes blood to the cerebrum, the eye, the forehead, nose, and internal ear.

internal carotid nerve (in·TUR·nul kuh·RAHT·ud NURV)—a sympathetic nerve serving the internal carotid artery and its branches.

internal jugular vein (in·TUR·nul JUG·yuh·lur VAYN)—the vein located at the side of the neck to collect blood from the brain and parts of the face and neck, (*See* jugular vein.)

internal respiration (in·TUR·nul res·pih·RAY·shun)—an exchange of gases between the blood and the capillaries and tissues of the body.

international color ring (in·tur·NASH·un·ul KUL·ur RING)—also called J and L color ring; a ring of color samples used to match hair colors, originated by Jacques Leclebort and accepted by the industry as standardization of colors for manufacturers of hair goods.

international unit (IU) (in·tur·NASH·un·ul YOO·nit)—the amount of a substance, such as a vitamin or antibiotic, that produces a biological effect and has had established an accepted measure of the activity or potency of the substance.

interosseous (in·tur·AHS·ee·us)—lying between or connecting bones.

interosseous artery, anterior (in·tur·AHS·ee·us ART·uh·ree, an·TEER·ee·ur)—artery that supplies blood to the muscles of the deep anterior part of the forearm.

interosseous artery, posterior (in·tur·AHS·ee·us ART·uh·ree, poh·STEER·ee·ur)—artery that supplies blood to the posterior forearm.

interosseous membrane of the forearm (in·tur·AHS·ee·us MEM·brayn UV THE FOR·arm)—pertaining to the strong, fibrous membrane between the radius and the ulna; forearm.

interosseous membrane of the leg (in·tur·AHS·ee·us MEM·brayn UV THE LEG)—the strong, fibrous sheet between the margins of the tibia and the fibula.

interosseous nerve (in·tur·AHS·ee·us NURV)—a somatic, sensory nerve distributed in the ankle joint.

interparietal (in·tur·puh·RY·eh·tul)—between walls; between parietal bones.

interpenetrate (in·tur·PEN·uh·trayt)—to pervade; permeate; penetrate thoroughly.

interpose (in·tur·POHZ)—to place or put between the parts.

interstice (in·TUR·stus)—a narrow opening between adjoining parts.

intertwist (in·tur·TWIST)—to join strands by twining or twisting together.

intervascular (in·tur·VAS·kyuh·lar)—situated between vessels.

interweave (in·tur·WEEV)—to blend small strands of hair into a pattern.

intestinal (in·TES·tin·ul)—pertaining to the intestines.

intestine (in·TES·tin)—the digestive tube from the stomach to the anus.

intra- (IN·truh)—a prefix meaning inside of; within.

intraarterial (in·truh·ar·TEER·ee·ul)—within or directly into an artery.

intraarticular (in·truh·ar·TIK·yuh·lar)—within a joint.

intracardiac (in·truh·KAR·dee·ak)—occurring within or situated in the heart.

intracellular (in·truh·SEL·yuh·lur)—occurring or within a cell or cells.

intracorneal (in·truh·KOR·nee·ul)—within the horny layer of the skin; also, within the cornea of the eye.

intracranial (in·truh·KRAY·nee·ul)—occurring within the cranium.

intracuticular (in·truh·kyoo·TIK·yuh·lur)—within the epidermis.

intradermal (in·truh·DUR·mul)—within the dermis.

intradermal nevus (in·truh·DUR·mul NEE·vus)—a skin lesion containing melanocytes located in the dermis.

intraepidermal (in·truh·ep·ih·DUR·mul)—within the epidermis.

intramuscular (in·truh·MUS·kyuh·lur)—affecting the inside of the muscle.

intraneural (in·truh·NUR·ul)—within a nerve.

intumesce (in·too·MES)—to swell, expand, or enlarge.

invasion (in·VAY·zhun)—the process in which bacteria or other microorganisms enter the body.

inventory (IN·ven·tor·ee)—a list of stock items; an accounting of products on hand; a record of supplies used and to be reordered.

inversion (in·VUR·zhun)—the act of turning inward.

inverted triangle (in·VUR·tud TRY·ang·gul)—a face shape having a narrow chin, broad cheeks, and broad forehead.

inverter (in·VUR·tur)—a device for converting direct current into alternating current.

invisible (in·VIZ·ih·bul)—not capable of being seen.

invisible light (in·VIZ·ih·bul LYT)—light that cannot be seen with the naked eye, but can be felt; examples are infrared and ultraviolet light.

involuntary (in·VAHL·un·tair·ee)—functioning or acting independently of the will or conscious control.

involuntary muscle (in·VAHL·un·tair·ee MUS·ul)—a muscle that functions automatically without the action of the will.

involute (IN·vuh·loot)—in hairdressing, having ends rolling upward; curving; spiraling.

inward (IN·ward)—toward the inside.

iodine tincture (EYE·uh·dyn TINK·chur)—a solution of iodine and sodium iodide in diluted alcohol; used as a local anti-infective.

iododerma (eye·oh·duh·DUR·muh)—a skin condition caused by the injection of iodine compounds.

iodoform (eye·OH·duh·form)—a yellow crystalline compound formed by the action of iodine on alcohol and potash, used as an antiseptic for wounds and sores.

ion (EYE·ahn)—an atom or group of atoms carrying an electric charge; when negatively charged, called "anions"; when positively charged, called "cations."

ionic bond (eye·AHN·ik BAHND)—the chemical bond between charged atoms or ions.

ionization (eye·ahn·ih·ZAY·shun)—the separating of a substance into ions.

ionto mask (eye·AHN·toh MASK)—a mask of spongy material that covers the face, and is used with a galvanic machine during the process of the ionization or disincrustation facial treatment.

iontophoresis (eye·ahn·toh·foh·REE·sus)—the process of introducing water soluble products into the skin with the use of electric current, such as the use of the positive and negative poles of a galvanic machine.

ionto rollers (eye·AHN·toh ROHL·urz)—metal rollers attached to a galvanic machine used to aid the penetration of creams or lotions into the skin during a facial treatment.

iridescence (ihr·ih·DES·ens)—the quality of being iridescent; a varied play of colors creating a sheen as in a soap bubble or mother of pearl.

iris (EYE·ris)—the colored muscular disklike diaphragm of the eye that regulates the size of the pupil.

iron (EYE·urn)—a metallic element with the symbol Fe, required in the human diet; recommended amount is approximately 10 milligrams daily.

iron heater (EYE·urn HEET·ur)—a small, compact electric heater used to heat thermal curling irons.

iron holder (EYE·urn HOL·dur)—an apparatus designed to hold a thermal curling iron.

irons (EYE·urnz)—heated implements designed to wave or curl the hair while it is dry.

irregular (ih·REG·yuh·lur)—lacking symmetry; unevenly shaped or arranged.

irreparable (ih·REP·uh·ruh·bul)—damaged beyond repair.

irreversible (ihr·ee·VUR·sih·bul)—not capable of being reversed.

irrigate (IHR·ih·gayt)—to flush with water; to spray; to refresh with water.

irritability (ihr·ih·tuh·BIL·ih·tee)—the quality or state of being readily excited or stimulated to annoyance.

irritability (ih·rit·uh·BIL·uh·tee)—the capability of muscles to react and receive stimuli.

irritant (IHR·ih·tent)—somthing that irritates, excites, or stimulates.

irritate (IHR·ih·tayt)—to make inflamed or sore.

irritation (ihr·ih·TAY·shun)—the reaction of tissues or nerves to overstimulation.

ischemia (is·KEE·mee·uh)—constricted blood flow in muscles.

ischemic pain (is·KEE·mik PAYN)—pain following an injury to muscle and tissue caused by increases in lactic acid in muscles.

isochromatic (eye·soh·kroh·MAT·ik)—having the same color throughout; matched in color.

isometric (eye·soh·MET·rik)—having equal measurements in several dimensions.

isometric exercise (eye·soh·MET·rik EKS·ur·syz)—an exercise for the muscles in which contractions are counteracted by equal force exerted by the opposing muscles, and the body part affected does not move.

isopropyl alcohol (eye·soh·PROH·pul AL·kuh·hawl)—a homologue of ethyl alcohol; used as a solvent and rubefacient.

isopropylamine (eye·soh·PROH·pil·uh·min)—a substance produced from acetone; an emulsifier used in many hair grooming creams and lotions.

isothermal (eye·soh·THUR·mul)—of equal temperature; without change in temperature.

isotonic contraction (eye·soh·TAHN·ik kahn·TRAK·shun)—contraction that occurs when a muscle contracts and the distance between the ends of the muscle changes.

itch (ICH)—an irritating sensation on the skin causing a desire to rub or scratch the affected area; any of various skin conditions such as scabies.

ithylordosis (ith·ih·lor·DOH·sis)—lordosis unaccompanied by lateral curvature of the spine.

itis (EYE·tis)—suffix meaning inflammation of a specific part; e.g., arthritis, dermatitis, inflammation of the skin or joint; such terms are often preceded by the word infectious, as in infectious dermatitis.

ive (IV)—a word termination signifying relating or belonging to, such as active.

ivory (eye·VUH·ree)—the smooth, yellowish-white dentine substance of tusks; the creamy, white color of ivory; a light skintone resembling ivory.

ize (YZ)—a word termination forming transitive verbs, such as sterilize.

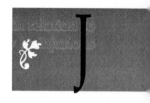

jack (JAK)—in electricity, a plug-in device used to make electrical contact.

jagged (JAG·ud)—having rough, uneven edges.

jasmine (JAZ·min)—a fragrant flowering plant of the olive family used in fragrances.

jaundice (JAHN·dus)—yellowness of the skin, tissues, and body fluids caused by deposits of bile pigments.

jaw (JAW)—either of two boney structures forming the framework of the mouth, the upper jaw (maxilla) and the lower jaw (mandible).

jawbone (JAW·bohn)—one of the bones forming the jaw, particularly the bone of the lower jaw of humans or animals.

jaw clamp (JAW KLAMP)—a hair clip with teeth to secure large sections of hair; also called a butterfly clamp.

jet (JET)—a sudden spurt or gush of liquid or gas emitted from a narrow orifice, such as a shower head or shampoo bowl attachment.

jet black (JET BLAK)—deep black resembling hard, black jet stone or marble.

joint (JOYNT)—a connection between two or more bones.

joint movement (JOYNT MOOV·ment)—the manipulating of a joint during massage.

jojoba (huh·HOH·buh)—an evergreen shrub that produces a bean from which oil is extracted for use in some cosmetic products.

jowl (JOWL)—the fleshy part of the lower jaw; a double chin.

jugal (JOO·gul)—pertaining to the cheek.

jugular (JOOG·yuh·lur, JUG·yuh·lur)—pertaining to the neck or throat or the large veins in the neck.

jugular bulb (JUG·yuh·lur BULB)—superior bulb of the internal jugular vein.

jugular fossa (JUG·yuh·lur FAHS·uh)—the depression or cavity between the carotid canal and the stylomastoid opening containing the superior bulb of the internal jugular vein.

jugular nerves (JUG·yuh·lur NURVZ)—pertaining to nerves in the jugular area.

jugular trunk (JUG·yuh·lur TRUNK)—one of two connecting lymph trunks on the right and left sides of the head and neck; the right drains into the right lympathic duct; the left drains into the thoracic duct.

jugular vein (JUG·yuh·lur VAYN)—one of the largest veins on either side of the neck that returns blood from the brain, neck, and parts of the face back to the heart.

jugular vein, anterior (JUG·yuh·lur VAYN, an·TEER·ee·ur)—vein located in the middle of the neck that drains the anterior part of the neck.

jugular vein, external (JUG·yuh·lur VAYN, eks·TUR·nul)—vein located parallel to arteries on the sides of the neck that returns blood to the heart from the face, head, and neck.

jugular vein, internal (JUG·yuh·lur VAYN, in·TUR·nul)—vein that returns blood to the heart from the brain, face, and neck.

jugular vein, posterior (JUG·yuh·lur VAYN, poh·STEER·ee·ur)—
vein situated in the occipital region that serves the skin and
muscles in the upper back area of the neck.

junction nevus (JUNK·shun NEE·vus)—a benign skin lesion
containing nerve cells and located at the junction of the
epidermis and dermis.

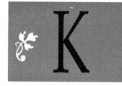

kaleidoscope (kuh·LY·duh·skohp)—a tube-shaped object used to show constantly changing colors and patterns; used to study color.

kaolin, kaoline (KAY·uh·lin)—fuller's earth; porcelain clay; used in some cosmetics, but chiefly in facial packs; mud pack.

karaya gum (kuh·RY·uh GUM)—Indian gum; a gum obtained in India and Africa from the trees of the genus Sterculia; used to make mucilages and wave set preparations.

keloid (KEE·loyd)—a thick scar resulting from excessive growth of fibrous tissue.

keloid acne (KEE·loyd AK·nee)—a follicular infection with pustules that causes keloidal scarring; frequently affects black sin.

keratic (kuh·RAT·ik)—pertaining to the cornea of the eye.

keratin (KAIR·uht·in)—a fiber protein characteristic of horny tissues: hair, nails, feathers, etc.; it is insoluble in protein solvents and has a high sulfur content; the principal constituent of hair and nails.

keratinization (kair·uh·tin·y·ZAY·shun)—the process of being keratinized; development of a horny quality in a tissue.

keratitis (kair·uh·TY·tis)—inflammation of the cornea of the eye.

keratoacanthoma (kair·uh·toh·ak·an·THOH·muh)—a skin nodule that usually occurs on hairy parts of the body and resembles squamous cell cancer of the skin.

keratoderma (kair·uh·tuh·DUR·muh)—a horny condition of the skin, especially of the palms of the hands and soles of the feet.

keratoid (KAIR·uh·toyd)—hornlike; horny tissue.

keratolytic (kair·uh·tuh·LIT·ik)—an agent that causes exfoliation of the epidermis, as in skin peeling processes.

keratoma (kair·uh·TOH·muh)—an acquired thickened patch of the epidermis commonly known as a callus.

keratonosis (kair·uh·toh·NOH·sis)—an anomaly in the horny structure of the epidermis.

keratoprotein (kair·uh·toh·PROH·teen)—the protein of the horny tissues of the body that make up such structures as the hair, nails, and epidermis.

keratosa, acne (kair·uh·TOH·puh, AK·nee)—a rare form of acne consisting of horny plugs projecting from the hair follicles, accompanied by inflammation, usually at the angles of the mouth.

keratosis (kair·uh·TOH·sis)—any disease of the epidermis that is marked by the presence of circumscribed overgrowths of the horny layer.

ketone body (KEE·tohn BAHD·ee)—one of three related substances (acetone, methyl, ethyl).

ketones (KEE·tohnz)—acetone, methyl, or ethyl; substances obtained by the oxidation of secondary alcohols; used as solvents in nail polish and polish removers.

khaki (KAK·ee)—a color between medium brown and tan.

kidney (KID·nee)—one of a pair of glandular organs that excretes urine.

kil (KIL)—a clay from the Black Sea region widely used as an ointment in the treatment of skin diseases.

kilo (KEE·loh)—a prefix meaning thousand.

kilocalorie (KIL·uh·kal·uh·ree)—the quantity of heat required to raise the temperature of one kilogram of water one degree centigrade.

kilowatt (KIL·uh·wat)—equals 1,000 watts.

kimono (kih·MOH·nuh)—a loose, Japanese-style robe or gown; used in salons to protect the client's clothing.

kinesics (kih·NEE·siks)—the study of body movements.

kinetics (kuh·NET·iks)—the branch of physics dealing with the effect of forces on the motion of physical objects or with changes on physical or chemical systems.

kinky (KINK·ee)—very curly or closely twisted.

kit (KIT)—in cosmetology, a case containing the implements the cosmetologist needs to perform services.

knead (NEED)—to work and press with the hands as in massage.

knee (NEE)—the joint of the human leg that articulates the tibia, fibula, and patella (knee cap).

knit (NIT)—to cause to draw together, as in the healing of bone.

knot (NAHT)—to intertwine and loop strands of hair, fabric, rope, etc., to form a flat or oval mass.

knotted hair (NAHT·id HAYR)—hair that has tangled, snarled lumps. (*See* trichonodrosis.)

knotting (ventilating) (NAHT·ing)—the process by which hair is attached to the foundation in the creation of a wig or hair piece; the actual knotting is also referred to as ventilating; there are two types of knotting generally used, single and double.

knotting gauze (NAHT·ing GAWZ)—a very light type of silk net that has not been stiffened; it is used for men's hair pieces and for knotted partings.

knotting hook holder (NAHT·ing HOOK HOHL·dur)—a steel, pencil-shaped holder with an adjustable top, used to hold the knotting or parting hooks used in wig making.

knuckle (NUK·ul)—one of the joints of the fingers; the joints connecting the fingers to the hands.

knuckling (NUK·ling)—a massage movement made by using the knuckles of the four fingers of the hand to lightly tap the skin.

kohl (KOHL)—a preparation used to darken the edges of the eyelids.

koilonychia (koy·loh·NIK·ee·uh)—a dystrophy of the fingernails associated with nutritional deficiencies, such as of iron and calcium; the nails become thin and concave in shape; also called "spoon nails."

kosmetikos (kahz·MET·ih·kohs)—a Greek word meaning skilled in use of cosmetics and from which the word cosmetology is derived.

kyphoscoliosis (ky·foh·skoh·lee·OH·sis)—backward and lateral curvature of the spinal column.

kyphosis (ky·FOH·sus)—backward curvature of the spine; humpback.

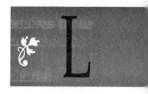

labdanum (LAB·duh·num)—a resin derived from the rockrose plant; used in some medicines, cosmetics, and perfumery.

labia (LAY·bee·uh); pl., **labium** (LAY·bee·um)—pertaining to the lips.

labial artery, inferior (LAY·bee·ul ART·uh·ree in·FEER·ee·ur)—artery that supplies blood to the lower lip.

labial artery, superior (LAY·bee·ul ART·uh·ree soo·PEER·ee·ur)—artery that supplies blood to the upper lip, septum, and wing of the nose.

labial nerve, inferior (LAY·bee·ul NURV in·FEER·ee·ur)—nerve that distributes stimuli to the lower lip.

labial nerve, superior (LAY·bee·ul NURV soo·PEER·ee·ur)—nerve that distributes stimuli to the skin of the upper lip.

labium (LAY·bee·um); pl., **labia** (LAY·bee·uh)—lip; a fleshy border or edge.

laboratory (LAB·uh·ruh·tor·ee)—a room containing apparatus for conducting experiments.

lac (LAK)—milk or a milklike substance.

lace (LAYS)—a very fine flesh-colored mesh that is used to blend hairlines where they meet the skin; this type of lace, which is used primarily in men's hair pieces, gives a natural effect to the hairline.

lacerate (LAS·uh·rayt)—to tear the skin or tissue.

laceration (las·uh·RAY·shun)—a tear of the skin or tissue.

lacing (LAYS·ing)—a delicate, even backcombing along an entire strand of hair, giving the hair a lacy quality.

lacing, French (LAYS·ing, FRENCH)—a style of braiding. (*See* French braid.)

lacquer (LAK·ur)—a liquid cosmetic used on the hair or nails.

lacrimal (LAK·ruh·mul)—pertaining to tears or weeping and the organs that secrete tears.

lacrimal artery (LAK·ruh·mul ART·uh·ree)—artery supplying blood to the eye and eyelid area.

lacrimal bone (LAK·ruh·mul BOHN)—small, thin bone resembling a fingernail; located in the anterior medial wall of the orbits (eye sockets).

lacrimal bones (LAK·ruh·mul BOHNZ)—fragile bones in eye sockets.

lacrimal duct (LAK·ruh·mul DUKT)—either of the two tear ducts of the eyes.

lacrimal glands (LAK·ruh·mul GLANDZ)—glands situated in the orbit of the eye in the depression of the frontal bone that secrete tears.

lacrimal nerves (LAK·ruh·mul NURVZ)—nerves distributed in the area of the upper eye and eyelid and affecting the tear glands.

lacteals (LAK·tee·ulz)—any one of the lymphatics of the intestines that take up chyle.

lactic acid (LAK·tik AS·ud)—a clear, syrupy organic acid; used in skin-freshening lotions.

lamina (LAM·uh·nuh)—a thin layer or scale.

lamp dry (LAMP DRY)—to style the hair and dry it at the same time under an infrared heat lamp.

lamp, hot quartz (LAMP HAHT KWORTZ)—a general all-purpose lamp used for skin tanning and other cosmetics and germicidal purposes.

lamp, infrared (LAMP IN·fruh·red)—a lamp producing infrared rays; used in skin care treatments.

lamp, magnifying (LAMP MAG·nih·fy·ing)—a lamp used to analyze the skin or scalp.

lamp, ultraviolet (LAMP ul·truh·VY·oh·let)—pertaining to the three types of lamps used in cosmetology practice: glass bulb, hot quartz, and cold quartz.

lamp, Wood's (LAMP, WOODZ)—a lamp developed by Robert W. Wood, an American physicist, to help diagnose skin and scalp conditions.

lancet (LAN·sut)—a small, sharp-pointed instrument; used by dermatologists to pierce a papule.

lank (LANK)—in cosmetology, describes hair that is long, lifeless; not curly.

lanolin (LAN·ul·un)—purified wool fat; used in some cosmetic preparations.

lanosterol (lan·oh·STAIR·awl)—the fatty alcohol derived from lanolin (oil from sheep wool); used as a softening agent in hand creams and lotions.

lanthionine (lan·THEE·oh·nyn)—a nonessential form of amino acid; bonding structure in the cortex resulting from processing with sodium hydroxide relaxer.

lanugo (luh·NOO·goh)—the fine hair that covers most of the body.

large intestine (LARJ in·TES·tin)—the distal portion of the intestine, which extends from the ileum to the anus, and consists of the cecum, colon, and rectum.

larynx (LAIR·inks)—the upper part of the trachea or windpipe; the organ of voice production.

laser (LAY·zur)—an instrument that emits radiation as a beam of great power; used in surgical procedures and in research.

lash (LASH)—the short, fine hair of the upper and lower eyelids.

lateral (LAT·ur·ul)—on or to the side.

lateral cutaneous nerve (LAT·ur·ul kyoo·TAY·nee·us NURV)—nerve that receives stimuli from the skin of the lateral side of the forearm.

lateral nasal cartilage (LAT·ur·ul NAYZ·ul KART·ul·ij)—the upper lateral cartilage of the nose.

lateral palpebral artery (LAT·ur·ul PAL·puh·brul ART·uh·ree)—artery that supplies blood to the eyelids and surrounding area.

lateral vibration (LAT·ur·ul vy·BRAY·shun)—a massage movement using the palms of the hands to press firmly on the muscles while moving them from side to side in a vibrating motion; primarily for shoulder and back massage.

lather (LATH·ur)—froth made by mixing soap and water.

lathering machine (LATH·ur·ing muh·SHEEN)—a machine used to produce lather or foam from soap and water that is used for shaving the face.

latissimus dorsi (lah·TIS·ih·mus DOR·see)—a broad, flat superficial muscle of the back.

lattice hair braid (LAT·us HAYR BRAYD)—a technique of crossing and interlacing strands of hair to resemble a lattice.

laurel (LOR·ul)—an evergreen tree or shrub of the genus laurus; including cinnamon, sassafras, and bay; used in some cosmetic and medicinal preparations.

lauric acid (LOR·ik AS·ud)—a fatty acid derived from laurel oil and coconut oil; used in the manufacture of some soaps and cosmetic products.

lauryl alcohol (LOR·ul AL·kuh·hawl)—an alcohol derived from laurel oil and used in detergent products.

lavender (LAV·un·dur)—a plant of the mint family producing pale violet flowers; the oils and dried flowers are used in perfumery.

layer (LAY·ur)—a single thickness, fold, or stratum.

layer cutting (LAY·ur KUT·ing)—cutting the hair into many thin layers by holding the hair at various angles from the head before cutting.

lecithin (LES·uh·thin)—a colorless, crystalline compound soluble in alcohol; found in animal tissue and yolk of egg; used as an emulsifier, natural antioxidant, and emollient in cosmetics.

left atrium (LEFT AY·tree·um)—upper thin wall chambers of the heart.

left ventricle (LEFT VEN·truh·kul)—lower, thick-walled chambers of the heart.

lemongrass (LEM·un·gras)—a tropical grass yielding a fragrant oil that is used in some cosmetic preparations.

lemon rinse (LEM·un RINS)—a product containing lemon juice or citric acid; formerly used to eliminate soap curd from hair; used as a bleach to slightly lighten hair.

lentigines (len·tih·JEE·neez); sing., **lentigo** (len·TY·goh)—the technical term for freckles.

lentigo (len·TY·goh)—a freckle; circumscribed spot or pigmentation in the skin.

lepid, lepido (LEP·id, LEP·ih·doh)—a word part meaning pertaining to scaly skin conditions.

lesion (LEE·zhun)—injury or damage that changes the structure of tissues or organs.

lesser multangular (LES·ur mul·TANG·gyuh·lur)—trapezoid; bone of the wrist.

lesser occipital (LES·ur ahk·SIP·ut·ul)—the nerve-supplying muscles at the back of the ear.

lesson plan (LES·un PLAN)—a detailed set of directions in logical sequence, for teaching a subject or a skill.

leuc, leuk, leuco, leuko (LOOK, LOOK·oh)—a combining form meaning white, colorless, weakly colored.

leucine (LOO·seen)—an essential amino acid produced by the breakdown of proteins.

leucocyte (LOO·koh·syt)—white blood corpuscle that performs the function of destroying disease-causing germs.

leuconychia (loo·koh·NIK·ee·ah)—a whitish discoloration of nails; white spots.

leukoderma (loo·koh·DUR·muh)—a skin disorder characterized by light abnormal patches, caused by a burn or congenital disease that destroys the pigment-producing cells.

leukotrichia (loo·koh·TRIK·ee·uh)—whiteness of the hair; canities.

levator (lih·VAYT·ur)—a muscle that elevates a part.

levator anguli oris (lih·VAYT·ur ANG·yoo·ly OH·ris)—caninus; muscle that raises the angle of the mouth and draws it inward.

levator labii superioris (lih·VAYT·ur LAY·bee·eye soo·peer·ee·OR·is)—quadratus labii superioris; muscle that elevates the upper lip and dilates the nostrils.

levator palpebrae (lih·VAYT·ur PAL·puh·bree)—muscle that raises the upper eyelid.

level (LEV·ul)—a unit of measurement, used to evaluate the lightness or darkness of a color, excluding tone; also called value or depth.

level system (LEV·ul SIS·tum)—a system colorists use to analyze the lightness or darkness of a hair color.

liability (ly·uh·BIL·ih·tee)—the state of being liable for one's products or services; the state of being obligated according to law; responsibility.

liability insurance (ly·uh·BIL·ih·tee in·SHUR·ans)—the act or system of insuring against personal damage.

lice (LYS)—plural of louse. (*See* pediculosis capitis.)

license (LYS·uns)—an official document granting permission to engage in a specified activity or to perform certain services.

lichen (LY·kun)—a type of skin lesion with solid papules.

lichenification (ly·kun·ih·fih·KAY·shun)—the process by which the skin becomes hard and leathery.

lichenoid eczema (LIK·uh·noyd EG·zuh·muh)—eczema characterized by papules on a reddened base, accompanied by a tingling and itching sensation.

lift (LIFT)—a term used in hair coloring to indicate the lightening action of a color or lightening product on the hair's pigment; to raise or cause to raise to a higher plane or position.

lift, face (LIFT, FAYS)—a technique used by a surgeon to lift the skin of the face to create a more youthful appearance. (*See* face lift and rhytidectomy.)

lift, hair (LIFT, HAYR)—a forklike comb employed in hair styling to raise the hair into a balanced position while combing.

ligament (LIG·uh·munt)—a tough band of fibrous tissue, serving to connect bones, or to hold an organ in place.

light (LYT)—radiant energy that can be seen and felt; less than usual in weight, amount, or force; not heavy.

lighten (LYT·un)—in hairstyling; to make the hair color lighter.

lightener (LYT·un·ur) (bleach)—the chemical compound that lightens the hair by dispersing, dissolving, and decolorizing the natural hair pigment. (*See* pre-lighten.)

lightening (LYT·un·ing)—*see* decolorize.

lightening retouch (LYT·un·ing REE·tuch)—the application of a lightening agent to the hair that has grown out since the first lightening application.

light therapy (LYT THAIR·uh·pee)—the application of light rays for treatment of disorders.

lilac (LY·lak)—the purple-pink flower used in perfumery; a purple-pink color.

lily of the valley (LIL·ee UV THE VAL·ee)—a perennial herb with oblong leaves and fragrant white, bell-shaped flowers; used in perfumes and some medicinal preparations.

lime (LYM)—a white powder containing calcium dioxide; a small oval-shaped green fruit of the citrus family.

limewater (LYM WAWT·ur)—a solution of calcium hydroxide that absorbs carbon dioxide from the air; used to neutralize acids and as an alkali in face masks and hair preparations.

limp (LIMP)—weak; lacking firmness or strength.

lineal albicantes (LYN·ee·ul al·bih·KAN·teez)—shiny white lines in the skin due to rupture of elastic fibers; often due to rapid weight loss or seen as stretchmarks following pregnancy.

linear (LIN·ee·ur)—pertaining to or resembling a line or lines; straight.

line, linea (LYN, LYN·ee·uh)—a thin, continuous mark used as a guide; a thin crease on the face or body.

linen (LIN·un)—a fiber made from flax; used in pure form or combined with other textiles.

line of demarcation (LYN UV dee·mar·KAY·shun)—a visible line of separation; an obvious difference between two colors on the hair shaft; line separating colored hair from regrowth; line created where makeup is not blended evenly; line separating healthy from diseased tissue.

liniment (LIN·uh·mint)—a medicated liquid applied to the skin to relieve sore or inflamed conditions.

linoleic acid (lin·uh·LEE·ik AS·ud)—an unsaturated fatty acid prepared from fats and oils; used as an emulsifier.

linseed (LIN·seed)—the dried seeds of flax; contains a mucilage that is used as an emollient in some cosmetic preparations.

liodermia (ly·oh·DUR·mee·uh)—a condition of abnormal smoothness and glossiness of the skin.

liparotrichia (LIP·uh·roh·trik·ee·uh)—abnormal oiliness of the hair.

lip color (LIP KUL·ur)—also called lipstick; a cosmetic in paste form, usually in a metal or plastic tube, manufactured in a variety of colors and used to color the lips.

lip color sealer (LIP KUL·ur SEEL·ur)—a product resembling fingernail base coat; used to keep lip color from seeping into fine lines around the lips.

lipectomy (lih·PEK·tuh·mee)—a surgical procedure to excise excessive fatty tissue.

lip gloss (LIP GLAWS)—a product formulated to add lubricating oil to the lips. Contains many of the same ingredients as lipsticks and is packaged in a small jar or lipstick tube.

lipid (LIP·ud)—any of a large class or organic substances insoluble in water, including fats, sterols, and waxes.

lip liner (LIP LYN·ur)—a colored pencil or brush used to outline the lips.

lipophilic (ly·puh·FIL·ik)—having an affinity or attraction to fat and oils.

liquefy (LIK·wuh·fy)—to reduce to a liquid state, said of both solids and gases.

liquefying cream (LIK·wuh·fy·ing KREEM)—a cream that becomes liquidlike upon contact with the warmth of the skin.

liquid (LIK·wud)—a substance that flows and is capable of being poured, as water or oil.

liquid dry cleaner (LIK·wud DRY KLEEN·ur)—a product used to clean wigs and hair pieces.

liquid dry shampoo (LIK·wud DRY sham·POO)—a dry cleansing fluid used to clean the hair without the use of shampoo and water.

liquid measure (LIK·wud MEZH·ur)—a unit or system of units used to measure liquids.

liquid tissue (LIK·wud TISH·oo)—body tissue that carries food, waste products, and hormones by means of blood and lymph.

liter (LEE·tur)—in the metric system, a measure of capacity equal to the volume of one kilogram of water at 4°C, or 1,056 liquid quarts.

litmus paper (LIT·mus PAYP·ur)—strips of chemically treated paper containing coloring matter used in testing acidity or alkalinity of a product; red turns blue to indicate alkalinity and blue turns red to indicate acidity.

livedo (lih·VEE·doh)—a bluish, mottled discoloration of the skin.

liver (LIV·ur)—an internal organ that secretes bile for digestion.

liver spots (LIV·ur SPAHTS)—*see* chloasma.

lobe (LOHB)—a curved or rounded projection of a bodily organ or part; ear lobe.

localize (LOH·kul·yz)—to confine to a specific area.

lock (LOK)—in hairstyling, a strand or ringlet of hair.

logarithm (LAWG·uh·rith·um)—the power to which a fixed number, the base, is raised in order to produce a given number; used as a measure of pH, indicating each change by one full digit equals a ten-fold change of acidity.

long face (LAWNG FAYS)—a face that is longer in proportion than an oval shape; a long oval- or rectangular-shaped face.

long stem roller (LAWNG STEM ROHL·ur)—in hairsetting, a roller that is placed completely off the base to create maximum movement and minimum volume.

loofah (LOO·fuh)—also luffa; a fibrous fruit of the gourd family; used as a sponge when bathing to stimulate circulation and to remove dead surface cells from the skin.

loose (LOOS)—free; not confined or restrained; not tight.

lordosis (lor·DOH·sis)—a forward curvature of the lumbar spine; swayback.

lotion (LOH·shun)—a liquid solution generally a cosmetic preparation for the hands, face, and body.

louse (LOWS); pl. **lice** (LYS)—an insect of the genus pediculus; an animal parasite infesting the hairs of the head.

low calorie (LOH KAL·uh·ree)—having a low-caloric value; having fewer than usual number of calories.

low elevation (LOH el·uh·VAY·shun)—hair cutting technique using slight layering.

low frequency (LOH FREE·kwen·see)—in electricity, pertaining to current characterized by a low rate of oscillation.

low lighting (LOH LYT·ing)—the technique of coloring strands of hair darker than the natural color.

low molecular weight (LOH muh·LEK·yuh·lur WAYT)—term used in cosmetology to indicate the ability of a substance to penetrate hair or skin tissue.

lubricant (LOO·brih·kent)—an oily or slippery, smooth substance used to lubricate a part.

lucid (LOO·sid)—clear; transparent.

lucid layer (LOO·sid LAY·ur)—the clear layer of the skin; the stratum lucidum; located below the stratum corneum and above the stratum granulosum.

lucidum (LOO·sih·dum)—the clear layer of the epidermis.

lukewarm (LOOK·warm)—tepid; not hot; approximately body temperature: 98.6°F (Fahrenheit) or 37°C (Celsius).

lumbar region (LUM·bur REE·jun)—the area of the back lying lateral to the lumbar vertebrae.

lumbar vertebrae (LUM·bar VUR·tuh·bree)—the bones that make up the vertebral column located in the lower part of the back; the five vertebrae associated with the lower part of the back.

luminous (LOO·muh·nus)—emitting or reflecting light; shiny.

lump (LUMP)—a small mass; a swelling or tumor.

lunate (LOO·nayt)—crescent-shaped.

lunate bone (LOO·nayt BOHN)—semilunar; a bone of the wrist.

lung (LUNG)—one of a pair of organs of respiration.

lunula (LOO·nuh·luh)—the whitish, half-moon shape at the root of a fingernail.

lupus (LOO·pus)—any chronic or progressive ulcerative skin lesion.

lupus vulgaris (LOO·pus vul·GAIR·is)—tuberculosis of the skin.

luster (LUS·tur)—radiance; glossiness.

lye (LYE)—a solution of sodium or potassium hydroxide; a strong alkali substance used in making soap and other cleansing products.

lymph (LIMF)—a clear, yellowish fluid that circulates in the lymph spaces (lymphatics) of the body; carries waste and impurities away from the cells.

lymphagogue (LIM·fuh·gahg)—a substance that stimulates the flow of lymph.

lymphatic (lim·FAT·ik)—pertaining to, containing, or conveying lymph.

lymphatic blockage (lim·FAT·ik BLAHK·ij)—obstruction of lymphatic drainage.

lymphatic glands (lim·FAT·ik GLANDZ)—lymph nodes; the glands that produce white corpuscles and filter the lymph as it passes through them.

lymphatic system (lim·FAT·ik SIS·tum)—consists of lymph flowing through the lymph spaces, lymph vessels, lacteals, and lymph nodes or glands.

lymph channels (LIMF CHAN·ulz)—the lymph sinuses around lymphatic glands and vessels; a lymph channel that surrounds a nerve trunk.

lymph drainage massage (LIMF DRAYN·ij muh·SAHZH)—a method of massage that works upon lymph vessels and glands to eliminate watery stagnation of tissues (edemas) and to stimulate the flow of body fluids.

lymph node (LIMF NOHD)—any of the glandlike bodies found in lymphatic vessels; also lymph glands.

lymphocytes (LIM·fuh·syts)—lymph cells that neutralize and filter harmful bacteria and toxic substances collected in lymph.

lymphoderma (lim·fuh·DUR·muh)—a disease of the lymphatics of the skin.

lymphoid tissue (LIM·foyd TISH·oo)—tissue found in nodes, tonsils, and adenoids.

lysine (LY·seen)—an amino acid essential in nutrition to ensure growth; used to improve protein content.

lysis (LY·sus)—a combining form meaning to dissolve or loosen; the gradual disappearance of the symptoms of a disease, especially an infectious disease or fever.

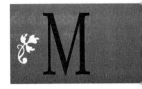

macassor oil (muh·KAS·ur OYL)—an oil obtained from Indonesia; used in some hairdressing preparations.

macerate (MAS·uh·rayt)—to reduce a solid to a soft mass by soaking in liquid.

maceration (mas·uh·RAY·shun)—a process used in perfumery in which the petals and parts of flowers are plunged into hot oil, which absorbs essential oils, from which fragrances are made.

machineless (muh·SHEEN·les)—work performed without the use of machines; in cosmetology, pertaining to methods of permanent waving and facial treatments that require no machines.

machine made (muh·SHEEN MAYD)—a term used to indicate that a wig or hair piece was made by machine and not by hand.

macro (MAK·roh)—large in size or duration.

macrofollicular (mak·roh·fah·LIK·yuh·lur)—pertaining to or having large follicles.

macronychia (mak·roh·NIK·ee·uh)—excessive size of the nails.

macroscopic (mak·ruh·SKAHP·ik)—visible to the naked eye.

macula (MAK·yuh·luh); pl., **maculae** (MAK·yuh·lee)—a spot or discoloration on the skin; a freckle; macule.

madarosis (mad·uh·ROH·sus)—loss of the eyelashes or eyebrows.

magenta (muh·JENT·uh)—the purplish-rose color produced from a fuchsin dye compound; fuchsia color.

magnesia (mag·NEE·zee·uh)—a skin freshener and an ingredient used in dusting powder; also used in some medicinal preparations, such as laxatives, and as an antacid.

magnesium carbonate (mag·NEE·zee·um KAR·buh·nayt)—perfume carrier and coloring material used in powders, shampoos, and in some medicinal preparations.

magnesium sulfate (mag·NEE·zee·um SUL·fayt)—an ingredient used in medicinal preparations and in some shampoos formulated for oily hair.

magnetic (mag·NET·ik)—pertaining to or having the properties of a magnet.

magnetic hair roller (mag·NET·ik HAYR ROHL·ur)—a plastic roller, either cylindrical or cone-shaped, used to shape and hold wet hair until it has been dried into the desired set.

magnetize (MAG·nuh·tyz)—convert into a magnet; to communicate magnetic properties to.

magnify (MAG·nuh·fy)—increase in fact or in appearance as by placement under a microscope; increase in size by use of a mirror or lens.

magnifying lamp (MAG·nuh·fy·ing LAMP)—an apparatus with a magnifying glass and source of light; used to examine the skin or scalp.

magnum (MAG·num)—the largest bone in the distal row of the carpus, located at the center of the wrist.

mahogany (muh·HAHG·uh·nee)—a reddish hard wood; a deep reddish-brown color.

maize (MAYZ)—in color, the deep shade of ripe yellow corn.

makeup (MAYK·up)—cosmetic products used to groom, color, or beautify the face.

makeup base (MAYK·up BAYS)—a clear or colored cosmetic in liquid or cream form, applied to the face as a foundation before the application of powder and cheek color.

makeup cape (MAYK·up KAYP)—a garment made of cloth or plastic designed to be draped across the chest and shoulders of a client to protect clothing during a makeup application or other salon service.

malady (MAL·uh·dee)—a disease, illness, or disturbed condition.

malar (MAY·lur)—of or pertaining to the cheek; the cheekbone.

malformation (mal·for·MAY·shun)—an abnormal or badly formed shape or structure, especially of the face or body.

malignant (muh·LIG·nent)—a growth or condition endangering health; not benign.

malleable (MAL·yuh·bul)—capable of being shaped or molded.

malleable block (MAL·yuh·bul BLAHK)—a head-shaped form, made of canvas and stuffed with sawdust, used for dressing-out and knotting the underside of a hair piece.

malnutrition (mal·noo·TRISH·un)—poor nutrition resulting from inadequate consumption of nutrients.

malpighian layer (mal·PIG·ee·un LAY·ur)—the stratum mucosum; the deepest layer of the epidermis.

malpractice (mal·PRAK·tis)—in cosmetology, the negligent or improper treatment of a client while performing a service.

mandible (MAN·duh·bul)—the lower jaw bone.

mandibular (man·DIB·yuh·lur)—pertaining to the lower jaw.

mandibular nerve (man·DIB·yuh·lur NURV)—the fifth cranial nerve, which supplies the muscles and skin of the lower part of the face.

manicure (MAN·ih·kyoor)—the artful treatment and care of the hands and nails.

manicure bowl (MAN·ih·kyoor BOHL)—a vessel shaped to fit the hand and fingers; warm, sudsy water is placed in the bowl and the fingers allowed to soak so that cuticles are softened before treatment.

manicure chair (MAN·ih·kyoor CHAYR)—a chair designed to allow the manicurist to sit comfortably during the manicure service.

manicure implements (MAN·ih·kyoor IM·pluh·ments)—the tools or equipment used for the manicuring procedure: nail file, cuticle pusher, cuticle scissor, cuticle nipper, emery board, buffer, etc.

manicure kit (MAN·ih·kyoor KIT)—a case or kit designed to carry the implements, equipment, and supplies used for the manicure service.

manicure lamp (MAN·ih·kyoor LAMP)—a flexible light fixture attached to the manicure table to provide adequate light during the manicure.

manicure machine (MAN·ih·kyoor muh·SHEEN)—a small electrically powered machine designed to aid in giving a manicure; the machine has attachments for various implements.

manicure oil heater (MAN·ih·kyoor OYL HEET·ur)—a thermostatically controlled electric heating cup used to heat the oil or cream used on the hands and nails during the manicure service.

manicure supplies (MAN·ih·kyoor suh·PLYZ)—products and materials that are used for the manicure service: cotton, cosmetics, etc.

manicure table (MAN·ih·kyoor TAY·bul)—a small table especially designed for the manicure service.

manicurist (MAN·ih·kyoor·ist)—one who professionally attends to the care of the hands and nails.

manikin: *see* mannequin.

manipulate (muh·NIP·yoo·layt)—to control; to handle skillfully.

manipulation (muh·nip·yuh·LAY·shun)—act or process of treating, working, or operating with the hands or by mechanical means, especially with skill.

mannequin; manikin (MAN·ih·kun)—in cosmetology, a model of the human head manufactured with hair, to be used for practice work; in fashion, a model of a human figure used for display purposes.

mannequin case (MAN·ih·kun KAYS)—a boxlike carrying case designed to hold the mannequin head and holder.

mannequin holder (MAN·ih·kun HOHL·dur)—a clamplike implement designed to be used to secure a mannequin head to a table top while it is in use.

mannequin slip-on (MAN·ih·kun SLIP·awn)—a glovelike mannequin form that can be slipped over another mannequin head to allow more varied practice routines.

mannitol (MAN·it·tawl)—a colorless, crystalline alcohol occurring in plants and animals; used as a humectant in creams and lotions.

mantle (MANT·ul)—nail mantle, the fold of the skin into which the nail root is lodged.

manual (MAN·yoo·ul)—done by hand or used by hand rather than by machines.

manus (MAN·us); pl., **mani** (MAN·eye)—the hand.

marbleizing (MAR·bul·yz·ing)—intertwining sections of light and dark shades of hair on one head.

marcel irons (mar·SEL EYE·urnz)—a curling (thermal) iron with a rod and groove attached to a handle that opens and closes; the iron is heated and strands of hair placed between the rod and groove to create curls or waves.

marcel wave (mar·SEL WAYV)—a wave resembling a natural hair wave, produced by a thermal iron; originated by Francois Marcel, a French hairdresser.

marginal blepharitis (MAR·jin·ul blef·uh·RY·tus)—inflammation of the sebaceous glands and hair follicles that line the margins of the eyelids.

marjoram (MAR·jur·um)—a perennial plant of the mint family with aromatic properties; used in soaps, perfumes, hair preparations, and cooking.

maroon (muh·ROON)—a deep, dark red color.

marrow (MAYR·oh)—a soft fatty substance filling the cavities of bone.

mascara (mah·SKAIR·uh)—a preparation used to darken the eyelashes.

mask; masque (MASK)—to hide or conceal; to apply a substance to the face as part of a facial treatment; a special cosmetic formula applied to the face to benefit and beautify the skin.

masotherapy (mas·oh·THAIR·uh·pee)—the treatment of the body by massage.

masque; mask (MASK)—a preparation, such as clay, paraffin wax, vegetables, fruits, gels, or other beneficial substances, applied to the face as part of a facial treatment.

mass (MAS)—a quantity of matter in any given body, relatively large in size with no particular shape.

massage (muh·SAHZH)—manual or mechanical manipulation of the body by rubbing, pinching, kneading, tapping, etc., to increase metabolism, promote absorption, relieve pain, etc.

massage compression (muh·SAHZH kahm·PRESH·un)—pressure used in massage movements.

massage cream (muh·SAHZH KREEM)—an emollient cream employed in skin treatment; designed to lubricate the skin; also referred to as tissue cream or nourishing cream.

massage equipment (muh·SAHZH ee·KWIP·munt)—implements used in massage manipulations.

massage movement direction (muh·SAHZH MOOV·ment dih·REK·shun)—in massage, the direction of movement toward the origin of a muscle in order to avoid damage to muscular tissue.

massage movements (muh·SAHZH MOOV·ments)—specific movements used in facial and body massage; basic movements include: friction, joint, percussion, petrissage, stroking, and vibration.

massage therapist (muh·SAHZH THAIR·uh·pist)—a professionally trained massage practitioner.

masseter (muh·SEET·ur)—one of the muscles of the jaw used in mastication.

masseteric artery (mas·uh·TAIR·ik ART·uh·ree)—the artery supplying blood to the muscles of the jaw (masseter).

masseteric nerve (mas·uh·TAIR·ik NURV)—a nerve in the face supplying the masseter muscle.

masseur (muh·SUR); fem., **masseuse** (muh·SOOZ)—man or woman who practices or gives massage.

masticate (MAS·tih·kayt)—to chew or to grind food with the teeth.

mastoid (MAS·toyd)—relating to the mastoid process; of or designating the projection of the temporal bone behind the ear.

mastoid process (MAS·toyd PRAH·ses)—a conical projection of the temporal bone.

materia medica (muh·TEE·ree·uh MED·ih·kuh)—a compilation of drugs and substances used in medicine; the branch of medical science that deals with the sources, propertie, and preparation of drugs and like substances.

matrix (MAY·triks)—the formative portion of a nail or a tooth; the intercellular substance of a tissue.

matte (MAT)—in makeup, a dull, nonshiny finish achieved by use of a special base or by applying face powder over foundation.

matter (MAT·ur)—a substance that occupies space and has weight. Forms: solid, liquid, and gas.

matting (MAT·ing)—tangling the hair into a thick mass; another term for back combing.

maturation (mach·uh·RAY·shun)—in skin care, the ripening or coming to a head of a pimple or other blemish.

maturity (muh·CHOOR·ih·tee)—the quality of being responsible, self-disciplined, and well-adjusted.

mauve (MOHV)—a coal tar dye of a purple-rose shade; a moderate purple, violet, or lilac color.

maxilla (mak·SIL·uh)—bone of the upper jaw.

maxillary (MAK·suh·lair·ee)—pertaining to the jaws.

maxillary artery (MAK·suh·lair·ee ART·uh·ree)—artery that supplies blood to the lower regions of the face.

maxillary nerves (MAK·suh·lair·ee NURVZ)—the nerves of the upper part of the face.

mayonnaise (MAY·uh·nayz)—a creamy salad dressing made of egg yolks, olive or other vegetable oils, lemon juice, or vinegar; used as a hair conditioner.

measure (MEZH·ur)—a standard or unit of measurement, as a foot, yard, gallon, pound, ounce, etc.

mechanical (muh·KAN·ih·kul)—relating to a machine; performed by means of some apparatus; not manual.

mechanism (MEK·uh·niz·um)—mechanical construction; parts of a machine.

medial; median (MEE·dee·ul; MEE·dee·un)—pertaining to the middle.

median nerve (MEE·dee·un NURV)—the nerve located in the center of the arm that supplies blood to the arm and hand.

medical gymnastics (MED·ih·kul jim·NAS·tiks)—application of gymnastics to treat disease.

medicamentosus (med·ih·kuh·men·TOH·sus)—a skin eruption caused by a drug.

medicate (MED·ih·kayt)—to treat a condition by use of drugs or other medications.

medicated ingredient (MED·ih·kayt·ud in·GREE·dee·ent)—a substance added to cosmetics to promote healing.

medicine (MED·ih·sin)—a drug or other healing substance; the science of preventing, treating, or curing diseases.

medium elevation (MEE·dee·um el·uh·VAY·shun)—a term used in hairdressing to indicate that hair is held at approximately a 45 degree angle to the head while it is being cut.

medium hair (MEE·dee·um HAYR)—a hair fiber neither especially large nor small in circumference, but of a thickness about halfway between fine and coarse.

medius (MEE·dee·us)—the middle finger.

medulla (muh·DUL·uh)—the center structure of the hairshaft, not present in every hair fiber; the marrow in the various bone cavities; soft inner portion of an organ.

medulla oblongata (muh·DUL·uh ob·lawng·GAY·tuh)—the lowest or posterior part of the brain, continuous with the spinal cord.

medullary (MED·yoo·lair·ee)—pertaining to marrow or medulla.

medullary space (MED·yoo·lair·ee SPAYS)—the cavity through the shaft of the long bones.

megalonychosis (meg·uh·lon·ih·KOH·sus)—noninflammatory hypertrophy of the nails.

melanin (MEL·uh·nin)—the tiny grain of pigment in the epidermis and hair cortex, and in the choroid or coat of the eye; creates natural color, and protects against strong light rays.

melanism (MEL·uh·niz·um)—excessive pigmentation of the hair, skin, eyes, tissues, or organs.

melanochroi (mel·uh·NAHK·ruh·wy)—a term used to describe very fair skin and very dark hair of Caucasians.

melanocyte (muh·LAN·uh·syt)—a melanin-forming cell in the hair bulb.

melanocytic nevi (mel·uh·noh·SIT·ik NEE·vye)—commonly called moles; brown spots sometimes having hair growing from them.

melanocytoma (mel·uh·noh·sy·TOH·muh)—a benign, heavily pigmented tumor.

melanoderma (mel·uh·noh·DUR·muh)—abnormal darkening of the skin, usually in patches caused by accumulation or deposits of melanin.

melanodermatitis (mel·uh·noh·dur·muh·TY·tis)—an inflamed skin condition characterized by increased skin pigmentation.

melanogenesis (mel·uh·noh·JEN·uh·sis)—the formation of melanin.

melanoid (MEL·uh·noyd)—having dark pigment.

melanoma (mel·uh·NOH·muh)—a black or dark brown pigmented tumor.

melanonychia (mel·uh·nuh·NIK·ee·uh)—darkening of the finger-nails or toenails.

melanophore (muh·LAN·uh·fohr)—a pigment cell containing melanin.

melanoprotein (mel·uh·noh·PROH·teen)—the protein coating of a melanosome.

melanosis (mel·uh·NOH·sis)—a condition in which pigment is deposited in the skin or other tissues.

melanosome (MEL·uh·noh·sohm)—protein-coated granule containing melanin.

melanotic sarcoma (mel·uh·NAHT·ik sar·KOH·muh)—a fatal skin cancer that starts with a mole.

membrane (MEM·brayn)—a thin sheet or layer of pliable tissue surrounding a part, separating adjacent cavities, lining a cavity, or connecting adjacent structures.

mental artery (MEN·tul ART·uh·ree)—artery that supplies blood to the lower lip and the chin.

mentalis (men·TAY·lis)—the muscle that elevates the lower lip and raises and wrinkles the skin of the chin.

mental nerve (MEN·tul NURV)—a nerve that supplies the skin of the lower lip and chin.

menthol (MEN·thawl)—an alcohol obtained from peppermint or other mint oils, often employed for its marked cooling effect.

menthyl salicylate (MEN·thil suh·LIS·ih·layt)—an organic compound that is used as a filtering agent in sunburn preventives; produces an even tan by removing the majority of the ultraviolet rays.

mentum (MEN·tum); pl., **menti** (men·EYE)—of or pertaining to the chin.

mercurochrome (mur·KYUR·uh·krohm)—a germicide, three to five percent solution of iodine, used for cuts.

mercury bichloride (MUR·kyuh·ree by·KLOH·ryd)—a powerful germicide; very poisonous.

mercury compound (MUR·kyuh·ree KAHM·pownd)—quicksilver; used in face masks, bleaching creams, hair tonics, and other cosmetics.

mesh (MESH)—an open weave foundation used to attach hair in a hair piece; a wig foundation or base made of a net material.

mesh hair roller (MESH HAYR ROHL·ur)—a roller covered with a woven mesh fabric, usually of nylon.

meso (MES·oh)—a prefix denoting in the middle; intermediate.

mesomorph (MES·uh·morf)—a body type characterized by a sturdy body structure and great strength.

mesorrhine (MES·uh·ryn)—pertaining to a broad, high-bridged nose.

mesothelium (mes·uh·THEE·lee·um)—smooth tissue that allows the movement of organs to take place with little or no friction.

meta (MET·uh)—a prefix signifying over; beyond; among; between change or transformation.

metabolism (muh·TAB·uh·liz·um)—the constructive and destructive life process of the cell.

metacarpal (met·uh·KAR·pul)—pertaining to the bones of the palm of the hand.

metacarpal, dorsal (met·uh·KAR·pul, DOR·sul)—the vein that draws blood from the back of the hand.

metacarpal, palmar (met·uh·KAR·pul, PAHL·mur)—the main vein that draws blood from the palm of the hand.

metacarpus (met·uh·KAR·pus)—the bones of the palm of the hand; the part of the hand containing five bones between the carpus and phalanges.

metallic (muh·TAL·ik)—relating to, or resembling metal.

metallic hair dye (muh·TAL·ik HAYR DYE)—a solution containing metal salts, such as copper, lead, silver, and bismuth, to change hair color gradually by progressive build-up and exposure to air.

metaphase (MET·uh·fayz)—in biology, in meiotic cell division, the middle stage of mitosis when the cell chromosomes lie nearly in a single plane at the equator of the spindle.

metastasis (muh·TAS·tuh·sus)—the migration or transference of a disease from one site in the body to another by the conveyance of cells in blood vessels or lymph channels.

metatarsus (met·uh·TAR·sus)—the bones that make up the instep of the foot; the part of the foot between the phalanges and the tarsus, containing five bones.

metatoluene-diamine (met·uh·TAHL·yoo·een-DY·uh·min)—an oxidation dye used to provide lighter shades of red and blond; an aniline derivative type dye.

meter (MEE·tur)—an instrument for measuring the strength of an electric current in amperes; the basic metric unit of length, equal to 39.37 inches.

methodology (meth·uh·DAHL·uh·jee)—principals, practices, and particular procedures applied to a field of learning.

methyl alcohol (METH·ul AL·kuh·hawl)—methanol, a solvent, flammable and toxic; used in the manufacture of formaldehyde and some disinfectants.

methyl salicylate (METH·ul suh·LIS·ih·layt)—the chief constituent of oil or wintergreen, used as a counter irritant, anesthetic, and disinfectant.

metric (MET·rik)—based on the meter as a unit of measurement; pertaining to the metric system. (*See* metric conversion chart.)

metric system (MET·rik SIS·tum)—a decimal system of weights and measures based on the gram, from which measures of weights and mass are derived, and the meter, from which measures of area, length, and volumes are derived.

mica (MY·kuh)—a mineral occurring in the form of thin, shining, transparent plates.

micro (MY·kroh)—a prefix denoting very small; slight; millionth part of.

microbicide (my·KROH·bih·syd)—an agent that destroys microbes.

microcirculation (my·kroh·sur·kyoo·LAY·shun)—pertaining to the microvasculature; circulation of blood in the body's system of five vessels (100 microns or less in diameter).

microfollicular (my·kroh·fah·LIK·yoo·lur)—characterized by very small follicles.

micron; mikron (MY·krahn)—a measurement equal to one thousandth of a millimeter or one millionth of a meter.

micronychia (my·kroh·NIK·ee·uh)—the presence of an abnormally small fingernail or toenail.

microorganism (my·kroh·OR·gah·niz·um)—microscopic plant or animal cell; bacterium; viruses; fungi.

microscope (MY·kruh·skohp)—an instrument for making enlarged views of minute objects.

microscopic (my·kroh·SKAHP·ik)—extremely small; visible only with the aid of a microscope; not visible to the naked eye.

mid (MID)—a prefix denoting the middle part.

middle ear (MID·ul EER)—the portion of the ear between the tympanic membrane and the opening of the eustachian tube.

middle temporal artery (MID·ul TEM·puh·rul ART·uh·ree)—the artery that supplies blood to the temporal muscles.

midfrontal (mid·FRUN·tul)—pertaining to the middle of the forehead.

milia (MIL·ee·uh)—white heads. (*See* milium.)

miliaria (mil·ee·AIR·ee·uh)—an eruption of minute vesicles due to retention of fluid at the mouths of the sweat follicles.

miliaria profunda (mil·ee·AIR·ee·uh proh·FUN·duh)—a skin reaction in the sweat retention syndrome, characterized by papules located at the sweat pores.

miliaria rubra (mil·ee·AIR·ee·uh ROOB·ruh)—prickly heat; burning and itching usually caused by exposure to excessive heat.

miliary fever (MIL·ee·air·ee FEE·vur)—sweating sickness; an infectious disease characterized by fever, profuse sweating, and the production of papular vesicular and other eruptions.

milium (MIL·ee·um); pl., **milia** (MIL·ee·uh)—a small, whitish pearl-like mass in the epidermis due to retention of sebum; a whitehead.

milli (MIL·ee)—thousand; a combining form meaning one thousandth part of.

milliameter (mil·ee·AM·uh·tur)—an instrument that registers electric current in milliamperes; used to measure the amount of current required for a given treatment.

milliampere (mil·ee·AM·peer)—one thousandth of an ampere.

milligram (MIL·ih·gram)—a unit of weight in the metric system equal to one thousandth of a gram.

milliliter (MIL·ih·lee·tur)—a unit of capacity in the metric system equal to one thousandth of a liter; equivalent to a cubic centimeter.

millimeter (MIL·ih·mee·tur)—one thousandth of a meter.

mineral (MIN·ur·ul)—any inorganic material found in the earth's crust.

mineral oil (MIN·ur·ul OYL)—white oil; oil found in the rock strata of the earth; a colorless, tasteless oil derived from petroleum and used in creams, lotions, moisturizing products, powders, lip and eye makeup, hairdressings, and many other cosmetics; it is a widely used cosmetic lubricant and binder.

mini (MIH·nee)—combination form meaning miniature or of small dimensions; smaller than average.

minibraid (MIH·nee·brayd)—thin strands of hair woven to form small braids.

minifall (MIH·nee·fawl)—a loose-hanging hair piece (shorter than a regular fall) that is attached at the crown.

minimize (MIN·ih·myz)—to reduce to the smallest possible degree.

minishears (MIH·nee·sheerz)—small scissors used to cut and layer hair in small graduations.

miniwig (MIH·nee·wig)—a very short wig or hair piece.

mink oil (MINK OYL)—an oil produced by the small mammal (genus mustela); used in some cosmetics for its softening properties.

mint (MINT)—any of several aromatic herbs used as a flavoring and in some cosmetic preparations.

minute (my·NOOT)—very small; tiny.

miscible (MIS·uh·bul)—the property of certain liquids to mix with each other in equal proportions.

mitosis (my·TOH·sis)—indirect nuclear division, the usual process of cell reproduction of human tissues.

mixed nerves (MIKST NURVZ)—nerves that contain both sensory and motor fibers and have the ability to both send and receive messages.

mixing (MIKS·ing)—the intermingling of hair of various shades and/or lengths.

mixture (MIKS·chur)—a preparation made by incorporating an insoluble ingredient in a liquid vehicle; sometimes used to identify an aqueous solution containing two or more solutes; a combination of two or more substances that are not chemically united.

mobility (moh·BIL·ih·tee)—the quality of being movable.

mode (MOHD)—a current style of fashion; a manner or method of doing something.

model (MAHD·ul)—an object used as an example of something to be made or already existing; one who is hired to display clothes, hairstyles, or merchandise.

moderate porosity (MAHD·ur·ut por·AHS·ih·tee)—category of normal hair in which the cuticle is close to the hair shaft.

modern blend (MAHD·urn BLEND)—descriptive of a basic perfume type that contains aldehydes (a class of organic chemical compounds) and has its own distinctive fragrance.

modifier (MAHD·ih·fy·ur)—anything that will change the form or characteristics of an object or substance; a chemical found as an ingredient in permanent hair colors, whose function is to alter the dye intermediates.

moist (MOYST)—slightly wet; damp.

moisture (MOYST·yur)—water or other liquid spread in very small drops in the air or on a surface.

moisture gradient (MOYST·yur GRAY·dee·unt)—the amount of moisture in the skin or hair.

moisturizer (MOYST·yur·yz·ur)—a product formulated to add moisture to dry skin or hair.

mold (MOHLD)—a fungus growth usually growing in dark, damp places; to form into a particular shape.

molded curl (MOHLD·ud KURL)—*see* carved curl.

molding (MOHLD·ing)—the act of forming or directing hair into a desired pattern.

mole (MOHL)—a small brownish spot on the skin; pigmented nevis.

molecular attraction (muh·LEK·yuh·lur uh·TRAK·shun)—the force that is exerted between two unlike molecules tending to draw them together and to resist separation.

molecular breakdown (muh·LEK·yuh·lur BRAYK·down)—the disrupting or disuniting of a molecular unit.

molecular weight (muh·LEK·yuh·lur WAYT)—the sum of the weights of the atoms of a molecule.

molecule (MAHL·uh·kyool)—the smallest possible unit of any substance that still retains its characteristics; two or more atoms joined chemically.

molluscum (mah·LUS·kum)—pertaining to a skin disease having waxy, dome-shaped nodules.

molluscum contagiosum (mah·LUS·kum kahn·tay·jee·OH·sum)—a viral disease of the skin, characterized by waxy, dome-shaped nodules.

molluscum fibrosum (mah·LUS·kum fy·BROH·sum)—a cutaneous tumor of the dermis, characterized by fibrous papules.

mongolism (MAHNG·goh·liz·um)—a congenital disease characterized by yellowness of the skin and slightly slanting eyes; Down syndrome.

monilethrix (mah·NIL·ee·thriks)—beaded hair; a condition in which the hairs show a series of constrictions, giving the appearance of fusiform beads.

mono (MAHN·oh)—a prefix denoting one; single.

monochromatic (mahn·uh·kroh·MAT·ik)—consisting of one color or color family; displaying shades and tints of the same color.

monochromatism (mahn·uh·KROH·muh·tiz·um)—total color blindness.

moons (MOONZ)—cresent-shaped areas at the base of the fingernails.

mordant (MORD·unt)—a substance, such as alum, phenol, aniline oil, that fixes the dye used in coloring.

morphology (mor·FAHL·uh·jee)—the branch of biology that deals with structure and form; it includes histology and cytology of the organism at any stage of its life history.

moth patches (MAWTH PACH·ez)—increased deposits of pigment in the skin.

motile (MOH·tul)—having the power of movement, as certain bacteria.

motor (MOH·tur)—of or relating to muscular movement.

motor nerves (MOH·tur NURVZ)—nerves that carry impulses from nerve centers to muscles.

motor oculi (MOH·tur AHK·yoo·ly)—third cranial nerve; the nerve controlling most of the eye muscles.

motor point (MOH·tur POYNT)—a point on the skin over a muscle where pressure or stimulation will cause contraction of that muscle.

motor units (MOH·tur YOO·nits)—muscle fibers that are controlled by nerve fibers.

mount (MOWNT)—that part of a wig (excluding the crown) or any hair piece made of foundation net, hair lace, or gauze, on which hair is knotted.

mousse (MOOS)—a light, airy, whipped hair setting and sculpturing product resembling shaving foam; the whipped dessert called mousse.

mousy (MOW·see)—hair color that is similar to the drab, gray-brown color of a mouse.

movement (MOOV·ment)—the change of place or position of hair; the rhythmic quality or motion of hair.

muco (MYOO·koh)—a combining form meaning mucus or mucous membrane.

mucosa (myoo·KOH·suh)—mucous membrane.

mucosum, stratum (myoo·KOH·sum STRAY·tum)—a membrane secreting mucus that lines passages and cavities communicating with the air.

mucous membrane (MYOO·kus MEM·brayn)—a membrane secreting mucous that lines passages and cavaties communicating with the air.

mucus (MYOO·kus)—a thick, slippery secretion produced by the mucous membranes to lubricate and cleanse the part.

mudpack (MUD·pak)—a thick, spreadable product, usually containing clay; used for facial and body treatments.

multi (MUL·tih)—many; more than one.

multicellular (mul·tih·SEL·yoo·lur)—having many cells.

multicolor (mul·tih·KUL·ur)—having many colors.

multidimensional (mul·tih·dih·MEN·shun·ul)—having several dimensions.

multidirectional (mul·tih·dih·REK·shun·ul)—extending in many directions.

multilayered (mul·tih·LAY·urd)—having several layers.

multiple (MUL·tih·pul)—consisting of more than one.

murky (MUR·kee)—thick, hazy in color; not clear.

muscle (MUS·ul)—the contractile tissue of the body by which movement is accomplished.

muscle-bound (MUS·ul-bownd)—having tight, inflexible muscles.

muscle energy technique (MUS·ul EN·ur·jee tek·NEEK)—technique utilizing neurophysiological muscle reflexes to improve functional mobility of joints.

muscle fatigue (MUS·ul fuh·TEEG)—cessation of muscle response to contraction.

muscle insertion (MUS·ul in·SUR·shun)—the distal point of muscle attachment.

muscle oil (MUS·ul OYL)—a vegetable oil in which either lecithin or cholestrin is dissolved; used in conjunction with massage to soften the skin and the help prevent fine lines.

muscle origin (MUS·ul OR·ih·jin)—the proximal point of muscle attachment.

muscle spasm (MUS·ul SPAZ·um)—a sudden involuntary contraction of muscles.

muscle strains (MUS·ul STRAYNZ)—torn or pulled muscles.

muscle strapping (MUS·ul STRAP·ing)—a heavy massage treatment used to reduce fatty deposits.

muscle tone (MUS·ul TOHN)—the normal degree of tension in a healthy muscle.

muscular (MUS·kyuh·lur)—relating to a muscle or the muscles.

muscular tissue (MUS·kyuh·lur TISH·oo)—contracted and moves various parts of the body.

musculi colli (MUS·kyoo·ly KOH·lih)—the anterior muscles of the neck.

musculi dorsi (MUS·kyoo·ly DOR·see)—the muscles of the back.

musk (MUSK)—a secretion with a penetrating odor, obtained from the male musk deer, and used in the making of some perfumes and medicines.

muslin (MUZ·lin)—any of several plain-weave cotton fabrics of varying fineness.

mustache (MUS·tash)—the growth of hair on the upper lip.

mustache brush (MUS·tash BRUSH)—a small brush designed to groom the mustache.

mustache comb (MUS·tash KOHM)—a small comb with fine teeth designed to groom the mustache.

mustache styles (MUS·tash STYLZ)—various designs of mustaches, some combined with beard and sideburn styles; usually styled to enhance the client's facial features or to conceal an undesired facial feature.

mutation (myoo·TAY·shun)—to change, as in quality, form, or nature.

mutton chop (MUT·un CHAHP)—a beard style with side whiskers, narrow at the temples, and widening at the lower cheeks.

myalgia (my·AL·jee·uh)—pain in the muscles.

myasthenia (my·us·THEE·nee·uh)—muscular weakness.

mycetoma (my·suh·TOH·muh)—any disease or infection caused by fungus.

myocardium (my·oh·KAR·dee·um)—cardiac muscle responsible for pumping of the heart.

myodystrophy (my·uh·DIS·truh·fee)—degeneration of muscles.

myoedema (my·oh·eh·DEE·muh)—edema of a muscle.

myofibrils (my·oh·FYB·rulz)—muscle fibers containing filaments give muscles their contractible ability.

myology (my·AHL·uh·jee)—the science of the nature, functions, structure, and diseases of muscles.

myomalacia (my·oh·muh·LAY·shee·uh)—degeneration with softening of muscle tissue.

myoneural (my·oh·NOO·rul)—relating to nerve endings in muscle tissue.

myopalmus (my·oh·PAL·mus)—twitching and quivering of muscles.

myopathic (my·oh·PATH·ik)—pertaining to disease of the muscles.

myoplasty (MY·oh·plas·tee)—plastic surgery on a muscle or group of muscles.

myosin (MY·oh·sin)—muscular filament, gives contractile ability.

myositis (my·oh·SY·tis)—inflammation of muscle tissue.

myotasis (MY·ot·uh·sis)—stretching and extending of muscle.

myotrophy (MY·ot·ruh·fee)—nutrition of the muscles.

myrrh (MUR)—an aromatic gum resin from the myrrh shrub; used in perfumery, in some medicinal preparations, and in skin tonics.

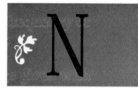

naevus; nevus (NEE·vus); pl., **naevi, nevi** (NEE·vy)—a birthmark; a congenital skin blemish.

nail (NAYL)—unguis; the horny protective plate located at the end of the finger or toe.

nail bed (NAYL BED)—that portion of the skin on which the body of the nail rests.

nail biting (NAYL BYT·ing)—the habit of biting off the tips of the nails to the nail bed. (*See* onychophagia.)

nail bleach (NAYL BLEECH)—a product used in manicuring to remove stains and to whiten the nails.

nail body (NAYL BAHD·ee)—the horny nail blade resting upon the nail bed.

nail brush (NAYL BRUSH)—a small brush used to clean under and around the nails.

nail buffer (NAYL BUF·ur)—an instrument made of leather or chamois; used with a polishing powder to polish the nails to a high luster.

nail cap (NAYL KAP)—an artificial nail attached to the natural nail to make the nail stronger and more attractive.

nail emery (NAYL EM·uh·ree)—a small, flat stick coated with finely ground emery; used as a manicuring instrument; emery board.

nail enamel (NAYL in·AM·ul)—a fingernail polish in liquid form, applied to protect and beautify the nails.

nail extender (NAYL ek·STEN·dur)—a product applied to the natural nail over a fingernail form; when the mixture hardens, it is shaped to resemble a longer natural nail.

nail file (NAYL FYL)—a metal instrument with a specially prepared surface used to file and shape the nails.

nail fold (NAYL FOHLD)—nail wall.

nail grooves (NAYL GROOVZ)—the slits or furrows on the sides of the nails upon which the nail moves as it grows.

nail lacquer (NAYL LAK·ur)—a thick liquid that forms a glossy film on the nail.

nail mantal (NAYL MAN·tul)—the fold of skin in which the nail root is embedded.

nail matrix (NAYL MAY·triks)—the portion of the nail bed extending beneath the nail root.

nail mold (NAYL MOHLD)—a form used in the creation of artificial nails.

nail plate (NAYL PLAYT)—the nail body.

nail polish remover (NAYL PAHL·ish ree·MOOV·ur)—a solution used to remove polish from the nails.

nail repair (NAYL ree·PAYR)—the use of a special tape and cement to mend a broken nail.

nail root (NAYL ROOT)—the part of the nail located at its base; embedded underneath the skin.

nail shaper (NAYL SHAYP·ur)—a disk made of emery; used to shape the nails.

nail skin (NAYL SKIN)—cuticle.

nail tips (NAYL TIPS)—preformed artificial nails that are applied to the tips of the natural fingernails.

nail transplant (NAYL TRANZ·plant)—the repairing of a broken nail by cementing the broken part to the natural fingernail.

nail wall (NAYL WAWL)—cuticle covering the lateral and proximal edge of the nail.

nail white (NAYL WHYT)—a nail cosmetic used to whiten the free edge of the nails.

nail wrapping (NAY RAP·ing)—a corrective treatment using tissue and sealer to form a protective coating for a damaged or fragile nail.

nape (NAYP)—the back part of the neck.

nape line (NAYP LYN)—the hairline at the nape of the neck; nape section.

naris (NAIR·is); pl., **nares** (NAIR·eez)—a nostril.

nasal (NAY·zul)—pertaining to the nose.

nasal bones (NAY·zul BOHNZ)—bones that form the bridge of the nose.

nasalis (nay·ZAY·lis)—a muscle of the nose.

nasal nerve (NAY·zul NURV)—nerve that receives stimuli for the skin on the sides of the nose.

nasitis (nay·ZYE·tus)—rhinitis; inflammation of nasal mucous membrane of the nose.

nasus (NAY·zus); pl., **nasi** (NAY·zye)—the nose.

natural bristle brush (NACH·uh·rul BRIS·ul BRUSH)—a brush with bristles made from the hairs of an animal, not from synthetic hair.

natural distribution (NACH·uh·rul dis·truh·BYOO·shun)—the direction hair assumes as it grows out from the scalp.

natural growth pattern (NACH·uh·rul GROHTH PAT·urn)—the direction in which hair grows naturally, usually in a large circle from the crown.

natural immunity (NACH·uh·rul im·YOO·net·ee)—natural resistance to disease.

natural neckline (NACH·uh·rul NEK·lyn)—haircutting technique that allows the hair to follow its natural growth tendency rather than forcing a pattern into the hair.

navicular (nuh·VIK·yuh·lur)—boat-shaped; a bone of the wrist.

neck (NEK)—the part of the body that connects the trunk and the head.

neck duster (NEK DUS·tur)—a brush used to remove hair from the neck after a haircut; in some states this procedure is prohibited as it is considered unsanitary.

neckline (NEK·lyn)—in haircutting, the line where the hair growth of the head ends and the neck begins; hairline.

neck strips (NEK STRIPS)—soft, flexible strips of paper placed around the client's neck to keep the shampoo cape from touching the skin while a service is being given.

negative pole (NEG·uh·tiv POHL)—the pole from which negative galvanic current flows.

negative skin test (NEG·uh·tiv SKIN TEST)—having no reaction to a skin test for allergy, indicating the safety of performing the service.

negative terminal (NEG·uh·tiv TUR·mih·nul)—the end of the conducting circuit of the electric current manifesting alkaline reaction; the zinc plate in a battery.

nerve (NURV)—a whitish cord, made up of bundles of nerve fibers, through which impulses are transmitted.

nerve cell (NURV SEL)—a neuron; the fundamental cellular unit of the nervous system.

nerve center (NURV SEN·tur)—an aggregation of neurons with a specific function for a part of the body; command center.

nerve fiber (NURV FY·bur)—threadlike processes (axons and dendrites) arising from a neuron, which make up a nerve.

nerve impulse (NURV IM·puls)—an electrical wave transmitted along a nerve that has been stimulated.

nerve tissue (NURV TISH·oo)—controls and coordinates all body functions.

nervous cutaneous (NUR·vus kyoo·TAY·nee·us)—a cutaneous nerve; any nerve supplying an area of the skin.

nervous system (NUR·vus SIS·tum)—the body system composed of the brain, spinal cord, nerves, ganglia, and other parts of the receptor; controls and coordinates all other systems and makes them work.

net (NET)—a fabric of thread or cord woven in an open pattern or meshwork; a fabric of this type used to cover the hair and hold the set in place while drying.

net foundation (NET fown·DAY·shun)—a mesh or other open-weave material used for a foundation of a hair piece.

nettle (NET·ul)—an herb (genus urtica) used for its astringent qualities.

neuralgia (noo·RAL·juh)—acute pain along the course of a nerve.

neurasthenia (nur·us·THEE·nee·uh)—a condition of weakness and depression due to exhaustion that affects the nervous system.

neuritis (nuh·RY·tus)—inflammation of a nerve.

neurology (nuh·RAHL·uh·jee)—the science of the structure, function, and pathology of the nervous system.

neuromuscular junction (nuh·roh·MUS·kyuh·lur JUNK·shun)—the point where the motor neuron and muscle join.

neuron (NOO·rahn)—the basic unit of the nervous system, consisting of a nucleus, its processes, and extensions; a nerve cell.

neutral (NOO·trul)—exhibiting no positive properties; indifferent; in chemistry, neither acid nor alkaline, pH of 7; a color balanced between warm and cool, which does not reflect a highlight of any primary or secondary color.

neutral blond (NOO·trul BLAHND)—a beige-blond that is neither gold nor ash.

neutralization (noo·truh·ly·ZAY·shun)—that process that counterbalances or cancels another action of an agent or color; in chemistry, reaction forming a substance that is neither alkaline nor acid; a chemical reaction between an acid and a base; rehardening the hair in cold waving or in chemical hair relaxing.

neutralize (NOO·truh·lyz)—to render ineffective; to effect neutralization; counterbalance of an action or influence.

neutralizer (NOO·trul·yz·ur)—an agent capable of neutralizing another substance.

neutralizing (NOO·truh·lyz·ing)—the process of stopping the action of a permanent wave solution and hardening the hair in its new form by the application of a chemical solution.

neutralizing headband (NOO·truh·lyz·ing HED·band)—an absorbent band placed around the client's hairline during a permanent to prevent dripping on the client's face during the neutralizing process.

nevus (NEE·vus)—a birthmark.

nevus pilosus (NEE·vus py·LOH·sus)—hairy nevus; a birthmark characterized by hair growing from the dark area.

new growth (NOO GROHTH)—the part of the hair shaft between the scalp and the hair that had previously received treatment.

ninth cranial nerve (NYNTH KRAY·nee·ul NURV)—the glossopharyngeal nerve.

nipper (NIP·ur)—a tool used in pedicuring and manicuring to trim the cuticle around fingernails or toenails.

nit (NIT)—the egg of a louse, usually attached to a hair.

nitrazine paper (NY·truh·zeen PAY·pur)—a form of paper used to test the acidity or alkalinity of products.

nitrocellulose (ny·troh·SEL·yuh·lohs)—pyroxylin; gun cotton; a granular, yellowish mass formed in the chemical reaction between cellulose and nitric acid; used in nail polishes.

nitrogen (NY·truh·jun)—a colorless gaseous element; tasteless and odorless; found in air and living tissue.

nitrous (NY·trus)—designating a compound of nitrogen.

no-base relaxer (NOH-BAYS ree·LAKS·ur)—a preparation used to straighten the hair that does not require application of a protective base.

node (NOHD)—a knot or knob; a circumscribed swelling; a knuckle or finger joint.

nodose (NOH·dohs)—having nodes or knotlike swellings.

nodule (NAHD·yul)—a small node.

noma (NOH·muh)—a sore or ulcer, usually of the mouth.

non (NAHN)—a prefix denoting not.

nonalkaline (nahn·AL·kuh·lin)—*see* acid.

nonallergenic cosmetic (nahn·al·ur·JEN·ik kahz·MET·ik)—a preparation formulated without certain ingredients that have been found to cause reaction in hypersensitive people.

nonconductor (nahn·kun·DUK·tur)—any substance that does not easily transmit electricity, light, heat, or sound.

noninfectious (nahn·in·FEK·shus)—not spread by contact; unable to spread disease.

nonpathogenic (nahn·path·uh·JEN·ik)—not harmful; not disease producing; organisms that perform useful functions.

nonresistant (nahn·ree·ZIS·ten)—porous hair; the condition of the hair that absorbs moisture readily.

nonstriated (nahn·STRY·ayt·ud)—without striations, as smooth muscle that acts involuntarily without the action of the will.

nonstripping shampoo (nahn·STRIP·ing sham·POO)—a shampoo that cleanses the hair without removing tint.

normal (NOR·mul)—regular; natural; conforming to some ideal norm or standard.

normal hair condition (NOR·mul HAYR kahn·DIH·shun)—an average condition in which hair is neither porous nor resistant, neither dry nor oily.

normal hair shampoo (NOR·mul HAYR sham·POO)—a shampoo formulated for hair that is neither too dry nor too oily.

normalize (NOR·mul·yz)—to make something conform to a norm or standard; to return the pH of the skin or hair to normal.

normalizer (NOR·mul·yz·ur)—a solution used to return the hair to its normal pH (4.5 to 5.5), or the skin to about 4.5 to 6.0.

normal skin (NOR·mul SKIN)—skin that is neither too dry nor too oily and is free of conditions such as blackheads, whiteheads, acne, or disease.

nose (NOHZ)—the organ of smell.

no stem (NOH STEM)—a type of curl or roller that is placed directly on its base for maximum volume and minimum mobility.

nostril (NAHS·trul)—one of the two external openings of the nose.

nourish (NUR·ish)—to feed; to furnish with whatever promotes growth.

nourishing cream (NUR·ish·ing KREEM)—a cream formulated to nourish the skin; used in massage and facial treatments.

nourishment (NUR·ish·ment)—anything that nourishes; nutriment; food.

novice (NAHV·is)—a beginner in any occupation; one who is learning a skill, trade, or craft.

noxious (NAHK·shus)—harmful; poisonous.

nucha (NOO·kuh)—the nape or back of the neck.

nucleic acid (noo·KLEE·ik AS·ud)—one of a group of compounds found in cell nuclei and cytoplasm involved in building the proteins necessary to the formation of living matter.

nucleus (NOO·klee·us); pl., **nuclei** (noo·klee·EYE)—the active center of cells; plays an important part in cell reproduction.

nutmeg (NUT·meg)—the hard, aromatic seed of the East Indian tree; used as a spice and to flavor mouthwashes and dentifrices.

nut oil (NUT OYL)—an oil from the kernels of walnuts often used in skin preparations.

nutrient (NOO·tree·unt)—a nourishing substance; nutritious.

nutriment (NOO·trih·ment)—that which nourishes; food.

nutrition (noo·TRISH·un)—the processes involved in taking in nutriments and assimilating and utilizing them.

nylon (NY·lahn)—a synthetic thermoplastic polyamide from which fibers and bristles are made.

nylon fiber (NY·lahn FY·bur)—a combination of clear polish with nylon fibers. It is first applied vertically and then horizontally on the nail plate.

O

O—chemical symbol for oxygen.

oatmeal (OHT·meel)—a cereal made from oats that is sometimes mixed with other ingredients and used as a facial cleanser or mask.

obese (oh·BEES)—extremely overweight; stout; corpulent; fat.

obesity (oh·BEE·sut·ee)—the condition of having excessive body weight over what is considered to be normal for one's height and bone structure.

objective (ub·JEK·tiv)—aim or goal; something observable or verifiable by scientific methods.

oblique (oh·BLEEK)—slanting or inclined.

oblong (AHB·lawng)—longer than broad; rectangle whose horizontal sides are longer than its vertical sides.

oblong face shape (AHB·lawng FAYS SHAYP)—a face characterized by a long, thin structure.

obsolete (ahb·suh·LEET)—out of date; no longer in use; not current.

occipita (ahk·SIP·it·uh)—the back of the head or skull.

occipital (ahk·SIP·it·ul)—pertaining to the back part of the head; the bone that forms the back and lower part of the cranium.

occipital artery (ahk·SIP·it·ul ART·uh·ree)—the artery that supplies blood to the skin and muscles of the scalp, back of the head, and the neck.

occipital bone (ahk·SIP·ih·tul BOHN)—the hindmost bone of the skull below the parietal bones.

occipital frontalis (ahk·SIP·it·ul frun·TAY·lus)—epicranius; the scalp muscle.

occipitalis (ahk·SIP·ih·tahl·is)—a muscle that draws the scalp backward.

occipital lobe (ahk·SIP·ih·tal LOHB)—one of the lobes of the cerebrum.

occipital nerve (ahk·SIP·ih·tul NURV)—major occipital nerve; nerve that receives stimuli for the skin of the posterior portion of the scalp.

occupational disease (ahk·yuh·PAY·shun·ul dih·ZEEZ)—illness resulting from conditions associated with an occupation such as coming in contact with certain chemicals, dyes, etc.

ocher (OH·kur)—a hydrated iron oxide mixture; a dark yellow color derived from or resembling ocher; yellow ocher.

ocular (AHK·yuh·lur)—pertaining to the eye; the eyepiece of a microscope; the lens at the upper end of the microscope.

oculist (AHK·yuh·list)—a specialist in diseases of the eye.

oculofacial (ahk·yuh·loh·FAY·shul)—pertaining to the eyes and face.

oculomotor (ahk·yuh·loh·MOHT·ur)—pertaining to movement of the eyeball.

oculomotor nerve (ahk·yuh·loh·MOHT·ur NURV)—third cranial nerve that controls the motion of the eye.

oculus (AHK·yoo·lus); pl., **oculi** (AHK·yoo·lye)—the eye.

odontic (oh·DAHN·tik)—pertaining to the teeth.

odor (OH·dur)—scent; the property of a substance that causes it to be perceptible to the sense of smell.

odorless (OH·dur·les)—having no odor.

off base (AWF BAYS)—in hairstyling, the position of a curl or a roller completely off its base for maximum mobility and minimum volume.

off-color (AWF-KUL·ur)—lacking the correct or acceptable standard of color.

off the scalp lightener (AWF THE SKALP LYT·un·ur)—generally a stronger hair lightener or bleach usually in powder form, not to be used directly on the scalp.

off-white (AWF-WHYT)—not pure white; white that has an undertone of gray or yellow.

ohm (OHM)—a unit for measuring the resistance of an electric current.

Ohm's law (OHMZ LAW)—the simple statement that the strength of a current in an electric circuit is equal to the electromotive force divided by the resistance.

oil (OYL)—a greasy liquid of vegetable, anima,l or mineral origin, soluble in alcohol and ether, but not in water; used in foods, cosmetics, and many other products.

oil bleach (OYL BLEECH)—a combination of sulphonated oil, ammonia water, and hydrogen peroxide.

oiled silk (OYLD SILK)—silk material treated with oil; used to protect those parts of a man's hair piece where adhesive is placed.

oil gland (OYL GLAND)—an oil-secreting gland; the sebaceous gland.

oily hair (OYL·ee HAYR)—hair that has an excessive amount of oil due to overactivity of the sebaceous glands.

oily hair shampoo (OYL·ee HAYR sham·POO)—a preparation formulated for cleansing excessive oil from the hair and scalp.

oily skin (OYL·ee SKIN)—skin that is excessively oily due to the overactivity of the sebaceous glands.

ointment (OYNT·ment)—a medicated mixture applied externally; a preparation for the skin or scalp.

ol (AWL)—a word termination denoting that the name of the substance to which the termination is added belongs to the series of alcohols or hydroxyl derivatives, such as glycerol.

oleaginous (oh·lee·AJ·un·us)—oily; greasy.

oleic acid (oh·LEE·ik AS·ud)—an oily acid used in soaps, shampoos, and some ointments.

oleum (OH·lee·um); pl., **olea** (OH·lee·uh)—oil.

olfaction (ahl·FAK·shun)—the sense of smell; the act or process of smelling.

olfactory (ahl·FAK·tuh·ree)—relating to the sense of smell; first cranial nerve; the special nerve of smell.

olfactory glands (ahl·FAK·tuh·ree GLANDZ)—serous glands found in the mucous membranes of the nose.

olfactory nerve (ahl·FAK·tuh·ree NURV)—the first cranial nerve; sensory nerve fibers of the mucous membrane of the nose.

olfactory organ (ahl·FAK·tuh·ree OR·gan)—the sense organ located in the nasal cavity responsible for the ability to detect pleasant or unpleasant odors.

oligocythemia (ahl·ih·goh·sy·THEEM·ee·uh)—a deficiency of red corpuscles.

oligotrichia (ahl·ih·goh·TRIK·ee·uh)—scantiness or thinness of hair.

olive (AHL·iv)—a small oily fruit from which a rich oil is obtained.

olive green (AHL·iv GREEN)—a yellow-green color resembling that of the green olive.

olive oil (AHL·iv OYL)—a light-yellow oil pressed from olives; used in some foods and in some cosmetic preparations.

oma (OH·muh)—a word termination properly added to words derived from Greek roots, denoting a tumor, such as cystoma.

on base curl (AWN BAYS KURL)—a curl placed directly on its base.

oncogenic (ahng·koh·JEN·ik)—tending to cause tumors; relating to tumor formation.

one application process (WUN ap·lih·KAY·shun PRAH·ses)—a hair coloring process that decolorizes and colors in a single application.

on the scalp lightener (AWN THE SKALP LYT·un·ur)—a liquid, cream, or gel form of lightener (bleach) that can be used directly on the scalp.

onych (AHN·ik)—prefix from the Greek word *onyx* meaning nail; the first syllable of many names for diseases and conditions affecting the nails.

onychatrophia (ahn·ih·kuh·TROH·fee·uh)—atrophy of the nails.

onychauxis (ahn·ih·KAHK·sis)—enlargement of the nails.

onychia (uh·NIK·ee·uh)—inflammation of the matrix of the nail with formation of pus and shedding of the nail.

onychitis (uh·nih·KY·tis)—inflammation of the area around the nails.

onycho (AHH·in·kuh)—a prefix meaning relating to the nails.

onychoclasis (ahn·ih·KAHK·lah·sis)—breaking of a nail.

onychocryptosis (ahn·ih·koh·krip·TOH·sis)—ingrowing nail.

onychogryposis (ahn·ih·koh·gry·POH·sis)—thickening and curvature of the nail.

onychohelcosis (ahn·ih·koh·hel·KOH·sis)—ulceration of a nail.

onycholysis (ahn·ih·KAHL·ih·sis)—loosening of the nail without shedding.

onychomadesis (ahn·ih·koh·muh·DEE·sis)—separation and falling off of a nail from the nailbed.

onychomycosis (ahn·ih·koh·my·KOH·sis)—disease of the nails due to fungi.

onychopathy (ahn·ih·KAHP·uh·thee)—any disease of the nails.

onychophagia (ahn·ih·koh·FAY·jee·uh)—the habit of biting the fingernails.

onychophosis (ahn·ih·kahf·OH·sis)—growth of horny epithelium in the nailbed.

onychophyma (ahn·ih·koh·FY·muh)—enlarged or thickened swelling of the nails.

onychoptosis (ahn·ih·kahp·TOH·sis)—periodic shedding of one or more nails; in whole or in part.

onychorrhexis (ahn·ih·koh·REK·sis)—abnormal brittleness with striation of the nail plate; fissures may or may not be present.

onychorrhiza (ahn·ih·koy·RY·zuh)—the root of the nail.

onychosis, onychonosus (ahn·ih·KOH·sis, ahn·ih·koh·NOH·sus)—any deformity or disease of the nails.

onychostroma (ahn·ih·koh·STROH·muh)—the matrix of the nail.

onychotrophy (ahn·ih·KAHT·ruh·fee)—nourishment of the nails.

onyx (AHN·iks)—a nail of the fingers or toes.

onyxis (AHN·ik·sis)—ingrowing toenail.

onyxitis (ahn·ik·SY·tis)—inflammation of the nail matrix.

ooze (OOZ)—to flow or leak out slowly; to gradually seep or trickle moisture.

opaque (oh·PAYK)—impervious to light rays; neither transparent nor translucent.

open end (OH·pen END)—the concave, indented end of a wave or shaping.

open mesh net (OH·pen MESH NET)—a wig net with large openings between the threads.

operator (AHP·ur·ay·tur)—one who is able to perform correctly any service rendered professionally in the care of the face, hair, etc.; term sometimes used to describe a cosmetologist.

ophthalmic (ahf·THAL·mik)—pertaining to the eye.

ophthalmic artery (ahf·THAL·mik ART·uh·ree)—the main branch of the carotid artery supplying the eye and nearby structures.

ophthalmic nerve (ahf·THAL·mik NURV)—a sensory nerve that innervates the skin of the forehead, the upper eyelids, and interior portion of the scalp, orbit, eyeball, and nasal passage.

ophthalmitis (ahf·thal·MY·tis)—inflammation of the eye.

ophthalmology (ahf·thal·MAHL·uh·jee)—the science dealing with the structure, functions, and diseases of the eye.

ophthalmoplasty (ahf·THAL·moh·plas·tee)—plastic surgery of the eye or its parts.

opponent muscles (uh·POH·nent MUS·ulz)—muscles in the palm that act to bring thumb toward the fingers.

optic (AHP·tik)—pertaining to the eye or to vision.

optical illusion (AHP·tih·kul ih·LOO·zhun)—an image that appears different from what actually exists.

optician (ahp·TISH·un)—one who makes eyeglasses.

optic nerve (AHP·tik NURV)—the second cranial nerve; the nerve of sight that conducts impulses from the retina of the eye to the brain.

optional (AHP·shun·ul)—left to one's discretion or choice; not compulsory.

optometrist (ahp·TAHM·uh·trist)—a person who examines eyes and fits or prescribes glasses to correct visual defects.

oral (OR·ul)—pertaining to the mouth.

orange (OR·enj)—a round, juicy fruit of the citrus family; a reddish-yellow color produced by mixing equal parts of the primary colors, red and yellow.

orange oil (OR·enj OYL)—a deep orange colored liquid from the fresh peel of a ripe orange; used in soaps and perfumery.

orangewood stick (OR·enj·wood STIK)—a stick made from the wood of the orange tree; used in manicuring procedures.

orbicular (or·BIK·yuh·lur)—circular; a term applied to a muscle whose fibers are circularly arranged.

orbicularis oculi (or·bik·yuh·LAIR·is AHK·yuh·lye)—orbicularis palpebrarum; the ring muscle of the eye.

orbicularis oris (or·bik·yuh·LAIR·is OH·ris)—orbicular muscle; muscle of the mouth.

orbicularis palpebrarum (or·bik·yuh·LAIR·is pal·puh·BRAIR·um)—a muscle of the face that closes the eyes.

orbit (OR·bit)—the bony cavity of the eyeball; the eye-socket.

orbital (OR·bih·tul)—pertaining to the orbits.

orchid (OR·kud)—a distinctive flower of temperate regions from which essences for perfumes are derived; orchid color, a delicate light rosy purple.

organ (OR·gun)—in plants and animals, a structure composed of specialized tissues and performing specific functions.

organic (or·GAN·ik)—relating to an organ; pertaining to substances having carbon-to-carbon bonds.

organic chemistry (or·GAN·ik KEM·is·tree)—chemistry of carbon-based compounds.

organic compound (or·GAN·ik KAHM·pownd)—a compound containing carbon exclusive of salts and carbonic acid.

organic cosmetics (or·GAN·ik kahz·MET·iks)—cosmetics made from animal or vegetable products.

organism (OR·gah·niz·um)—any animal or plant with organs that function to maintain life.

oriental blends (or·ee·EN·tul BLENDZ)—a basic perfume type usually including amber, musk, civet oils, and special spices.

Oriental hair (or·ee·EN·tul HAYR)—hair from Asian countries; used in the manufacture of wigs and hair pieces.

orifice (OR·uh·fus)—an opening; a mouth.

origin (OR·ih·jin)—the beginning; the starting point of a nerve; the place of attachment of a muscle to a bone.

original (uh·RIJ·ih·nul)—something that is new, different and creative.

originate (uh·RIJ·ih·nayt)—to produce as new; to create.

ornament (ORN·uh·ment)—in hairdressing, a ribbon, comb, pin, or other accessory added to the finished hairstyle.

orris root (OR·is ROOT)—a special powder used to give a dry shampoo.

orthopedics (or·thuh·PEED·iks)—the branch of surgery that deals with prevention and correction of problems of the skeletal system.

os (AHS)—a bone.

oscillate (AHS·ul·ayt)—to swing back and forth like a pendulum; to vibrate.

oscillation (ahs·uh·LAY·shun)—movement like a pendulum; a swinging or vibration.

oscillator (AHS·uh·layt·ur)—an apparatus that produces vibrating movements used in massage.

osis (OH·sis)—a word termination denoting an abnormal or a diseased condition.

os magnum (AHS MAG·num)—bone in the lower row of the carpus.

osmidrosis (ahz·mih·DROH·sis)—bromidrosis; foul-smelling perspiration.

osmosis (ahz·MOH·sis)—the diffusion of a fluid or solution through a semipermeable membrane; especially the passage of a solvent through a membrane from a dilute solution into a more concentrated one.

osseous; osseus (AHS·ee·us)—bony.

osteoarthritis (ahs·tee·oh·arth·RY·tis)—age-related arthritis; affects joints that have experienced wear and tear or trauma; results in bone thickening and progressive joint immobilization.

osteodermia (ahs·tee·oh·DUR·mee·uh)—a condition characterized by bony formations in the skin.

osteology (ahs·tee·AHL·uh·jee)—science of the anatomy, structure, and function of bones.

osteoporosis (ahs·tee·oh·puh·ROH·sis)—a thinning of bones, leaving them fragile and prone to fractures.

otoplasty (AH·toh·plas·tee)—plastic surgery of the external ear.

ounce (OWNS)—a unit of measure of weight; one sixteenth of a pound.

outcrop (OWT·krahp)—in cosmetology, a new growth of hair.

outer ear (OW·tur EER)—the flared outer portion of the ear.

outer perimeter (OW·tur puh·RIM·ih·tur)—in cosmetology, the outer area of the hair length.

outgrowth (OWT·grohth)—*see* new growth.

outline (OWT·lyn)—the line that defines a shape; the boundary of a figure or a body; the defining of the eyes or lips by use of a cosmetic pencil.

outmoded (owt·MOH·dud)—outdated; no longer in fashion.

outside curve (OWT·syd KURV)—the convex, curving outward curve in which hair may be cut.

outside design line (OWT·syd dee·ZYN LYN)—the nape and face framing design of a hairstyle.

outside movement (OWT·syd MOOV·ment)—the volume, height, or mass of hair that creates the outer silhouette of the hairstyle.

oval (OH·vul)—egg-shaped; shaped like an ellipse; something having an oval shape; oval facial type.

oval design (OH·vul DE·zyn)—a hair design shaped like an ellipse; a hair design having an oval shape.

overdirected (oh·var·dih·REK·tud)—in excess of the normal amount of direction.

overgrowth (OH·vur·grohth)—excessive or abnormal growth.

overhydration (oh·vur·hy·DRAY·shun)—the presence of excess fluids in the tissues of the body.

overlap (oh·vur·LAP)—to extend over and cover a part of something; when color or lightener is allowed to run onto the previously tinted or lightened hair during application.

overlapping (oh·vur·LAP·ing)—in cosmetology, applying a chemical solution, such as tint or lightener, beyond the limits of the new growth of hair.

overlapping curl (oh·vur·LAP·ing KURL)—a pincurl that partially covers its adjacent curl.

overload principle (OH·vur·lohd PRIN·sih·pul)—training where stresses to the body are greater than what the body is accustomed to.

overporosity (oh·vur·puh·RAHS·ih·tee)—excessive ability of the hair to absorb moisture; undesirable stage of porosity requiring correction.

overprocessing (oh·vur·PRAH·ses·ing)—overexposure of the hair to the chemical action of the wave solution, usually resulting in weakened or damaged hair.

ovular (AHV·yuh·lur)—egglike in shape; pertaining to the ovum, or egg.

o/w—abbreviation for oil in water.

oxidation (ahk·sih·DAY·shun)—the act of combining or causing an element or compound to combine with oxygen; the loss of an electron in a chemical reaction; in hair coloring, the reaction of dye intermediates with hydrogen peroxide found in hair coloring developers; or the interaction of hydrogen peroxide on the natural pigment.

oxidation dye (ahk·sih·DAY·shun DYE)—aniline derivative dye; hair tint. (*See* dye intermediate.)

oxidation-reduction reactions (ahk·sih·DAY·shun-ree·DUK·shun ree·AK·shuns)—among the most common types of chemical reactions, prevalent in all areas of chemistry.

oxidative hair color (ahk·sih·DAY·tiv HAYR KUL·ur)—a product containing oxidation dyes that require hydrogen peroxide to develop the permanent color.

oxide (AHK·syd)—a compound of oxygen with another element or radical.

oxidize (AHK·sih·dyz)—to combine or to cause an element or radical to combine with oxygen.

oxidizing agent (AHK·sih·dyz·ing AY·jent)—a substance that releases oxygen, causing a chemical reaction; an example in hydrogen peroxide.

oxygen (AHK·sih·jin)—a gaseous element, essential to animal and plant life.

oxygenation (ahk·sih·juh·NAY·shun)—saturation with oxygen; to combine a substance with oxygen; the aeration of the blood with oxygen.

oxygen debt (AHK·sih·jin DET)—an accumulation of lactic acid after strenuous activity.

oxyhemoglobin (ahk·sih·HEE·muh·gloh·bin)—the combination of hemoglobin with oxygen.

oxymelanin (ahk·sih·MEL·uh·nin)—a compound formed by a combination of an oxidizing agent with the dark melanin (color) pigments in the hair; generally found in the red to yellow shades.

oz—symbol for ounce.

ozone (OH·zohn)—a pale blue gas that is another form of oxygen; used as a deodorizing and bleaching agent; a form of oxygen used as a disinfectant.

ozone spray (OH·zohn SPRAY)—a fine mist produced by the combination of ozone and water.

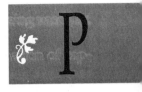

pack (PAK)—a special cosmetic formula used to benefit the skin. (*See* mask.)

packet (PAK·it)—a small package used for samples of skin and hair care products.

packing (PAK·ing)—heavy back combing, matted at the scalp and extended along the hair strand, giving the strand of hair almost a rigid quality.

pad (PAD)—a small, soft cushionlike item, usually of cotton or sponge; used to apply makeup, to remove nail polish, etc.

pageboy style (PAYJ·boy STYL)—a hairstyle in which the ends of the hair are turned under.

pain (PAYN)—a body sensation that warns of tissue damage.

pain receptors (PAYN ree·SEP·turz)—sensory nerve fibers that respond to pain-causing stimuli.

painting (PAYNT·ing)—a technique in hair coloring in which the hair is darkened or lightened in thin strands with a brush.

palate (PAL·ut)—the roof of the mouth and the floor of the nose.

palatine (PAL·uh·tyn)—referring to the roof of the mouth or palate.

palatine bones (PAL·uh·tyn BOHNZ)—bones form the floor and outer wall of the nose, roof of the mouth, and floor of the orbits.

pale (PAYL)—deficient in color; light shade of any color; lacking brightness.

palette (PAL·it)—a thin board with a hole for the thumb upon which the artist places an assortment of paint colors; the selection of colors for an individual.

palid (PAL·id)—weak and lacking color.

pallor (PAL·ur)—paleness; deficiency of color, especially of the face.

palm (PAHM)—the inner surface of the hand between the wrist and base of the fingers.

palmar (PAHL·mur)—of or pertaining to the palm or hollow of the hand.

palmar arch (PAHL·mur ARCH)—the branches of arteries in the palm that supply blood to the bones, joints, muscles, and skin of the palm of the hand and fingers.

palmar friction (PAHL·mur FRIK·shun)—a massage movement using the palm of the hand to apply pressure and a rubbing movement over underlying structures.

palmar kneading (PAHL·mur NEED·ing)—a massage movement in which the flesh is grasped with palms and fingers, squeezed, and released.

palmar manus (PAHL·mur MAN·us)—the palm of the hand.

palmar rotation (PAHL·mur roh·TAY·shun)—a massage movement in which the palms are moved in a circle over underlying tissues.

palmar stroking (PAHL·mur STROHK·ing)—a massage movement in which the palms are used to stroke large areas of the skin; also called effleurage.

palm oil (PAHM OYL)—palm butter; oil obtained from the fruit and seeds of the palm tree; used in soaps and lubricants.

palpebra (pal·PEE·bruh); pl., **palpebrae** (pal·PEE·bree)—the eyelid or eyelids.

palpebral artery (PAL·puh·brul ART·uh·ree)—the lateral artery that supplies blood to the upper and lower eyelids.

palpebral nerve, inferior (PAL·puh·brul NURV, in·FEER·ee·or)— nerve that receives stimuli from the lower eyelid.

palpebral nerve, superior (PAL·puh·brul NURV, soo·PEER·ee·or)— nerve that receives stimuli from the upper eyelid.

palpebrarum (pal·puh·BRAY·rum)—of or pertaining to the eyelids.

panacea (pan·uh·SEE·uh)—a remedy that is claimed to be curative for all diseases; a universal remedy; a cure-all.

pancreas (PANG·kree·us)—a gland located in the abdomen that secretes an enzyme that digests proteins, fats, carbohydrates, and the hormone insulin.

panel (PAN·ul)—in hairdressing, the area between two parallel partings.

panhidrosis (pah·hy·DROH·sis)—generalized perspiration.

papain (puh·PAY·in)—enzyme from the juice of papaya; used as a digestant and in some facial preparations.

papaya (puh·PY·uh)—a fruit from the carico papaya tree from which papain is extracted; used in skin care preparations.

paper curl (PAY·pur KURL)—a curl rolled up on a stick, encased in a triangle of special paper and pressed with a warm iron.

paper curling (PAY·pur KURL·ing)—producing curls by dividing hair into strands that are formed into flat circle curls, covered with folded paper, and heated by a pressing iron.

papilla (puh·PIL·uh); pl., papillae (puh·PIL·ee)—a small cone-shaped projecting body part.

papilla, hair (puh·PIL·uh, HAYR)—a small, cone-shaped elevation at the bottom of the hair follicle in the dermis.

papillary (PAP·uh·lair·ee)—relating to, resembling, or provided with papillae.

papillary layer (PAP·uh·lair·ee LAY·ur)—the outer layer of the dermis.

papilloma (pap·uh·LOH·muh); pl., **papillomata** (pap·uh·LOH·muh·tuh)—an epithelial tumor formed by hypertrophy of the papillae of the skin.

papular (PAP·yuh·lur)—characterized by papules.

papule (PAP·yool)—a pimple; a small circumscribed elevation on the skin containing no fluid.

papulosis (pap·yuh·LOH·sis)—a condition involving multiple papules.

papulous (PAP·yuh·lus)—covered with papulae or pimples.

para (PAYR·uh)—a prefix denoting alongside of; beyond; beside; against or near. (*See* paraphenylenediamine.)

parabens (PAYR·uh·beenz)—parabens (methyl-, propyl-, and parahydroxybenzoate) are preservatives that are the most commonly used in cosmetics; they are safe to use, non-poisonous, and nonirritating.

paradye (PAYR·uh·dye)—an aniline derivative hair tint.

paraffin (PAYR·uh·fin)—a white mineral wax consisting of hydrocarbons and extracted from petroleum; used in hair removal products and in some types of facial masks.

paraffin wax mask (PAYR·uh·fin WAKS MASK)—a specially prepared facial mask containing paraffin and other beneficial ingredients.

parallel (PAYR·uh·lel)—extending, as two lines, in the same direction and maintaining a constant distance apart.

paralysis (puh·RAL·ih·sis)—loss of muscle function or of sensation through injury to or disease of the nerves or neurons.

para-phenylene-diamine (payr·uh-FEEN·ih·leen-dye-AM·in)—an aniline derivative used in oxidation dye, most permanent hair colors, often abbreviated at P.P.D.

parasite (PAYR·uh·syt)—a vegetable or animal organism that lives in or on another organism and draws its nourishment from that organism.

parasitic (payr·uh·SIT·ik)—pertaining to parasites.

parasitical (payr·uh·SIT·ih·kul)—pertaining to living organisms that live upon or within some other living being.

parasympathetic nervous system (payr·uh·sim·puh·THET·ik NUR·vus SIS·tum)—functions to conserve energy and reverse action of the sympathetic nervous system.

parathyroid (payr·uh·THY·royd)—an endocrine gland located near the thyroid.

para tint (PAYR·uh TINT)—a tint made from an aniline derivative; oxidation dyes.

para-toluene-diamine (PAYR·uh-TAHL·yoo·en-dye·AM·in)—a variety of aniline derivative dyes commonly used in preparations compounded to provide red and blond tones.

parietal (puh·RY·ut·ul)—pertaining to the wall of a cavity; a bone at the side of the head.

parietal artery (puh·RY·ut·ul ART·uh·ree)—the artery that supplies blood to the side and crown of the head.

paronychia (payr·uh·NIK·ee·uh)—felon; an inflammation of the tissues surrounding the nail.

parotid (puh·RAHT·ud)—near the ear; a gland near the ear.

parsley oil (PARS·lee OYL)—oil obtained from the ripe seeds of the herb of the parsley family; used as a fragrance and a preservative.

part (PART)—a line dividing the hair to the scalp.

part base (PART BAYS)—the part or line in the hair toward which the hair is rolled or curled.

parting silk (PART·ing SILK)—strong, fine (white or flesh-colored) silk; used in wiggery for making drawn-through partings.

passive (PAS·iv)—inactive; inert; acted upon by causes from without.

passive massage (PAS·iv muh·SAHZH)—a massage movement in which the part (hand, foot, finger, toe) is bent up, down, or forward to flex the joints.

pastel (pas·TEL)—a soft, delicate color or tint.

paste on (PAYST AWN)—any item such as a jewel, flower, artificial lash, or nail that can be glued or pasted on the skin, hair, or nails as a decoration.

pat (PAT)—to tap lightly; to apply makeup by pressing lightly to the skin.

patch (PACH)—a blotch; an irregular spot or area.

patch test (PACH TEST)—FDA required test for determining allergy to a specific substance; made by applying a small amount of the substance to the skin and observing the reaction.

pate (PAYT)—top of the head.

patella (puh·TEL·uh)—the kneecap.

pathogenesis (path·uh·JEN·uh·sis)—the origin of and course of development of a disease.

pathogenic (path·uh·JEN·ik)—causing disease; disease-producing.

pathological (path·uh·LAHJ·ih·kul)—relating to pathology; morbid; diseased; due to disease.

pathology (puh·THAHL·uh·jee)—the science that treats modifications of the functions and changes in structure caused by disease.

pattern (PAT·urn)—in hairstyling, a diagram showing where and in which direction hair rollers or pincurls are placed in order to achieve the finished style; a head shape or design from which a hair piece is constructed.

peak (PEEK)—a point formed by the hair growth at the center of the forehead; also called a widow's peak, named after a bonnet styled with a center point at the forehead; worn by widows in the 19th century.

peanut oil (PEE·nut OYL)—arachis oil; oil obtained from the seeds of the peanut; used in many cosmetics such as hair preparations, face creams, shampoos, and emollients.

pear-shaped face (PAYR-SHAYPT FAYS)—a facial structure characterized by a wide jaw and a narrow forehead.

pectin (PEK·tin)—a carbohydrate contained in the cell walls of some fruits and vegetables, such as lemons, apples, and carrots, and used as the basis of gels; a substance used in facial masks.

pectoralis (pek·tor·AL·is)—a muscle of the chest.

pectoralis major (pek·tor·AL·is MAY·jor)—the muscle that flexes and rotates the arm forward and inward.

pectoralis minor (pek·tor·AL·is MY·nur)—the muscle that draws the shoulder forward and rotates the scapula (shoulder blade) downward.

pectoral nerve (PEK·tuh·rul NURV)—lateral pectoral nerve; the nerve that stimulates the pectoralis major and minor.

pedi (PED·ee)—pertaining to the feet.

pedicare (PED·ih·kayr)—care of the feet.

pediculosis (puh·dik·yuh·LOH·sis)—a skin disease caused by infestation of lice.

pediculosis capitis (puh·dik·yuh·LOH·sis KAP·ih·tus)—infestation of the hair of the head with lice.

pediculous (puh·DIK·yuh·lus)—infested by pediculi; lousy.

pedicure (PED·ih·kyoor)—the care of the feet and toenails.

peel (PEEL)—a technique in facial treatments in which a product is applied to the face to remove dead cells from the surface of the skin.

peeling treatment (PEEL·ing TREET·ment)—a facial treatment using a chemical agent to remove the surface layer of skin, the epidermis, to eliminate lines and acne scars.

pelada (puh·LAH·duh)—a disease of the hair causing circumscribed patches of baldness; alopecia areata.

pelage (PEL·ij)—the hair covering of the body of humans and animals.

pellagra (puh·LAG·ruh)—a syndrome due to niacin deficiency; characterized by dermatitis, and in later stages, by nervous and mental disorders.

pencil sharpener (PEN·sil SHARP·un·ur)—a tool designed to sharpen writing pencils or makeup pencils.

pencils, makeup (PEN·silz, MAYK·up)—pencils manufactured with a wide assortment of colored leads; used for making up the eyes, lips, and for facial contouring.

penetrate (PEN·uh·trayt)—to pass into or through; to enter by overcoming resistance.

penetrating tint (PEN·uh·trayt·ing TINT)—a hair color that enters or penetrates into the cortex and deposits color.

penetration (pen·uh·TRAY·shun)—act or power of penetrating.

pep bag (PEP BAG)—a trade term that designates a product that speeds up the action of a lightener and hydrogen peroxide.

peppermint oil (PEP·ur·mint OYL)—an aromatic plant of the mint family whose leaves produce an oil used in flavorings, toothpaste, mouthwashes, and various lotions.

pepsin (PEP·sin)—an enzyme that digests protein.

peptide (PEP·tyd)—a compound of two or more amino acids containing one or more peptide groups; continuous filaments in the case of fiber protein or keratin.

peptide bond (PEP·tyd BAHND)—the joining together of amino acids.

peptones (PEP·tohnz)—any of various water-soluble products of partial hydrolysis of proteins.

per (PUR)—a prefix denoting through; throughout; by; for.

percussion (pur·KUSH·un)—a form of massage consisting of repeated light blows or taps of varying force.

perforate (PUR·fuh·rayt)—to pierce with holes.

perfume (PUR·fyoom)—a fragrant substance, usually a volatile liquid, which emits a pleasant odor or scent.

peri (PAYR·ih)—a prefix denoting about; near; around.

pericardium (payr·ih·KAR·dee·um)—the membranous sac around the heart.

perimeter (puh·RIM·ih·tur)—the outer line of a hairstyle, the silhouette line.

perimysium (payr·ih·MIS·ee·um)—the sheath that encases bundles of muscle fibers.

perionychium (payr·ee·uh·NIK·ee·um)—the epidermis surrounding a nail.

periosteum (payr·ee·AHS·tee·um)—the fibrous membrane covering the surface of the bones.

peripheral nervous system (puh·RIF·uh·rul NUR·vus SIS·tum)—system of nerves an ganglia that connect the peripheral parts of the body to the central nervous system; it has both sensory nerves and motor nerves.

periphery (puh·RIF·ur·ee)—the part of the body away from the center; the outer part or surface.

peristalsis (payr·ih·STAWL·sis)—muscular movements of the digestive tract.

periwig (PAYR·ih·wig)—an old-fashioned name for a wig.

perm (PURM)—a permanent wave or a straightening treatment.

permalite (PUR·muh·lyt)—a light for drying the permanent wave after the wave has been set.

permanent (PUR·muh·nent)—lasting; enduring; not changing. (*See* permanent wave.

permanent, cold wave (PUR·muh·nent, KOHLD WAYV)—a system of permanent waving employing chemicals rather than heat.

permanent color (PUR·muh·nent KUL·ur)—permanent tint; a hair color mixed with developer that is enduring and remains in the hair until the new growth of hair.

perm cap (PURM KAP)—a plastic head covering used during the processing time of a permanent wave to help speed up the action of the product being used.

permeable (PUR·mee·uh·bul)—permitting the passage of liquids.

perm rod (PURM RAHD)—a cylindrical or concave rod used for winding the hair for permanent waves.

peroneal brevis (payr·uh·NEE·ul BREH·vis)—muscle that allows the foot to be flexed downward and outward.

peroneal longus (payr·uh·NEE·ul LAWNG·gus)—muscle that flexes the foot and supports the arches.

peroneal muscle (payr·uh·NEE·ul MUS·ul)—muscle located on the outer portion of the lower leg that assists in turning the foot downward and outward.

peroneal nerve (payr·uh·NEE·ul NURV)—nerve that receives stimuli from the skin of the lateral aspect of the leg.

peroxide (pur·AHK·syd)—common term for hydrogen peroxide. (*See* hydrogen peroxide.

peroxide residue (pur·AHK·syd RES·ih·doo)—traces of peroxide left in the hair after treatment with lightener or tint.

peroxometer (pur·ahks·AHM·ih·tur)—a device that measures the strength of hydrogen peroxide.

perpendicular (pur·pen·DIK·yuh·lur)—being perfectly upright; being at right angles to a given line on a plane.

personality (pur·sun·AL·ih·tee)—the distinctive characteristics or qualities of a person.

perspiration (pur·spih·RAY·shun)—sweat; the fluid excreted from the sudoriferous glands of the skin.

perspire (pur·SPYR)—to emit perspiration from the pores of the skin; to sweat.

persulfate (pur·SUL·fayt)—in hair coloring, a chemical ingredient commonly used in activators; it increases the speed of the decolorizing process. (*See* activator.)

peruke (puh·ROOK)—a wig popular from the 17th-19th century.

peruquer; perukier (pur·OOK·ur)—a wig maker.

petrissage (PEH·treh·sahzh)—the kneading movement in massage.

petrolatum (peh·truh·LAYT·um)—petroleum jelly; a purified, yellow mixture of semisolid hydrocarbons obtained from petroleum.

petroleum (peh·TROH·lee·um)—an oily liquid coming from the earth and consisting of a mixture of hydrocarbons.

pH—symbol of hydronium-ion concentration in water; the relative degree of acidity or alkalinity; pH values are arranged on a scale from 1 to 14; above 7, represents alkalinity, below 7, represents acidity. A pH of 7 is neutral.

phalanx (FAY·langks); pl., **phalanges** (fuh·LAN·jeez)—one of the bones of the fingers or toes.

pharmacologist (far·muh·KAHL·uh·jist)—one versed in the science of the nature and properties of drugs.

pharynx (FAYR·inks)—the upper portion of the digestive tube, behind the nose and mouth.

phenol (FEE·nohl)—carbolic acid; caustic poison; in dilute solution is used as an antiseptic and disinfectant.

pheomelanin (fee·oh·MEL·uh·nin)—naturally occurring red/yellow pigment.

phlebitis (fluh·BYT·us)—inflammation of a vein.

pH number (PEE·AYCH NUM·bur)—also pH factor a measure of the degree of acidity or alkalinity of a solution.

phoresis (fuh·REE·sis)—a combining form meaning transmission; the process of introducing solutions into tissues through the skin by use of galvanic current.

phosphoric (fahs·FOR·ik)—pertaining to or derived from phosphorus.

phosphorous (FAHS·for·us)—an element found in the bones, muscles, and nerves; a mineral element required in the diet of humans.

photodermatitis (foh·toh·dur·muh·TY·tis)—a skin condition caused by exposure to light, cosmetics, drugs, or irritants.

photooxidative effect (foh·toh·ahk·sih·DAY·tiv ee·FEKT)—damage or chemical changes caused by sunlight.

pH paper (PEE·AYCH PAY·pur)—a special type of paper used to test the pH factor in a product; the paper changes color according to the degree of acidity or alkalinity, thus indicating its pH factor.

pH pencil (PEE·AYCH PEN·sil)—a pencil used to indicate the degree of acidity or alkalinity of a solution or product.

pH scale (PEE·AYCH SKAYL)—scale numbered from 0 to 14; used to indicate the degree of acidity or alkalinity of a solution; 7.0 indicates neutral, below 7 indicates acid and above 7 indicates alkaline.

phyma (FY·muh); pl., **phymata** (FY·muh·tuh)—a circumscribed swelling on the skin, larger than a tubercle.

physi; physio (FIZ·ee; FIZ·ee·oh)—combining form indicating relationship to nature.

physical (FIZ·ih·kul)—relating to the body, as distinguished from the mind.

physical change (FIZ·ih·kul CHAYNJ)—altering or changing the form or appearance of a substance without changing its chemical composition.

physics (FIZ·iks)—the branch of science that deals with matter, energy, motion, light, heat, electricity, sound, mechanics, and their interactions.

physiognomical haircutting (fiz·ee·uh·NAHM·ih·kul HAYR·kut·ing)—cutting and styling hair in accordance with the facial features of the client.

physiognomy (fiz·ee·AHG·nuh·mee)—the physical appearance of a person; especially his or her facial features thought to reveal certain traits or characteristics.

physiological (fiz·ee·uh·LAHJ·ih·kul)—of or relating to the functions of an organism and its parts during life.

physiology (fiz·ee·AHL·uh·jee)—the science of the function of living things and their parts.

physiotherapy (fiz·ee·oh·THAIR·uh·pee)—the use of physical means, such as light, heat, air, water, and exercise, in the treatment of diseases and injuries.

phytotherapy (fy·toh·THAIR·uh·pee)—treatment by use of plants; herbal therapy.

picealis (pis·eh·AH·lis)—a type of acne caused by an allergy to tar products.

picric acid (PIK·rik AS·ud)—an organic acid used as an antiseptic.

pie shape (PY SHAYP)—the triangular shape of the subsections used when setting hair with conoid rollers, and for curls when it is necessary to avoid splits in the finished style.

piggyback (PIG·ee·bak)—the double-rod method used in perming long hair; two rods are used for a strand of hair.

pigment (PIG·ment)—any organic coloring matter; as that of the red blood cells, of the hair, skin, iris, etc. Any substance or matter used as coloring; natural or artificial hair color.

pigmentary (PIG·men·tair·ee)—pertaining to producing or containing pigment.

pigmentation (pig·men·TAY·shun)—the deposition of pigment in the skin or tissues.

pileous (PY·lee·us)—pertaining to hair; hairy.

pili; pilar (PY·leh; PIH·lur)—hair; related to hair.

piliation (pih·lee·AY·shun)—the formation and production of hair.

pili incarnati (PY·leh in·kar·NAY·tye)—ingrown hairs.

pili multigemini (PY·leh mul·tih·JEM·ih·nye)—several hairs growing from a single follicle opening.

pili tactiles (PY·leh TAK·tih·leez)—tactile hairs; associated with the sense of touch.

pili torti (PY·leh TOR·tye)—a congenital deformity of the hair, characterized by short, broken hairs that resemble stubble.

pilocarpine (py·luh·KAR·peen)—an alkaloid obtained from the leaves of pilocarpus; a syrupy liquid; stimulates the tissues and increases secretion of the glands.

piloerection (py·luh·ih·REK·shun)—the condition known as gooseflesh, characterized by erection of hair and a bump around the follicle.

pilomotor (py·luh·MOH·tur)—causing movement of the hair; as the pilomotor muscles.

pilomotor muscle (py·luh·MOH·tur MUS·ul)—the arrector pili muscle.

pilomotor nerve (py·luh·MOH·tur NURV)—a nerve causing contraction of one of the arrectores pilorum muscles.

pilomotor reflex (py·luh·MOH·tur REE·fleks)—erection of hairs of the skin (gooseflesh) as a response to cold or emotional stimuli.

pilonidal (py·luh·NY·dul)—pertaining to hair growing within a cyst.

pilose (PY·lohs)—covered with hair; hairy.

pilosebaceous (py·luh·seh·BAY·shus)—pertaining to the hair follicles and the sebaceous glands.

pilosis (py·LOH·sis)—abnormal or excessive development of hair.

pilosity (py·LAHS·ih·tee)—the state of being pilose or hairy.

pilous gland (PY·lus GLAND)—the sebaceous gland of a hair follicle.

pilus (PY·lus); pl., **pili** (PY·lye)—a hair.

pilus cuniculatus (PY·lus kuh·nik·yuh·LAY·tus)—a burrowing hair.

pilus incarnatus (PY·lus in·kar·NAY·tus)—ingrown hair.

pilus incarnatus recurvus (PY·lus in·kar·NAY·tus ree·KUR·vus)—caused by a curved hair re-entering the skin; ingrown hair.

pimple (PIM·pul)—any small, pointed elevation of the skin; a papule or small pustule.

pin (PIN)—a small curved device designed to hold the hair in place; bobpins; hairpins.

pincurl (PIN·kurl)—a strand of hair combed smooth and wound into a circle with the ends on the inside of the curl; a flat curl.

pincurl base (PIN·kurl BAYS)—the area of the scalp where a pincurl is secured; the base may be sectioned into a square, a slanted oblong, or an arc or C-shaped base.

pincurl direction (PIN·kurl dih·REK·shun)—the line in which a pincurl is moved or designed to move.

pincurl foundation (PIN·kurl fown·DAY·shun)—the area at the scalp where the pincurl is secured; pincurl base.

pincurling (PIN·kurl·ing)—the forming of circles or ringlets by winding the hair and fastening the circles in place with clips.

pincurl permanent wave (PIN·kurl PUR·muh·nent WAYV)—a cold wave achieved by setting the hair in pincurls instead of rollers.

pincurl stem (PIN·kurl STEM)—the part of the pincurl between the base and the first arc of the circle of hair.

pincurl wave (PIN·kurl WAYV)—the technique of alternating the direction of the rows of pincurls to form a wave when the hair is combed.

pineal body (PY·nee·ul BAHD·ee)—a ductless gland attached to the brain.

pine tar (PYN TAR)—tar obtained from the wood of the palm tree; used in soaps, shampoos, and medications for skin ailments.

pink (PINGK)—a pale hue of crimson.

pinkeye (PINGK·eye)—an acute, highly contagious conjunctivitis marked by redness of the eyeball.

pinna (PIN·uh)—the external ear, exclusive of meatus.

pint (PYNT)—a liquid or dry measure, equal to half a quart.

pipette (py·PET)—a slender tube used for measuring liquids.

pisiform (PY·suh·form)—pea-shaped; a bone of the wrist.

pit (PIT)—a surface depression or hollow.

pith (PITH)—center; the marrow of the bones; the center of the hair.

pit scar (PIT SKAR)—a scar that heals with a hollow pit; usually caused by acne.

pituitary (puh·TOO·uh·tair·ee)—a ductless gland located at the base of the brain.

pityriasis (pit·ih·RY·uh·sus)—dandruff; an inflammation of the skin characterized by the formation and flaking of fine, thin scales.

pityriasis capitis simplex (pit·ih·RY·uh·sus KAP·ih·tis SIM·pleks)— a scalp inflammation marked by dry dandruff or thin scales.

pityriasis pilaris (pit·ih·RY·uh·sus py·LAYR·is)—a skin disorder characterized by an eruption of papules surrounding the hair follicles: each papule pierced by a hair and tipped with a horny plug or scale.

pityriasis steatoides (pit·ih·RY·uh·sis stee·uh·TOY·deez)—a scalp inflammation marked by fatty type of dandruff; characterized by yellowish to brownish waxy scales or crusts on the scalp.

pityroid (PIT·ih·royd)—pertaining to a condition of the skin or scalp characterized by thin scales.

pityrosporum ovalli (pit·ih·roh·SPOH·rum oh·VAY·lee)—a species of fungus found on the skin or hair follicle and associated with infectious seborrheic dermatitis.

pivot point (PIV·ut POYNT)—pivot hair shaping; the exact point from which the hair is directed in forming a curvature or shaping.

placental extract (pluh·SEN·tul EK·strakt)—the nourishing substance surrounding an embryo or fetus; after birth; used in some facial preparations.

plait (PLAYT)—to interweave strands of hair into an intricate pattern; to braid.

plankton extract (PLANGK·tun EK·strakt)—the microscopic animal and plant life found in the oceans and in fresh water; algae or seaweed; used in certain cosmetic preparations, usually in facial and body treatment preparations.

planta pedis (PLAN·tuh PEE·dis)—the under-surface or sole of the foot.

plantar (PLANT·ur)—pertaining to the sole of the foot.

plantar arterial arch (PLANT·ur ART·eer·ee·ul ARCH)—the arch in the sole of the foot made by the lateral plantar artery and branch of the dorsalis pedis artery.

plantar flexion (PLANT·ur FLEK·shun)—bending the foot or toes downward toward the sole of the foot.

plantar flexor (PLANT·ur FLEK·sur)—muscle that bends the foot downward.

plantar reflex (PLANT·ur REE·fleks)—flexing of the toes in response to stroking massage movements on the outer sides of the soles.

plant extracts (PLANT EK·strakts)—organic substances extracted from leaves, roots, and flowers of various plants for use in such products as perfumes and grooming aids.

plasma (PLAZ·muh)—the fluid part of the blood an lymph.

plastic applicator (PLAS·tik AP·lih·kay·tur)—a squeeze bottle used for applying tints and lighteners.

plastic cap (PLAS·tik KAP)—a cap made of plastic employed as a head covering to help retain body heat during a number of cosmetology techniques, such as permanent waving and coloring.

plasticizer (PLAS·tih·sy·zur)—a compound that keeps a substance soft and thick, as in nail polishes.

plastic surgeon (PLAS·tik SUR·jun)—a surgeon who builds up or molds tissue and bones to repair physical defects.

plastic surgery (PLAS·tik SUR·jur·ee)—surgical repair of defects or deformities.

platelets (PLAYT·lets)—blood cells that aid in the forming of clots.

platinum (PLAT·ih·num)—a heavy steel-gray metal; the color resembling platinum; a silver-gray.

platinum blond (PLAT·ih·num BLAHND)—very light, almost white blond hair.

platysma (plah·TIZ·muh)—a broad thin muscle of the neck.

pledget (PLEJ·et)—a compress or small, flat mass of absorbent cotton.

plexus (PLEK·sus)—a network of nerves or veins.

pliability (ply·uh·BIL·ut·ee)—flexibility.

pluck (PLUK)—to pull with sudden force.

plume (PLOOM)—a cluster of feathers or hair generally seen in showy headdresses.

plump (PLUMP)—full, rounded; as a plump, full face or figure.

podiatrist (puh·DY·uh·trust)—one who treats diseases of the feet.

point (POYNT)—a sharp end or apex; an abcess, the wall of which becomes thin and is about to break.

point knotting (POYNT NAHT·ing)—a method of attaching hair; in the formation of a hair piece, which ensures that only the points of the hair remain as part of the finished work.

point of distribution (POYNT UV dis·trih·BYOO·shun)—radial motion; the central point from which hair is distributed in a preplanned manner.

point of origin (POYNT UV OR·ih·jen)—in hairdressing, place where a motion starts or the beginning of a design.

points (POYNTS)—wigpoints; headless nails used for attaching the wig foundation to the wooden block in order to ensure a custom fit.

poison (POY·zun)—a substance that when taken internally is injurious to health or dangerous to life.

poisoning, blood (POY·zun·ing BLUD)—septicemia; the invasion of pathogenic bacteria into the blood, causing infection.

poison ivy (POY·zun EYE·vee)—a climbing plant that produces an irritating oil that may cause an intensely itching skin rash.

poisonous (POY·zun·us)—having the quality or effects of poison.

polarity (poh·LAYR·ut·ee)—the property of having two opposite poles, as that possessed by a magnet or galvanic current; the negative and positive state of electric current.

polarity therapy (poh·LAYR·ut·ee THAYR·uh·pee)—therapy using massage, exercises, and thinking practices to balance the body physically and energetically.

pole (POHL)—an electrical terminal.

poliomyelitis (poh·lee·oh·my·uh·LY·tus)—a disease affecting the motor neurons and resulting in paralysis of the related muscle tissue.

poliosis (poh·lee·OH·sus)—a condition characterized by absence of pigment in the hair.

polish (PAHL·ish)—nail enamel formulated to strengthen, protect, and beautify the nails; clear or colored lacquer.

polish dryer (PAHL·ish DRY·ur)—a chemical preparation that speeds the drying process of freshly applied nail polish.

polish remover (PAHL·ish ree·MOOV·ur)—a product that is used to dissolve and remove nail polish.

polish thinner (PAHL·ish THIN·ur)—a chemical preparation formulated to thin nail polish that has become too thick.

pollex (PAHL·eks)—the thumb.

polychromatic (pahl·ee·kroh·MAT·ik)—having many colors.

polyglycerol (pahl·ee·GLIS·ur·awl)—a substance prepared from fats, oils, and esters; derived from vegetables such as corn soy beans and from peanuts, palm, sesame, tallow, and pure lard.

polymer (PAHL·uh·mur)—substance formed by combining many small molecules (monomers) usually in a long chainlike structure; examples are hair, plastic, rubber, and human tissue.

polyp (PAHL·up)—a smooth growth extending from the surface of the skin; polyps may also grow within the body.

polypeptide bonds (pahl·ee·PEP·tyd BAHNDZ)—bonds that link peptide chains together to form protein.

polypeptide chain (pahl·ee·PEP·tyd CHAYN)—amino acid chains joined together by peptide bonds; the prefix "poly" meaning many.

polyunsaturated (pahl·ee·un·SACH·uh·rayt·ud)—pertaining to any of a class of fats having more than two double bonds in its molecule, or to fats used in diets to reduce blood cholesterol.

pomade (poh·MAYD)—a perfumed ointment for the hair or scalp.

pompadour (PAHM·puh·dor)—a hairstyle that is combed up from the forehead; a style using a pad or roller to create a puffed arrangement of the hair above the forehead.

pomphus (PAHM·fus)—a whitish or pinkish elevation of the skin; a wheal.

pons (PAHNZ): also **pons varolii** (PAHNZ vuh·ROH·lee·eye)—a broad band of nerve fibers that connects the cerebrum, cerebellum, and medulla oblongata.

poppy oil (PAHP·ee OYL)—an oil obtained from the seeds of the poppy plant; used as a lubricant and in emulsions.

pore (POR)—a small opening of the sweat glands of the skin.

porosity (puh·RAHS·ut·ee)—ability of the hair to absorb moisture.

porous (PAW·rus)—full of pores.

porous hair (PAW·rus HAYR)—hair that is characterized by lifted cuticle scales that allow faster absorption of moisture or chemicals into the hair.

portable (POR·tuh·bul)—easily carried or moved from one place to another.

portable hair dryer (POR·tuh·bul HAYR DRY·ur)—a compact hair dryer in a case that can be carried from place to place.

positive (PAHZ·ih·tiv)—affirmative; not negative; the presence of abnormal conditions; having a relative high potential in electricity.

positive pole, P or + (PAHZ·ih·tiv POHL)—the pole from which positive electricity flows.

positive skin test (PAHZ·ih·tiv SKIN TEST)—direct proof that the substance involved in a test is hostile to the body; having a reaction to a skin test for allergy; showing signs of redness, swelling, irritation.

positive terminal (PAHZ·ih·tiv TUR·mih·nul)—the end of a conducting circuit manifesting acid reaction; the carbon plate in a battery.

post (POHST)—a prefix denoting back; after.

posterior (poh·STEER·ee·ur)—situated behind; coming after or behind.

posterior auricular artery (poh·STEER·ee·ur aw·RIK·yuh·lur ART·uh·ree)—the artery that supplies blood to the scalp.

posterior auricularis (poh·STEER·ee·ur aw·rik·yuh·LAYR·us)— muscle that draws the ear backward.

posterior auricular nerve (poh·STEER·ee·ur aw·RIK·yuh·lur NURV)—nerve that supplies stimuli to muscles in the posterior surface of the ear.

posterior cerebral artery (poh·STEER·ee·ur suh·REE·brul ART·uh·ree)—artery that supplies blood to the cortex and the temporal and occipital bones.

posterior cutaneous nerve (poh·STEER·ee·ur kyoo·TAY·nee·us NURV)—nerve that stimulates the skin of the posterior aspect of the forearm.

posterior interosseous artery (poh·STEER·ee·ur in·tur·AHS·ee·us ART·uh·ree)—artery that supplies blood to the muscles and skin of the forearm.

posterior tibial artery (poh·STEER·ee·ur TIB·ee·ul ART·ur·ee)—artery that supplies blood to ankles and dorsum of the foot.

postiche (paw·STEESH)—artificial hair piece; curls, braids, or other extra hair piece used in creating coiffures.

posticheur (puh·stesh·OOR)—one who designs and dresses hairpieces.

postnasal (pohst·NAY·zul)—situated behind the nose.

posture (PAHS·choor)—the position of carriage of the body when standing, sitting, walking, or posing.

potassium (puh·TAS·ee·um)—an element, the salts of which are used in medicine; an essential mineral found in vegetables and fruits and necessary to the health of the skin; potassium and sodium regulate the water balance within the body.

potassium bromate (puh·TAS·ee·um BROH·mayt)—a metallic element of the alkali group; used in medicines as a sedative.

potassium carbonate (puh·TAS·ee·um KAR·buh·nayt)—a white salt that forms a highly alkaline solution; used to make soap and other cleansing products.

potassium chloride (puh·TAS·ee·um KLOH·ryd)—a colorless, crystalline salt; used as a buffer in solid perfumes and in some eye washes.

potassium hydroxide (puh·TAS·ee·um hy·DRAHK·syd)—a powerful alkali, used in the manufacture of soft soaps.

potassium permanganate (puh·TAS·ee·um pur·MANG·guh·nayt)—a salt of permanganate acid, used as an antiseptic and deodorant.

potential (poh·TEN·shul)—indicating possibility of power; tension in an electrical source enabling it to do work under suitable conditions.

poultice (POHL·tus)—a soft mass of some substance mixed with water, sometimes medicated; applied to the skin to supply heat and moisture.

powder (POW·dur)—a finely ground substance forming a mass of loose particles; used as a cosmetic and in some medicines.

powder base (POW·dur BAYS)—term sometimes used to describe a foundation cream or lotion that is applied to the face before powder.

powder bleach (POW·dur BLEECH)—a strong fast-acting bleach in powdered form; used for off-the-scalp lightening.

powder dry shampoo (POW·dur DRY sham·POO)—a substance composed of a mixture of orris root, borax, etc., which is employed to clean hair without using soap or water.

powder lightener (POW·dur LYT·un·ur)—*see* powder bleach, off-the-scalp lightener.

powder puff (POW·dur PUF)—a small fluffy circle or square of cotton, sponge, or silk used to apply powder.

prebleaching (pree·BLEECH·ing)—*see* prelightening.

precaution (pree·KAW·shun)—a written or verbal warning with the purpose is to prevent harm and to ensure safety.

precipitate (pree·SIP·ih·tayt)—in chemistry, to cause a substance in a solution to settle in solid particles; to separate from solution or suspension by chemical or physical change.

precipitation (pree·sip·ih·TAY·shun)—in chemistry, the process of separating the constituents of a solution by reagents or by mechanical means; the process of precipitating.

precision (pree·SIZH·un)—the state or quality of being accurate and precise; exactness.

predispose (pree·dis·POHZ)—to make susceptible; to render vulnerable to a disorder or disease.

predisposition (pree·dis·puh·ZISH·un)—a condition of special susceptibility to disease; allergy.

predisposition test (pree·dis·puh·ZISH·un TEST)—*see* patch test.

prelightening (pree·LYT·un·ing)—a decoloring process, preliminary to the application of toner. Generally the first step of double-process hair coloring, used to lift or lighten the natural pigment. (*See* decolorize.)

preliminary (pree·LIM·ih·nayr·ee)—introductory; preparatory.

premature (pree·muh·CHOOR)—happening, arriving, existing, or performed before the usual time.

premature canities (pree·muh·CHOOR kuh·NISH·eez)—premature graying of the hair.

preocrus (PREE·uh·krus)—muscle that covers bridge of nose.

prescribe (pree·SKRYB)—to set or lay down, authoritatively, a course or a rule to be followed.

presenile (pree·SEN·yl)—prematurely old.

presoften (pree·SOF·un)—in hair coloring, the process of treating gray or very resistant hair to allow for better penetration of color.

presoftener (pree·SOF·un·ur)—a chemical solution applied to the hair in order to make easier the penetration of additional chemicals to the hair.

pressing (PRES·ing)—a temporary method of straightening over-curly hair with a heated comb or iron.

pressing irons (PRES·ing EYE·urns)—an implement resembling a curling iron; used to straighten hair.

pressure receptors (PRESH·ur ree·SEP·turz)—nerves supplying the skin that register pressure or touch; nerve fibers that respond to pressure.

prickle cell layer (PRIK·ul SEL LAY·ur)—the layer the cells between the granular cell layer and the basal cell layer of the epidermis.

prickly heat (PRIK·lee HEET)—also called miliaria rubra; a cutaneous eruption of red vesicles accompanied by burning and itching; usually caused by overexposure to heat.

primary (PRY·mayr·ee)—first; basic; fundamental; principal.

primary colors (PRY·mayr·ee KUL·urz)—pigments or colors that are fundamental and cannot be obtained from a mixture; primary colors are red, yellow, and blue.

primary hair (PRY·mayr·ee HAYR)—the baby-fine hair that is present over almost the entire smooth skin of the body.

primer (PRIH·mur)—*see* filler.

prism (PRIZ·um)—a transparent glass or crystal solid with triangular ends and two converging sides; it breaks up white light into its component colors; the spectrum.

procedure (proh·SEE·jur)—a series of definite steps to follow in a certain order to achieve desired results.

procerus (pruh·SEE·rus)—pyramidalis nasi muscle.

process (PRAH·ses)—a course of development; a series of actions to bring about a particular result or condition.

processed hair (PRAH·sest HAYR)—hair that has been lightened, stripped, tinted, permanently waved, or chemically relaxed.

processing (PRAH·ses·ing)—the action of a chemical solution in cold waving, hair straightening, or hair coloring.

processing time (PRAH·ses·ing TYM)—the time or period required for the chemical solution to act upon the hair.

profession (pruh·FESH·un)—an occupation that requires a liberal, scientific, or artistic education, or related equivalent.

professional (pruh·FESH·un·ul)—one who pursues as a business or livelihood, a particular occupation or vocation.

profile (PROH·fyl)—the outline of a face, head, figure, or an object seen in a side view.

profile base (PROH·fyl BAYS)—a profile section of a hairform used in practical exercises.

prognosis (prahg·NOH·sis)—the probable course of a disease.

progressive dye (pruh·GRES·iv DYE)—color that develops gradually; metallic dye. Color products that deepen or increase absorption over a period of time during processing. A coloring system that produces increased absorption with each application.

projection angle (pruh·JEK·shun ANG·gul)—the angle at which the hair is held while cutting.

proliferate (pruh·LIF·ur·ayt)—to grow by reproduction of new parts, cells, or offspring.

prominence (PRAHM·ih·nents)—a projection.

prominent (PRAHM·ih·nent)—especially noticeable or conspicuous.

prong (PRAWNG)—the round rod of the marcel iron; a slender pointed or projecting part of an implement.

pronounced (proh·NOWNST)—strongly marked or clearly indicated.

properties (PRAHP·ur·teez)—the identifying characteristics of a substance that are observable; a peculiar quality of anything such as color, taste, smell, etc.

prophase (PROH·fayz)—the first stage in mitosis.

proportion (pruh·POR·shun)—a harmonious relationship between parts or things; balance or symmetry; comparative relation of one thing to another.

propylparaben (proh·pil·payr·A·been)—esters of p-hydroxybenzoate are widely used in cosmetics as a preservative and to destroy bacteria and fungus.

protantors (proh·TAN·turz)—muscles found in the forearm that turn hand in and down.

protective cream (proh·TEK·tiv KREEM)—a base cream applied to the skin to protect it against chemicals used during a perm, color, or straightening treatment.

protein (PROH·teen)—a complex organic substance present in all living tissues, such as skin, hair, and nails; necessary to sustain life; also used in some skin and hair conditioners.

proteinaceous (proht·un·AY·shus)—pertaining to or resembling protein.

protein filler (PROH·teen FIL·ur)—a conditioning filler.

protinator (PROH·tin·ay·tur)—an agent that accelerates the release of oxygen in hair lightening.

protoplasm (PROHT·uh·plaz·um)—the material basis of life; a substance found in all living cells.

proximal (PRAHK·sih·mul)—nearest; located near the center of the body.

pruritus (proo·RYT·us)—itching.

psoriasis (suh·RY·uh·sis)—a skin disease characterized by red patches; covered with adherent white-silver scales.

pterygium (teh·RIJ·ee·um)—a forward growth of the eponychium with adherence to the surface of the nail.

ptyalin (TY·uh·lun)—a starch-splitting enzyme found in the saliva.

pull burn (PUL BURN)—scalp irritation resulting from uneven winding of the hair during permanent waving.

pull test (PUL TEST)—a test to determine the degree of elasticity of the hair.

pulmonary (PUL·muh·nayr·ee)—relating to the lungs.

pulmonary circulation (PUL·muh·nayr·ee sur·kyoo·LAY·shun)—blood circulation from heart to lungs to be purified and back to heart.

pumice (PUM·us)—hardened volcanic substance, white or gray in color; also called pumice stone; used for smoothing and polishing.

punctata, acne (punk·TAH·tuh, AK·nee)—a form of acne in which the lesions are pointed papules with a comedone in the center.

pungent (PUN·jent)—acrid; of odors, sharp or irritating.

pupil (PYOO·pul)—the small opening in the iris of the eye through which light enters.

purple (PUR·pul)—any of a variety of colors combining equal or unequal portions of red and blue; a secondary color produced by combining equal parts of red and blue.

purpura (PUR·puh·ruh)—a disease characterized by the formation of purple patches on the skin and the mucous membranes.

pus (PUS)—a fluid product of inflammation, consisting of a liquid containing leucocytes and the debris of dead cells and tissue elements.

pusher (PUSH·ur)—a steel instrument used to loosen the cuticle from the nail.

push wave (PUSH WAYV)—a wave that is pushed into place with the hands.

pustular (PUS·tyuh·lur)—pertaining to or characterized by pustules.

pustule (PUS·chool)—an inflamed pimple containing pus.

pustulosa, acne (pus·tyuh·LOH·suh, AK·nee)—a form of acne characterized by pustules.

putrefaction (pyoo·truh·FAK·shun)—decomposition; decay; the splitting up of the molecule of a protein into less complex substances by bacteria and fungi along with the formation of foul-smelling products.

PVP abbreviation for polyvinyl pyrrolidone (pahl·ee·VY·nul pir·ROHL·ih·dahn)—a synthetic polymer incorporated in hair sprays and some conditioning products.

pyogenic (py·oh·JEN·ik)—pus-forming.

pyosis (py·OH·sis)—the formation of pus.

pyramidal bone (pih·RAM·ih·dul BOHN)—the wedge-shaped bone of the carpus.

pyramidalis nasi (pih·ram·ih·DAY·lis NAY·sye)—procerus; muscle of the nose.

pyrogallol (py·roh·GAL·awl)—pyrogallic acid; antiseptic hair dye for hair restorers; used medicinally in the treatment of psoriasis, ringworm, and other skin infections.

pyrogenic granuloma (py·roh·JEN·ik gran·yoo·LOH·muh)—a severe inflammation of the nail in which a lump of red tissue grows up from the nail bed to the nail plate.

quadrant (KWAHD·rent)—a quarter of a circle, subtending an arc of 90°; anything resembling the quarter section of a circle.

quadratus (kwah·DRAY·tus)—a square-shaped muscle; a muscle of the lower jaw.

quadratus labii inferioris (kwah·DRAY·tus LAY·bee·eye in·feer·ee·OR·is)—a muscle of the lower lip.

quadratus labii superioris (kwah·DRAY·tus LAY·bee·eye soo·peer·ee·OR·is)—a muscle of the upper lip.

quadriceps femoris (KWAHD·ruh·seps FEM·uh·rus)—the large extensor muscle of the thigh.

quality of hair (KWAHL·ut·ee UV HAYR)—the form, length, elasticity, size, and texture of the hair.

quantitative analysis (KWAHN·tih·tay·tiv uh·NAL·ih·sis)—the process of finding the amount of percentage of an element or ingredient present in a material or compound.

quart (KWORT)—a measure of capacity; the fourth part of a gallon, or two pints; the dry quart is equal to 1.10 liters and a liquid quart is equal to 0.946 liter.

quarter (KWOR·tur)—one of four equal parts.

quartz lamp (KWORTZ LAMP)—a glass bulb lamp used for cosmetic purposes; the cold quartz lamp produces mostly short ultraviolet rays, and the hot quartz lamp is an all-purpose lamp used for tanning and for germicidal purposes.

quaternary ammonium compounds (quats) (KWAT·ur·nayr·ee uh·MOH·nee·um KAHM·powndz)—a group of compounds of organic salts of ammonia employed very effectively as disinfectants, conditioners, and other surface-active agents.

quaternium (kwah·TAYR·nee·um)—pertaining to a quaternary ammonium compound; used as an ingredient in hair conditioners.

quince seeds (KWINTS SEEDZ)—the dried seeds of Pyrus Cydonia, which yield a mucilage used in the making of hand lotions.

quinine (KWY·nyn)—an alkaloid from cinchona bark that enters into the composition of some hair lotions and medicines.

quininoderma (kwin·ih·noh·DUR·muh)—a form of dermatitis caused by the ingestion of quinine.

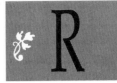

radial artery (RAY·dee·ul ART·ur·ee)—artery that supplies blood to the muscles of the skin, of the hands and fingers, and to the wrist, elbow, and forearm.

radial motion (RAY·dee·ul MOH·shun)—*see* point of distribution.

radial nerve (RAY·dee·ul NURV)—a nerve that affects the arm and hand.

radial pulse (RAY·dee·ul PULS)—the pulse in the radial artery as felt at the wrist near the base of the thumb.

radiation (ray·dee·AY·shun)—the process of giving off light or heat rays; energy radiated in the form of waves or particles.

radiation burn (ray·dee·AY·shun BURN)—a burn resulting from overexposure to radiant energy, such as X rays, radium, or strong sunlight.

radiation therapy (ray·dee·AY·shun THAYR·uh·pee)—the treatment of disease and skin conditions by any type of radiation, most commonly with ionizing radiation such as beta and gamma rays and by X rays.

radical (RAD·ih·kul)—extreme; in chemistry, a group of atoms passing as such from one compound to another, acting thus like a single atom.

radium (RAY·dee·um)—a radioactive metallic element; the rays from this metal are used in the treatment of some skin diseases.

radius (RAY·dee·us)—a line extending or radiating from a center point to the circumference or outer limit of a circle; the outer and smaller bone of the thumb side of the forearm.

ragged (RAG·ud)—having an irregular edge or outline; uneven.

raise (RAYZ)—to make higher; to elevate or lift.

raised scar (RAYZD SKAR)—scar tissue that has healed and formed above the level of the surrounding skin.

rake (RAYK)—a high-frequency electrode used in scalp treatments.

rake comb (RAYK KOHM)—a large-toothed comb designed to remove tangles.

range of motion (RAYNJ UV MOH·shun)—the action of a joint through the entire extent of its movement.

rash (RASH)—a skin eruption having little or no elevation; a superficial, often localized condition of the skin.

rat (RAT)—a cushion or small pad over which the hair is combed to create body and volume.

ratio (RAY·shee·oh)—a proportion; the relationship between two items with respect to quantity, size, or amount.

rat-tail comb (RAT-tayl KOHM)—a comb designed with teeth on one end and a long, slender tail at the other; used to section and subsection the hair; also called "fantail" comb.

ratting (RAT·ing)—the technique of back combing sections of hair from ends toward the scalp forming a cushion or base over which longer hair is combed.

raw (RAW)—irritated; chafed; abraded.

ray (RAY)—a beam of light or heat.

razor (RAY·zur)—an instrument with a keen cutting edge used for shaving and haircutting; hair shaper.

razor blade (RAY·zur BLAYD)—the cutting edge of part of the razor; disposable blade for insertion into the back of the razor.

razor hone (RAY·zur HOHN)—a rectangular block of abrasive material such as a fine grained hard stone used to sharpen razor blades.

razor strop (RAY·zur STRAHP)—a straplike device made of leather and/or canvas; used to bring the razor blade to a smooth, whetted edge.

re (REE)—a prefix denoting again; back to the original or former state or position.

reactant (ree·AK·tunt)—a substance that is affected or altered during the course of a chemical reaction.

reaction (ree·AK·shun)—a response.

reagent (ree·AY·jent)—a substance used in detecting, examining, or measuring other substances because of its chemical or biological activity.

real (REE·ul)—genuine; not artificial; as real hair.

rebuild (ree·BILD)—in treating hair; to replace damaged protein structure by conditioners.

recede (ree·SEED)—to move back; to slope backward as a receding hairline.

receptacle (ree·SEP·tuh·kul)—a container used for storage; a basin.

receptive (ree·SEP·tiv)—able or inclined to receive; open or responsive to ideas or suggestions.

receptor (ree·SEP·tur)—a cell or group of cells that receive stimuli, as a pain or sensation receptor of the skin.

recess (REE·ses)—a hollow, depression, or indentation.

recline (ree·KLYN)—to lie down or back; to cause to assume a recumbent position.

recognize (REK·ug·nyz)—to avow knowledge of; identify.

recondition (ree·kahn·DIH·shun)—in cosmetology, to restore the hair to its natural healthy state by conditioning.

reconditioner (ree·kahn·DIH·shun·ur)—a product formulated to improve the condition of hair by replacing lost protein, moisture, oil, etc.

reconditioning (ree·kahn·DIH·shun·ing)—the application of a special product to the hair in order to improve its condition.

reconstructing (ree·kahn·STRUKT·ing)—in cosmetology, replacing internal and external protein structure in the hair.

reconstruction perm (ree·kahn·STRUK·shun PURM)—permanent wave procedure that first removes excessive curl and then reconstructs desired curl pattern.

reconstructive surgery (ree·kahn·STRUK·tiv SUR·jur·ee)—plastic surgery and cosmetic surgical procedures to build and repair facial and body structures damaged by accidents and disease; surgery to correct and beautify.

record card (REK·urd KARD)—card designed with a special form to keep a record of the services rendered, formulas, supplies used, and any condition pertaining to the client.

recover (ree·KUV·ur)—to bring back; to be restored to normal condition.

rectangle (REK·tang·gul)—a four-sided figure with two sets of parallel sides.

rectangular (rek·TANG·yoo·lur)—having edges or surfaces that meet at right angles.

rectifier (REK·tih·fy·ur)—an apparatus to change an alternating current of electricity into a direct current.

rectum (REK·tum)—the terminal portion of the digestive tube.

rectus (REK·tus)—straight; any of several straight muscles.

rectus capitis anterior (REK·tus KAP·ih·tis an·TEER·ee·ur)—the muscle that flexes the head.

rectus capitis lateralis (REK·tus KAP·ih·tis lat·uh·RAY·lis)—muscle that assists in lateral movements of the head.

rectus capitis posterior (REK·tus KAP·ih·tus puh·STEER·ee·ur)—muscle that functions to extend the head.

red (RED)—the color of the spectrum farthest from violet; one of the primary colors; a warm hue.

red corpuscle (RED KOR·pus·ul)—the blood cell that to carries oxygen to the cells; called erythrocyte.

redhead (RED·hed)—a person having red hair.

red-on-red (RED-awn-RED)—the technique of prelightening strands of red hair to orange, then toning to produce a lighter, medium, or deeper red color.

reduce (ree·DOOS)—to diminish in amount, extent, or number.

reducing agent (ree·DOOS·ing AY·jent)—a substance that is capable of adding hydrogen to a chemical compound or subtract oxygen as a cold wave solution.

reduction (ree·DUK·shun)—the subtraction of oxygen from or the addition of hydrogen to a substance; to make smaller; to lessen; realigning the bone that is dislocated.

refined hair (ree·FYND HAYR)—hair that has been chemically treated to make it more pliable.

reflect (ree·FLEKT)—to project back a light or image.

reflex (REE·fleks)—an involuntary nerve reaction; an automatic response to a stimulus that does not involve the conscious mind.

reflexology (ree·flexs·AHL·uh·jee)—the study of body reflexes; the study of the various areas of the feet as they affect and are affected by other parts of the body.

refresh (ree·FRESH)—to restore to normal or previous vitality.

regimen (REJ·uh·mun)—a systematic course of action or a plan to improve health or a particular condition.

regrowth (ree·GROHTH)—*see* new growth.

rehydration (ree·hy·DRAY·shun)—the restoration of water to the skin or other parts of the body when it has become dehydrated.

rejuvenate (ree·JOO·vuh·nayt)—to make young or vigorous again.

relapse (REE·laps)—the return of symptoms and signs of a disease or condition after apparent recovery has taken place.

relax (ree·LAKS)—to loosen or slacken; to make less tense or rigid.

relaxation (ree·lak·SAY·shun)—the act of relaxing.

relaxer (ree·LAK·sur)—a chemical applied to the hair to remove the natural curl.

relaxer testing (ree·LAK·sur TEST·ing)—checking the action of the relaxer in order to determine the speed at which the natural curl is being removed.

release (ree·LEES)—to free; to let go; a form signed by the client before a service for insurance purposes.

remedy (REM·uh·dee)—a medicine or treatment that relieves or cures a condition.

remover (ree·MOOV·ur)—hair color remover; a chemical compound formulated to remove color from the hair; tint stain remover, a product to remove tint stains from the skin; nail polish remover, a product formulated to remove nail polish.

renal (REE·nul)—relating to the kidney.

reprocess (ree·PRAH·ses)—to repeat a chemical service due to unsatisfactory results.

reproductive (ree·pruh·DUK·tiv)—pertaining to reproduction or the process by which plants and animals produce offspring.

research (REE·surch)—a careful search for facts and principles.

residue (REZ·ih·doo)—that which remains after a part is taken; remainder.

resilience (ree·ZIL·yens)—property of the hair enabling it to retain curl formation and spring back into curled shape after being extended.

resin (REH·zin)—mixture or organic compounds used in hair sprays and setting preparations, for their holding properties.

resistance (ree·ZIST·ens)—an opposing or slowing force; the characteristics of the hair shaft that makes penetration by moisture or chemicals difficult.

resistive massage (ree·ZIS·tiv muh·SAHZH)—a massage movement to develop strength in the joints of the client's hands and wrists.

resorcinal (ruh·ZOR·sin·awl)—a chemical obtained from various resins; chiefly used as an external antiseptic in psoriasis, eczema, seborrhea, and ringworm.

respiration (res·puh·RAY·shun)—the act of breathing; the process of inhaling air into the lungs and expelling it.

respiratory (RES·puh·ruh·tor·ee)—relating to respiration.

respiratory system (RES·puh·ruh·tor·ee SIS·tum)—the system of organs consisting of the nose, pharynx, larynx, trachea, bronchi, and lungs, that assist in breathing.

restorative (ruh·STOR·uh·tiv)—a food or medicine given to restore health and vigor.

restorative art (ruh·STOR·uh·tiv ART)—the craft of restoring the features of a deceased person through corrective and artistic techniques. (*See* desairology.)

restore (ree·STOR)—to bring back to former strength; repair; rebuild; to heal or cure.

restructuring (ree·STRUK·chur·ing)—rebuilding and bringing back into alignment the structural layers of the hair.

retard (ree·TARD)—to hinder or delay.

retention (ree·TEN·shun)—keeping; maintaining.

retention papers (ree·TEN·shun PAY·purz)—special papers used to control the ends of the hair in wrapping, e.g., in winding hair on rods or rollers.

reticular (ruh·TIK·yuh·lur)—spongelike structure associated with the medulla of the hair and the lower layer of the dermis.

reticular layer (ruh·TIK·yuh·lur LAY·ur)—the deeper layer of the derma, which contains cells, vessels, glands, and follicles and supplies the skin with oxygen and nutrients.

retina (RET·un·uh)—the sensitive membrane of the eye which receives the image formed by the lens.

retina acid (RET·un·uh AS·ud)—a prescription cream for acne.

retouch (ree·TUCH)—application of hair color, lightener, or chemical hair relaxer to new growth of hair.

retral (REE·trul)—posterior; situated toward the back.

retro (RET·roh)—a prefix denoting backward or located behind.

reverse (ree·VURS)—to go in the opposite direction.

reverse back hand (ree·VURS BAK HAND)—a hand position with the palm up using a downward stroke when shaving the face.

reverse curl (ree·VURS KURL)—a curl formed for a style to move away from the face.

reverse elevation (ree·VURS el·uh·VAY·shun)—a haircut in which hair is shortest at the top of the head and longest at the lower hairline.

reverse free hand (ree·VURS FREE HAND)—a hand position with upward palm and upward stroke, used when shaving the face.

reverse graduation (ree·VURS graj·oo·AY·shun)—down-angle cutting of the hair.

reverse stack wave (ree·VURS STAK WAYV)—permanent wave wrap pattern with rods at top of each section wrapped to the scalp, and subsequent rods wrapped further from the scalp.

reversible (ree·VURS·ih·bul)—capable of going through a series of changes in either direction, forward or backward, as a reversible chemical reaction.

revert (ree·VURT)—to return to a previous condition.

rewave (REE·wayv)—in permanent waving, giving a permanent wave to a head of hair that still retains some of the former permanent.

Rhazes (RHAH·zees)—an Islamic Persian physician who advocated diet/exercise/massage in the treatment of disease.

rheostat (REE·uh·stat)—a resistance coil; an instrument used to regulate the strength of an electric current or intensity of light.

rheumatism (ROO·muh·tiz·um)—a painful disease of the muscles and joints, accompanied by swelling and stiffness.

rheumatoid arthritis (ROO·muh·toyd ar·THRY·tus)—a chronic inflammatory disease in which cartilage of joints erodes causing them to calcify and become immovable.

rhinitis (ry·NYT·us)—inflammation of the nasal mucous membrane.

rhinocheiloplasty (ry·noh·KY·loh·plas·tee)—plastic surgery of the nose and upper lip.

rhinokyphosis (ry·noh·ky·FOH·sus)—the condition of having an abnormal hump or bump in the bridge of the nose; a prominent bridge.

rhinophyma (ry·noh·FY·muh)—a form of acne rosacea characterized by redness and swelling of the skin of the nose, sometimes accompanied by nodules.

rhinoplasty (RY·noh·plas·tee)—plastic surgery of the nose.

rhinothrix (RY·noh·thriks)—hair growth in the nostrils.

rhysema (ry·SEE·muh)—a wrinkle line or corrugation of the skin.

rhythm (RITH·um)—regularly recurring movement.

rhythmic (RITH·mik)—movements marked by regular recurrence; moving in a definite rhythm.

rhytidectomy (rit·ih·DEK·tuh·mee)—the excision of the skin to eliminate wrinkles; facelift.

ribboning (RIB·un·ing)—hair-setting technique in which hair is forced between thumb and back of comb to create tension.

ribcage (RIB·kayj)—the skeletal framework of the chest made up of the sternum, the ribs, and the thoracic vertebrae.

riboflavin (RY·boh·flay·vin)—the heat stable factor of the vitamin B complex; a water-soluble vitamin and essential nutrient; used in emollients and conditioning agents.

ribonucleic acid (RNA) (ry·boh·noo·KLEE·ik AS·ud)—a nucleic acid of high molecular weight found in the cytoplasm and nuclei of cells; aids synthesis of cell proteins.

ribs (RIBZ)—the twelve pairs of bones forming the wall of the thorax.

ridge (RIJ)—crest of a wave.

ridge curl (RIJ KURL)—a pincurl placed immediately behind or below a ridge to form a wave.

right angle (RYT ANG·gul)—a 90° (degree) angle; an angle formed by intersection of two perpendicular lines.

right atrium (RYT AY·tree·um)—upper thin wall chambers of the heart.

right ventricle (RYT VEN·trih·kul)—lower thick-walled chambers of the heart.

rigid (RIJ·ud)—inflexible; fixed; not moving; resisting change of form.

rim (RIM)—the border or edge.

ringed hair (RINGD HAYR)—a variety of canities in which the hair appears white or colored in the rings.

ring finger (RING FING·gur)—the third finger, next to the little finger of the left hand, on which a wedding ring is customarily worn.

ringlet (RING·lut)—a small curl.

ringworm (RING·wurm)—a vegetable parasitic disease of the skin and its appendages that appears in circular lesions and is contagious.

rinse (RINS)—to cleanse with a second or repeated application of water after washing; a prepared rinse water; a solution that temporarily tints or conditions the hair.

rinse, color (RINS, KUL·ur)—*see* color rinse.

rinse, temporary (RINS, TEM·puh·rayr·ee)—an artificial coloring for the hair that coats the shaft and is removed with a single shampoo.

risorius (rih·ZOR·ee·us)—muscle at the side of the mouth.

RNA—abbreviation for ribonucleic acid.

rod (RAHD)—the round, solid prong of a waving iron; curler used for permanent waving.

rod selector chart (RAHD suh·LEK·tur CHART)—a chart designed for the selection of the proper size and circumference of permanent wave rods.

rolfing (RAHLF·ing)—a method of massage manipulating connective tissue using heavy pressure from the knuckles and elbows on areas of the body.

roll (ROHL)—to move forward or on a surface by turning over and over; to form by turning over.

rolled cotton (ROHLD KAHT·un)—cotton of the absorbent type packaged in rolls for use in cosmetology service procedures.

roller (ROHL·ur)—a cylindrical object varying in diameter and length, around which hair may be wound.

roller clip (ROHL·ur KLIP)—a metal pin, about three inches in length, used to secure a hair roller.

roller control (ROHL·ur kun·TROHL)—the size of the base, in relation to the diameter of roller to be used, and the position of the roller to the base.

roller curl (ROHL·ur KURL)—a means of setting hair by winding a damp strand around a cylindrical object in croquignole fashion and securing it in that position until the hair is dry.

roller direction (ROHL·ur dih·REK·shun)—the direction or line in which a roller is moved.

roller pick (ROHL·ur PIK)—also called a roller pin; a plastic pin about three inches in length, used to secure a hair roller to the scalp.

roller placement (ROHL·ur PLAYS·munt)—the positioning of a roller in relation to its base; 1/2 off or on base.

roller set (ROHL·ur SET)—setting the hair entirely with rollers.

roller tray (ROHL·ur TRAY)—an open-plastic receptacle with bins or trays on different levels, used to hold an store various-sized hair rollers.

rolling (ROHL·ing)—a massage movement in which the tissues are pressed and twisted.

root (ROOT)—the base; the foundation or beginning of any part.

root of hair (ROOT UV HAYR)—structure of the hair below the scalp.

root of the nail (ROOT UV THE NAYL)—base of the nail embedded underneath the skin.

root sheath (ROOT SHEETH)—the tough membrane covering the root of a hair.

ropy (ROH·pee)—pertaining to hair that is stringy, sticky, and resembles a rope or cord.

rosacea, acne (roh·ZAY·see·uh, AK·nee)—a chronic dermatitis appearing primarily on the cheeks, nose, and forehead.

rose color (ROHZ KUL·ur)—a pinkish-red or purplish-red.

rosemary (ROHZ·mayr·ee)—an essence made from an evergreen shrub of the mint family; used in conditioning rinses and tonics for the skin.

rose oil (ROHZ OYL)—attar of roses; an essential oil distilled from fresh roses; used in perfumes and powders.

roseola (roh·zee·OH·luh)—pertaining to a rose-colored eruption such as rubella or German measles.

rose water (ROHZ WAW·tur)—a fragrant preparation made from the oil distilled from rose petals and pure water.

rotary (ROH·tuh·ree)—turning on an axis like a wheel; moving in a circular pattern; a movement used in massage.

rotate (ROH·tayt)—to turn; to revolve.

rotation (roh·TAY·shun)—a massage movement for the joints using circular movements; used for fingers, hands, arms, toes, and ankles.

rouge (ROOZH)—a pink to red cosmetic used to color the skin, especially the cheeks; cheek color.

rough (RUF)—not smooth or polished; having an uneven texture; coarse.

round (ROWND)—spherical; having a contour that is circular or nearly ring-shaped; not flat or angular.

round brush (ROWND BRUSH)—a hairbrush with a circular row of bristles on a round handle, designed for styling hair with a hand-held hair dryer; styling brush.

round-shaped face (ROWND-SHAYPT FAYS)—a facial structure characterized by fullness at the cheekbones and jawline but shorter than an oval.

row (ROH)—an arrangement or series of items or people in a continuous line; a series of pincurls or rollers placed one after the other in a line.

royal jelly (ROY·ul JEL·ee)—a white, concentrated food produced in the stomachs of worker honeybees, and used as an ingredient in some cosmetic preparations.

rub (RUB)—to move or pass over a surface with pressure and friction.

rubber (RUB·ur)—a resinous, elastic material obtained from the latex of the rubber tree and used in various products such as elastic bands and fabrics.

rubbing alcohol (RUB·ing AL·kuh·hawl)—a preparation containing denatured ethyl alcohol or isopropyl alcohol; used as a rubefacient to stimulate the tissues of the skin.

rubedo (roo·BEE·doh)—any redness of the skin.

rubefacient (roo·buh·FAY·shunt)—an agent, such as rubbing alcohol that stimulates blood to the surface of the skin, causing a reddish color.

ruffing (RUF·ing)—back combing; teasing of the hair.

ruffle (RUF·ul)—to comb back the shortest hairs.

rupia (ROO·pee·uh)—thick, dark, raised crusts on the skin.

russet (RUS·ut)—a reddish or yellowish-brown color.

sable (SAY·bul)—the hair from the sable (marten); animal used for fine-quality makeup brushes; the color sable brown, a dark brown-black.

Sabouraud, Rousseau (SA·boo·roh, roo·SOA)—a discoverer of a 24-hour skin test used in hair coloring to determine whether a client can tolerate an aniline-derivative hair tint.

sacral (SAY·krul)—pertaining to or located near the sacrum; the five fused vertebrae in humans.

sacular (SAK·yuh·lur)—shaped like a sac, such as oil glands.

safety razor (SAYF·tee RAY·zur)—a straight razor or shaper with a removable guard for the cutting edge of the blade.

safflower (SAF·low·ur)—a thistlelike herb from which oil is expressed for use in creams and lotions to soften the skin.

saffron (SAF·rahn)—an old world plant of the iris family; the dried, aromatic stigmas are used as coloring matter in cosmetics; also used as a food flavoring; saffron yellow, an orange-yellow color.

safrole (SAF·rohl)—a substance found in the oil of sassafras; used in medicinal and fragrant preparations.

sage oil (SAYJ OYL)—an oil obtained from a plant of the mint family, reputed to have healing powers; used in skin freshening lotions and in some types of hair rinses.

sagittal plane (SAJ·ut·ul PLAYN)—divides body into left and right ports.

salad oil (SAL·ud OYL)—an edible vegetable oil such as olive oil and corn oil; used in many cosmetic preparations including: cleansers, creams, hair dressings, shampoos, and setting lotions.

salicylic acid (sal·uh·SIL·ik AS·ud)—white crystalline acid used as an antiseptic, and its salts in some medicinal preparations.

saline (SAY·leen)—salty; containing salt.

saliva (suh·LY·vuh)—the secretion of the salivary glands; spittle.

salivary gland (SAL·ih·veh·ree GLAND)—a gland in the mouth that secretes saliva.

sallow (SAL·oh)—a yellowish hue or complexion.

salmon (SAM·un)—a reddish or pinkish-orange color named after the color of the flesh of a fresh salmon; salmon pink.

salon (suh·LAHN)—an establishment or shop devoted to a specific service or purpose, as a beauty salon.

salt (SAWLT)—the union of a base with an acid; sodium chloride.

salt and pepper (SAWLT AND PEP·ur)—a mixture of pigmented and gray or white hair.

salve (SAV)—a thick ointment that heals and soothes the skin.

sample (SAM·pul)—a portion, piece, or part to use in testing or as an example of the whole.

sandalwood oil (SAN·dul·wood OYL)—oil expressed from the wood of a type of evergreen tree; used in perfumes.

sandpaper (SAND·pay·pur)—paper coated with fine sand; used for smoothing and polishing; used to make emery boards for manicuring.

sanitary (SAN·ih·teh·ree)—pertaining to cleanliness in relation to health, or to the absence of any agent that may be injurious to health.

sanitation (san·ih·TAY·shun)—the maintenance of sanitary conditions to promote hygiene and the prevention of disease.

sanitize (SAN·uh·tyz)—to make sanitary.

sanitizer (SAN·ih·tyz·ur)—a chemical agent or product used to sanitize implements; a tall glass or plastic jar filled with a sanitizing agent in which implements are kept in a sanitary condition.

saphena (sah·FEE·nuh)—either of two large superficial veins of the leg.

saphenous nerve (sah·FEE·nus NURV)—supplies impulses to the leg and foot.

saponification (sah·pahn·uh·fuh·KAY·shun)—act, process, or result of converting into soap.

saponify (sah·PAHN·uh·fy)—to make into soap.

saponin (SAP·uh·nun)—any of a group of glucosides, found in soapwort or soapbark, which form a soapy foam when dissolved in water; used as detergents and in shampoos.

saprophyte (SAP·ruh·fyt)—a microorganism that grows normally on dead matter, as distinguished from a parasite.

sarcoid (SAR·koyd)—resembling flesh.

sarcoplasmic reticulum (sar·koh·PLAZ·mik rih·TIK·yuh·lum)—plays a role in the contraction of muscles.

sarcothlasis (sar·koh·THLAY·sus)—a bruise or hematoma.

sarcous (SAR·kus)—pertaining to flesh or muscle.

saturate (SACH·uh·rayt)—to cause to become soaked or completely penetrated; to absorb all that is possible to hold.

saturated solution (SACH·uh·rayt·ud suh·LOO·shun)—a solution that contains the maximum amount of substance able to be dissolved.

saturation (sach·uh·RAY·shun)—the degree of concentration or amount of pigment in a color.

S-bonds—*see* sulfur bonds.

scab (SKAB)—a crust of hardened blood, serum, and dead cells formed over the surface of a wound.

scabies (SKAY·beez)—a skin disease caused by an animal parasite, attended with intense itching.

scald (SKAWLD)—to burn with hot liquid or steam.

scale (SKAYL)—any thin plate of epidermal flakes, dry or oily; regular markings used as a standard in measuring and weighing. (*See* imbrications.)

scaling (SKAYL·ing)—the sectioning and subsectioning of the hair to obtain the desired proportions; loss of dead epidermal cells.

scalp (SKALP)—the skin covering the cranium.

scalp antiseptic (SKALP ant·uh·SEP·tik)—a liquid used to relieve itching scalp and arrest the growth of microorganisms.

scalp conditioner (SKALP kun·DISH·un·ur)—a product used to improve the health of the scalp.

scalp electrode (SKALP ih·LEK·trohd)—a rake-shaped electrode used in some scalp massage procedures.

scalpette (skal·pet·AY)—a hair piece designed to cover an irregularly shaped bald area on the front and/or the crown of the head.

scalpial (SKAL·pee·ul)—the technical term for general all-around treatment of the scalp.

scalp lotion (SKALP LOH·shun)—a liquid solution used to treat a dry scalp and/or dandruff.

scalp massage (SKALP muh·SAHZH)—circular movements of the fingertips on the scalp to stimulate blood to the surface.

scalp movement (SKALP MOOV·ment)—a procedure that moves the scalp gently as part of a treatment.

scalp steamer (SKALP STEEM·ur)—an apparatus used to steam the scalp.

scalp treatment (SKALP TREET·munt)—a procedure to improve the health of the scalp.

scaly (SKAY·lee)—covered with or having scales.

scaphoid bone (SKAF·oyd BOHN)—the boat-shaped bone of the tarsus and the carpus.

scapula (SKAP·yuh·luh)—one of a pair of shoulder blades; a large, flat triangular bone of the shoulder.

scar (SKAR)—a mark remaining after a wound has healed.

scarfskin (SKARF·skin)—the epidermis or cuticle.

scarlet (SKAR·let)—a brilliant red-orange color.

scarlet fever (SKAR·let FEE·vur)—a contagious disease accompanied by fever and a red rash.

scent (SENT)—a distinctive odor or fragrance given off by a substance.

schedule (SKED·yul)—a timetable for a preplanned program.

sciatica (sy·AT·ik·uh)—a painful inflammation of the nerve running down the back of the leg, called the sciatic nerve.

science (SY·ens)—a body of knowledge arranged and systemized; based on observation and experiment to determine the basic nature or principles of the subject studied.

scientific (sy·en·TIF·ik)—pertaining to, or used in science.

scissors (SIZ·urz)—a two-bladed instrument used to cut and trim.

scleroderma (sklayr·uh·DUR·muh)—a disease of the skin characterized by hard, thick patches.

scleroid (SKLEER·oyd)—hard or bony in texture.

sclerosis (skluh·ROH·sus)—pathological hardening of tissues, especially by outgrowth of fibrous tissues.

scoliosis (skoh·lee·OH·sus)—abnormal lateral curvature of the spine.

scratch (SKRACH)—a slight wound in the form of a tear on the surface of the skin.

scratch patch test (SKRACH PACH TEST)—a test that consists of application of the test patch to an abraded skin area rather than to normal skin.

scrub (SKRUB)—to rub briskly.

scrupulous (SKROO·pyuh·lus)—extremely exact; careful and painstaking.

sculpture curl (SKULP·chur KURL)—a curl placed close to the head to appear as if it were carved; another term for pincurl.

sculptured nails (SKULP·churd NAYLZ)—artificial nails made by combining a liquid and powder mixture and painting it over a nail form attached to the natural nail; the new nail is then shaped to the desired length.

sculpturing (SKULP·chur·ing)—the formation of a hair shape and silhouette by creating volume or volume and indentation.

scurf (SKURF)—thin, dry scales or scabs on the body, especially on the scalp; dandruff.

scurvy (SKUR·vee)—a nutritional disorder caused by deficiency of vitamin C (ascorbic acid); characterized by extreme weakness, spongy gums, and bleeding under the skin.

scutellum (skoo·TEL·um)—a large scab often observed in favus; a fungal infection of the scalp.

seam (SEEM)—in hairstyling, an overlapping of two ends, as in a French twist.

seaweed (SEE·weed)—a plant growing in the sea; used in cosmetic preparations for its protein content.

sebaceous (sih·BAY·shus)—pertaining to or having the nature of oil or fat.

sebaceous cyst (sih·BAY·shus SIST)—a distended oily or fatty follicle or sac.

sebaceous gland (sih·BAY·shus GLAND)—oil glands of the skin connected to hair follicles; any glands in the corium of the skin that secrete sebum.

seborrhea (seb·uh·REE·uh)—an abnormal increase of secretion from the sebaceous glands.

seborrhea capitis (seb·uh·REE·uh KAP·ih·tis)—seborrhea of the scalp, commonly called dandruff; pityriasis.

seborrhea oleosa (seb·uh·REE·uh oh·leh·OH·suh)—excessive oiliness of the skin, especially of the forehead and nose.

seborrhea sicca (seb·uh·REE·uh SIK·uh)—an accumulation, on the scalp, of greasy scales or crusts, due to overaction of the sebaceous glands; dandruff or pityriasis.

seborrheic (seb·uh·REE·ik)—seborrheal; pertaining to the over-activity of the sebaceous glands.

seborrheic, alopecia (seb·uh·REE·ik, al·uh·PEE·shuh)—baldness caused by diseased sebaceous glands.

sebum (SEEB·um)—the fatty or oily secretions of the sebaceous glands, lubricates hair and skin.

secondary (SEK·un·deh·ree)—second in rank, importance, or value, or in the order of time or development.

secondary color (SEK·un·deh·ree KUL·ur)—a color obtained by mixing equal parts of two primary colors. Green, orange, and violet are secondary colors.

secondary hair (SEK·un·deh·ree HAYR)—the stiff, short, coarse hair found on eyelashes, eyebrows, and within the openings or passages of the nose and ears.

second degree burn (SEK·und duh·GREE BURN)—a burn characterized by pain, blistering, and destruction of the epidermis.

secrete (suh·KREET)—to separate from blood, form into new materials and emit as a secretion.

secretion (sih·KREE·shun)—the process by which materials are separated from the blood, usually by glandular function, and formed into new substances used to carry out special functions.

secretory (seh·KREET·uh·ree)—relating to secretion or to the secretions.

section (SEK·shun)—to divide the hair by parting into separate areas for control.

sedative (SED·uh·tiv)—tending to quiet or allay nervous excitement; any drug that produces a quieting effect on the central nervous system.

sedentary (SED·un·teh·ree)—settled; inactive.

seep (SEEP)—to ooze out slowly.

segment (SEG·munt)—to separate into constituent parts; one of the constituent parts of something.

selector switch (suh·LEK·tur SWICH)—an apparatus used to select the kind of current desired for a treatment.

selenium (suh·LEE·nee·um)—in nutrition, an essential mineral found in cereals, vegetables, and fish; preserves tissue elasticity and aids in promotion of body growth.

selenium sulphide (suh·LEE·nee·um SUL·fyd)—a bright-orange powder used in preparations for the treatment of seborrheic dermatitis and common dandruff.

SEM abbreviation for scanning electron microscope (SKAN·ing ih·LEK·trahn MY·kroh·skohp)—an analytical instrument that bombards an object with electrons to produce an image; an instrument capable of magnification from 50 to 75,000 or more.

semilunar bone (sem·ee·LOO·nur BOHN)—a crescent-shaped bone of the wrist.

semipermanent hair coloring (sem·ee·PUR·muh·nent HAYR KUL·ur·ing)—the process of hair coloring that is formulated to last through four to six shampoos. It penetrates the hair shaft and stains the cuticle layer, slowly fading with each shampoo.

semipermanent rinse (sem·ee·PUR·muh·nent RINS)—a nonpermanent hair rinse that is removed after several shampoos.

semipermanent shampoo hair color (sem·ee·PUR·muh·nent sham·POO HAYR KUL·ur)—a shampoo that imparts a semipermanent color that lasts several weeks.

semistand-up curl (sem·ee·STAND-up KURL)—the placement of a curl on its base in such a manner as to allow it to partially stand away from the scalp; this produces a slightly directional volume in the combout; also known as a flare curl.

semitransformation (sem·ee·trans·for·MAY·shun)—a frontal hair piece extending to just above or behind the ear.

senile (SEE·nyl)—relating to, or characteristic of old age or the infirmities of old age; exhibiting loss of mental faculties associated with old age.

senile canities (SEE·nyl kuh·NIT·eez)—grayness of the hair in elderly people.

sensation (sen·SAY·shun)—a feeling or impression arising as the result of the stimulation of an afferent nerve.

sense (SENS)—the faculty of sensation by which an individual perceives impressions such as taste, touch, smell, sight, and hearing.

sense organ (SENS OR·gan)—a living structure that receives sense impressions (the eye, ears, nose, skin, tongue, and mouth).

sensitive (SEN·sih·tiv)—easily affected by outside influences.

sensitive skin (SEN·sih·tiv SKIN)—skin that is easily damaged or reactive to substances.

sensitivity (sen·sih·TIV·ih·tee)—the state of being easily affected by certain chemicals or external conditions.

sensory (SEN·suh·ree)—relating to or pertaining to sensation.

sensory nerve (SEN·suh·ree NURV)—nerve carrying impulses from sense organs to the brain.

sentient (SEN·chunt)—sensitive; capable of sensation; feeling.

sepia (SEE·pee·uh)—a reddish-brown color.

sepsis (SEP·sis)—the presence of various pus-forming and other pathogenic organisms, or their toxins, in the blood or tissues; septicemia.

septal artery (SEP·tul ART·uh·ree)—the artery that supplies the nostrils.

septic (SEP·tik)—relating to or caused by sepsis.

septicemia (sep·tuh·SEE·mee·uh)—the condition that exists when pathogenic bacteria enter the bloodstream and circulate throughout the body, causing a general infection.

septum (SEP·tum)—a dividing wall; a partition, especially between bodily spaces or masses or soft tissue.

sequence of massage (SEE·kwens UV muh·SAHZH)—the pattern or design of massage.

sequestering agent (sih·KWES·tur·ing AY·jent)—a preservative used to prevent changes in the chemical and physical composition of certain products.

seratonin (sayr·uh·TOH·nin)—a vasoconstrictor that causes vascular spasm to temporarily close the blood vessel.

serous (SIR·us)—relating to or containing serum. Serous membranes act as a lubricant.

serrated (sur·RAYT·ud)—having sawlike notches along the edge.

serratus anterior (ser·RAT·us an·TEER·ee·ur)—a muscle of the chest assisting in breathing and in raising the arm.

serum (SEE·rum)—the clear portion of any bodily fluid; the fluid portion of the blood obtained after coagulation; an antitoxin as prepared for therapeutic use.

sesame oil (SES·uh·mee OYL)—the emollient produced from the seed of an East Indian herb.

set (SET)—to form and secure the hair into a pattern of curls or waves to meet the requirements of a specific hairstyle.

setting (SET·ing)—an arrangement of the hair to meet the requirements of a specific hairstyle.

setting gel (SET·ing JEL)—a semisolid holding agent used to set the hair.

seventh (facial) cranial nerve [SEV·enth (FAY·shul) KRAY·nee·ul NURV]—the chief motor nerve of the face.

shade (SHAYD)—the gradation in color value by adding black to a color; a color slightly but visibly different from the one under consideration. A term used to describe a specific color.

shading (SHAYD·ing)—adding depth of color to strands of hair; in makeup, shadowing a feature to create the illusion of receding or becoming less prominent.

shadow (SHAD·oh)—the low area of a circle in a hairstyle.

shadow wave (SHAD·oh WAYV)—a shaping that resembles the outline of a finger wave but does not have a definite ridge and formation.

shaft (SHAFT)—slender stemlike structure; the long, slender part of the hair above the scalp.

shaking (SHAYK·ing)—in massage, a vibrating movement in which the hand is pressed on the body part and firmly moved from side to side.

shampoo (sham·POO)—to subject the scalp and hair to washing and massaging with some cleansing agent such as soap or detergent; a product formulated for cleansing the hair and scalp.

shampoo bleach (sham·POO BLEECH)—a hair lightener containing peroxide and shampoo.

shampoo bowl (sham·POO BOHL)—a specially designed basin with a "U" shaped construction to allow the client to lie back in a comfortable position during the shampoo.

shampoo brush (sham·POO BRUSH)—a firm-bristled brush used to section the hair and apply shampoo near the scalp.

shampoo cape (sham·POO KAYP)—a plastic or cloth cape used to protect the client's clothing during the shampoo procedure.

shampoo comb (sham·POO KOHM)—a large, wide-toothed comb used to comb shampoo or other products through the hair and to remove tangles; rake.

shampooing (sham·POO·ing)—the act of cleaning the hair and scalp.

shampoo station (sham·POO STAY·shun)—the area where shampoo chairs and equipment are located.

shampoo tint (sham·POO TINT)—a shampoo product that cleans and adds color to the hair.

shape (SHAYP)—the contour of an object; in hair sculpture, shape implies two dimensions.

shaper (SHAYP·ur)—a razorlike device used for shaping or cutting hair.

shaping (SHAYP·ing)—the molding of a section of hair in a circular movement, in preparation for the formation of curls or a finger wave.

shaping, haircutting (SHAYP·ing HAYR·kut·ing)—the process of shortening and thinning the hair to a particular style or to the contour of the head.

shaping, hairstyling (SHAYP·ing HAYR·styl·ing)—the formation of uniform arcs or curves in wet hair, thus providing a base for various patterns in hairstyling.

shaping, pivot (SHAYP·ing PIV·ut)—*see* pivot, hair shaping.

shark-liver oil (SHARK-LIV·ur OYL)—a brown, fatty oil obtained from the livers of sharks; a rich source of vitamin A; used in some types of creams and lotions.

shave (SHAYV)—to cut hair or beard close to the skin; to remove hair from an area by use of a razor.

shaving (SHAYV·ing)—the technique of removing unwanted hair from the face or other part of the body using a razor.

shaving brush (SHAYV·ing BRUSH)—a brush with a handle and long, soft bristles, used to lather the face before shaving.

shaving cream (SHAYV·ing KREEM)—an emollient cream used to soften the beard before shaving.

shaving soap (SHAYV·ing SOHP)—a soap formulated to soften the beard before shaving.

shears (SHEERZ)—an instrument that is used for cutting hair.

sheath (SHEETH)—a covering enclosing or surrounding some organ.

sheen (SHEEN)—gloss; shininess.

shellac (shuh·LAK)—a resinous substance dissolved in alcohol that was used in hair sprays.

shiatsu (shee·AH·tsoo)—a Japanese therapeutic massage technique similar to acupuncture, except the thumbs and tips of the fingers are used on the special areas instead of needles.

shift (SHIFT)—to move the hair away from its natural fall position.

shin (SHIN)—the frontal part of a leg below the knee; the shinbone.

shine (SHYN)—to reflect light; gloss or sheen.

shingle (SHING·gul)—a short haircut, particularly at the nape area, where the haircut starts at the hairline from zero length, becoming gradually longer toward the crown.

short (SHORT)—low; brief; not long.

short circuit (SHORT SUR·kit)—to shut or break off an electric current before it has completed its course.

shorten (SHORT·un)—to reduce in length or duration.

shortwave (SHORT·wayv)—a form of high-frequency current used in permanent hair removal.

shoulder (SHOHL·dur)—the part of the body that connects the arms to the trunk.

shoulder length (SHOHL·dur LENGTH)—the length of the hair that reaches the top part of the shoulder.

shrink (SHRINK)—to contract into a smaller area.

shrivel (SHRIV·ul)—to shrink into wrinkles, especially due to loss of moisture.

siccant; siccative (SIH·kant; SIK·uh·tiv)—drying; tending to make dry.

side (SYD)—the right or left half of a body or object.

sideburn (SYD·burn)—continuation of the hairline in front of the ears.

side height (SYD HYT)—that area of the hair from the end of the sideburns up to the point at which the vertical and horizontal bone structures meet.

side part (SYD PART)—a part in the hair that is on the side, not the center.

sienna (see·EN·uh)—an earth pigment containing iron and maganese oxides; it is yellowish-brown in the raw state and when burned turns a deep reddish-brown; used as a coloring ingredient.

silhouette (sil·oo·ET)—an outline or outer dimension.

silica (SIL·ih·kuh)—dioxide of silicon.

silicon (SIL·ih·kahn)—a very abundant nonmetallic element.

silicone (SIL·ih·kohn)—a water-resistant lubricant for the skin.

silicote (SIL·ih·koht)—a silicone oil used in some cosmetic products.

silk (SILK)—a strong, glossy, natural fiber used in making better-quality wigs and hair pieces.

silk gauze (SILK GAWZ)—a fine gauze silk material used in toupee work or for ventilated parts of hair pieces.

silking (SILK·ing)—hair pressing.

silver hair (SIL·vur HAYR)—hair that has grayed to resemble the metallic white of silver metal; silver-gray hair.

silver nitrate (SIL·vur NY·trayt)—a white, crystalline salt; used as an antiseptic, germicide, and astringent in cosmetics and as a coloring agent in hair dyes.

simplex (SIM·pleks)—common; simple; single.

simplex, acne (SIM·pleks, AK·nee)—common pimple.

simulated (SIM·yoo·layt·ud)—fake; made to look genuine.

sinew (SIN·yoo)—a fibrous cord; a tendon.

singe (SINJ)—in hairdressing, to burn the hair ends; to burn lightly on the surface.

singeing (SINJ·ing)—process of lightly burning hair ends with a lighted wax taper.

single application coloring (SING·gul ap·lih·KAY·shun KUL·ur·ing)—a process that lightens and colors the hair in a single application. Also called single process. (*See* oxidative hair color.)

single application tints (SING·gul ap·lih·KAY·shun TINTS)—products that lighten and add color to the hair in a single application; also called one-process tints or one-step tints.

single floral (SING·gul FLOR·ul)—a basic type of perfume containing the fragrance of one flower, such as rose, gardenia, violet, or carnation.

single-process haircolor (SING·gul-PRAH·ses HAYR·kul·ur)—an oxidative tint solution that lifts or lightens while also depositing color in one application. (*See* oxidative haircolor.)

single-prong clip (SING·gul-PRAWNG KLIP)—a clip having only one prong, designed to hold small curls on thin hair.

sinus (SY·nus)—a cavity or depression; a hollow in bone or other tissue.

sinusoid (SY·nuh·soyd)—resembling a sinus; a blood space in certain organs, as the liver pancreas, etc.

sinusoidal current (sy·nuh·SOYD·ul KUR·unt)—an induced, interrupted current similar to faradic current, used during scalp and facial manipulations.

sizing (SYZ·ing)—the fitting of a wig to the client's head size.

skeletal muscles (SKEL·uh·tul MUS·ulz)—muscles connected to the skeleton.

skeleton (SKEL·uh·tun)—the bony framework of the body.

skill (SKIL)—the mastery of an art or technique; dexterity in doing learned physical tasks.

skin (SKIN)—the external covering of the body.

skin abrasion peel (SKIN uh·BRAY·zhun PEEL)—a process that rubs or wears away the surface of the skin, usually done with pumice stone powder; must be done only by a qualified professional person.

skin analysis (SKIN uh·NAL·ih·sis)—the examination and study of the skin to determine the appropriate treatment.

skin antiseptic (SKIN ant·uh·SEP·tik)—a liquid product formulated to relieve excessive oiliness or irritations.

skin astringent (SKIN uh·STRIN·jent)—a liquid product formulated to contract organic tissue; used to help control excessive oiliness and to invigorate the skin.

skin bleach (SKIN BLEECH)—a preparation formulated to lighten dark pigmentation spots on the skin.

skin care equipment (SKIN KAYR ih·KWIP·munt)—apparatus used during a facial treatment procedure (lamps, atomizer, receptacles, machines, etc.).

skin color (SKIN KUL·ur)—the color of skin as determined by the four types of pigment that determine skin color: melanin, hemoglobin (oxygenated and reduced), and carotenes.

skin freshener (SKIN FRESH·un·ur)—a liquid product used to invigorate the skin following the use of cleansing cream or lotion; a mild astringent.

skin graft (SKIN GRAFT)—skin taken from one part of the body to replace damaged skin on another part of the body; a service performed by a surgeon.

skin peel (SKIN PEEL)—mechanical skin peel; the use of rotating brushes to remove dead surface cells and debris from the skin.

skin peel (SKIN PEEL)—product peel; a procedure using a mild product to remove dead surface cells from the skin; also called epidermabrasion and not to be confused with dermabrasion.

skin peel product (SKIN PEEL PRAH·dukt)—a product such as vegetable enzymes in creams or lotions that give the face a mild surface peeling treatment.

skin pigmentation (SKIN pig·men·TAY·shun)—the deposition of pigment by the cells; color pigment.

skin scope (SKIN SKOHP)—a magnifying glass-lamp combination used to analyze skin conditions; a magnifying lamp.

skin test (SKIN TEST)—a test to determine the existence or non-existence of extreme sensitivity to certain things: foods, chemicals, etc., which do not adversely affect most individuals.

skin texture (SKIN TEKS·chur)—the general feel and appearance of the skin, such as coarse, fine, smooth, rough, etc.

skin toner (SKIN TOH·nur)—a preparation that serves to freshen and tone the skin.

skin treatment (SKIN TREET·munt)—a procedure, such as a massage, to improve the health and appearance of the skin of the face and neck.

skip waving (SKIP WAYV·ing)—a setting method featuring a ridge following a shaping, against which is placed a series of overlapping pincurls, then repeating the shaping and curl placement.

skull (SKUL)—the bony case or the framework of the head.

slack (SLAK)—loose; not tight.

slant (SLANT)—at an angle or incline; in hairdressing, to make a hair parting on an angle.

slap (SLAP)—a movement in massage using the open hand, palm side down, to strike a part of the body abruptly.

sleek (SLEEK)—smooth and glossy.

slicing (SLYS·ing)—carefully removing a section of hair from a shaping in preparation for making a pincurl (the remainder of the shaping is not disturbed).

slim (SLIM)—small in thickness; slender, as a human figure, a hair, or thread.

slip (SLIP)—a smooth and slippery feeling imparted by talc to face powder.

slip on (SLIP AWN)—a hollow rubber or plastic head with facial features and hair that can be slipped over a slip on mannequin head form; used to practice hairstyling techniques.

slippage (SLIP·ij)—the shifting and changing of position of sulfur bonds.

slithering (SLITH·ur·ing)—tapering the hair to graduated lengths by sliding down the surface of hair with scissors.

slough (SLUF)—to separate, a dead matter from living tissue; to discard.

smacking (SMAK·ing)—a massage movement in which the palm of the hand is used to slap the skin.

smaller occipital nerve (SMAWL·ur ahk·SIP·ut·ul NURV)—sensory nerve affecting skin behind the ear.

small intestine (SMAWL in·TES·tin)—the part of the intestine lying between the stomach and the colon, consisting of the duodenum, jejunum, and ileum.

smock (SMAHK)—a loose, lightweight garment worn to protect other clothing.

smocking (SMAHK·ing)—in wig making, a length of weft sewn in triangles, diamonds, or loops to create a flat, airy base.

smooth (SMOOTH)—continuous and unroughened; lacking blemishes; being without hair; lacking irregularities.

smooth face (SMOOTH FAYS)—a shaven face or face that is unblemished.

smooth muscle (SMOOTH MUS·ul)—muscle having nonstriated fibers.

smudge (SMUJ)—to spread or blur makeup or nail polish; to stain or smear.

snarls (SNARLZ)—tangles, as of hair.

soak (SOHK)—to place in a liquid to saturate or soften.

soap (SOHP)—a compound of fatty acid, derived from fats and oils, chemically combined with an alkaline base; used as a cleaning agent.

soap cap (SOHP KAP)—a combination of prepared tint and shampoo that is applied to the hair like a regular shampoo; this is used to add some color and brightness to faded hair.

soapless shampoo (SOHP·les sham·POO)—a shampoo made with a synthetic detergent; it can be formulated at nearly any pH but is usually slightly acidic in reaction.

sodium (SOH·dee·um)—a metallic element of the alkali metal group.

sodium carbonate (SOH·dee·um KAR·buh·nayt)—washing soda; used to prevent corrosion of metallic instruments when added to boiling water.

sodium chloride (SOH·dee·um KLOR·yd)—table salt (NaCL).

sodium hydroxide (SOH·dee·um hy·DRAHK·syd)—a powerful alkaline product used in some chemical hair relaxers; caustic soda; powerful alkali used in the manufacture of liquid soaps.

sodium hypochlorite (soh·DEE·um hy·puh·KLOR·yt)—disinfectant used to sanitize implements.

sodium lauryl sulfate (soh·DEE·um LOR·ul SUL·fayt)—a metallic compound of the alkaline group, in white or light yellow crystals; used in detergents; a detergent, wetting agent, and emulsifier; used in shampoos for its degreasing qualities.

sodium nitrate (SOH·dee·um NY·trayt)—a clear, odorless crystalline salt used to manufacture nitric acid; sodium nitrite; used as an oxidizing agent.

sodium perborate (SOH·dee·um pur·BOR·ayt)—a compound formed by treating sodium peroxide with boric acid; on dissolving the substance in water, peroxide of hydrogen is generated; used as an antiseptic and bleaching agent.

sodium sulphite (SOH·dee·um SUL·fyt)—a soft, white metallic salt of sulphurous acid; antiseptic, preservative, and antioxidant used in hair color.

sodium thiosulphate (SOH·dee·um thy·uh·SUL·fayt)—a compound used in solutions for impetiginous conditions and parasitic alopecias of the beard.

soft (SAWFT)—pliable; malleable; easily worked.

softener (SAWF·un·ur)—something that softens, as a compound added to water; in hairdressing, a term for a product applied before a permanent wave or color to lower cuticle resistance; a presoftener.

softening (SAWF·un·ing)—the application of a chemical product to hair, making it more receptive to hair coloring or permanent waving.

softening agent (SAWF·un·ing AY·jent)—a mild alkaline product applied prior to treatment to increase porosity, swell the hair's cuticle, and increase absorption. In hair coloring, tint that has not ben mixed with developer is frequently used. (*See* presoften.)

soft press (SAWFT PRES)—pressing the hair to remove 50 to 60 percent of the curl.

soft soap (SAWFT SOHP)—fluid or semifluid soap.

soft water (SAWFT WAWT·ur)—water that readily lathers with soap; water that is free from calcium or magnesium compounds.

sole (SOHL)—the bottom surface of the foot.

solid (SAHL·ud)—any substance that does not flow; form of matter with definite shape, volume, and weight.

solid form (SAHL·ud FORM)—in hairdressing, an unbroken surface; unactivated texture.

solid peroxide (SAHL·ud pur·AHK·syd)—sodium perborate and mild acid in tablet form that is dissolved in water before using.

solubility (sahl·yuh·BIL·ih·tee)—the extent to which a substance (solute) dissolves in a liquid (solvent) to produce a homogeneous system (solution).

soluble (SAHL·yuh·bul)—capable of being dissolved.

solute (SAHL·yoot)—the dissolved substance in a solution.

solution (suh·LOO·shun)—a blended mixture of solid, liquid, or gaseous substances; the act or process by which a substance is homogeneously mixed with a liquid, gas, or solid.

solvent (SAHL·vunt)—a liquid that dissolves another substance without any change in chemical composition.

sorbic acid (SOR·bik AS·ud)—a white crystalline solid from the berries of the mountain ash; also produced synthetically; used in a wide variety of cosmetics as a binder, humectant and preservative.

soybean (SOY·been)—a leguminous herb that produces oil used in the manufacture of soaps, shampoos, and bath oils.

sparse (SPARS)—thinly diffused; not dense; consisting of a few or scattered elements; thin, irregular eyebrows, balding areas of the head.

spasm (SPAZM)—an involuntary muscular contraction.

spasmodic (spaz·MAHD·ik)—pertaining to spasm; convulsive; intermittent.

spat (SPAT)—a slight blow or slap on the skin, used in some massage procedures.

spatula (SPACH·uh·luh)—a flexible implement with a blunt blade, used for removing creams from their containers.

spearmint oil (SPEER·mint OYL)—a fragrant plant of the mint family; used as a flavoring agent, in perfumes and in toothpastes.

specialist (SPESH·uh·list)—one who devotes himself or herself to some special branch of learning such as art, cosmetology, or business.

spectrum (SPEK·trum)—an arrangement of colored bands produced by the passage of white light through a prism.

speed (SPEED)—a rate of motion: fast, medium, slow; fast speed: the closest rate of motion from its point of origin within its shape; medium speed: the rate of motion in the middle are of a shape, between fast and slow; slow speed: the furthest rate of motion from its point of origin within its shape.

sphenoid (SFEE·noyd)—wedge-shaped; the wedge-shaped bone at the base of the skull, joins together all bones of the cranium.

sphere (SFEER)—a geometric figure generated by the revolution of a semicircle about its diameter.

spherical (SFEER·ih·kul)—relating to or having the shape of a sphere.

spinal (SPY·nul)—pertaining to the spine or vertebral column.

spinal accessory (SPY·nul ak·SES·uh·ree)—eleventh cranial nerve.

spinal column (SPY·nul KAHL·um)—the backbone or vertebral column.

spinal cord (SPY·nul KORD)—the portion of the central nervous system contained within the spinal or vertebral canal.

spinal nerves (SPY·nul NURVZ)—the nerves arising from the spinal cord.

spindle-shaped (SPIN·dul-SHAYPT)—shaped like a spindle; tapering toward each end.

spine (SPYN)—a sharp process of bone; the backbone.

spiral (SPY·rul)—coil; winding around a center, like a watch spring.

spiral curl (SPY·rul KURL)—also called helical wind; a method of curling hair by winding a strand around a rod; spiral winding.

spiral perm (SPY·rul PURM)—a method in permanent waving in which hair is wound on perm rods from the scalp toward the ends.

spiral rod (SPY·rul RAHD)—a rod upon which the hair is wound in a spiral manner for a permanent wave.

spirillum (spy·RIL·um); pl., **spirilla** (spy·RIL·uh)—spiral bacterium, causing diseases such as syphilis.

spirit gum (SPEER·it GUM)—gum used to attach false hair to skin or scalp.

splash neutralizer (SPLASH NOO·truh·ly·zur)—a chemical agent capable of stopping the action of the cold waving solution and setting or hardening the hair in its new form.

split end (SPLIT END)—visible separation at the end of the hair due to cuticle damage.

sponge (SPUNJ)—an elastic, porous substance that serves as an absorbent; the skeleton of an aquatic organism (phylum) cultivated for use as cosmetic and cleansing pads.

spongy hair (SPUN·jee HAYR)—hair that is overporous, due to overbleaching or abuse.

spool rod (SPOOL RAHD)—a straight cold wave rod.

spore (SPOHR)—a tiny bacterial body having a protective wall to withstand unfavorable conditions.

sports massage (SPORTS muh·SAHZH)—massage used to prepare athletes for upcoming events and to aid in bodily restoration following competitions.

spot bleaching or lightening (SPAHT BLEECH·ing OR LYT·un·ing)—applying bleach (lightener) to areas insufficiently lightened in order to produce even results.

spot tinting (SPAHT TINT·ing)—applying tint to areas insufficiently colored in order to achieve even results.

sprain (SPRAYN)—injury to a joint resulting in stretching or tearing of ligaments.

spray (SPRAY)—to discharge liquid in the form of fine vapor.

spray gun (SPRAY GUN)—an applicator used to spray a fine mist.

spray machine (SPRAY muh·SHEEN)—a device employed to apply a very fine spray or mist of astringent to massage the nerve ends in the skin.

spring grip irons (SPRING GRIP EYE·urnz)—thermal curling irons with a spring to enable it to close automatically.

springs; wig springs (SPRINGZ)—springs inserted into a wig or hair piece foundation that are designed to hold it close to the head.

spur (SPUR)—a pointed, horny outgrowth usually found on the feet.

squama (SKWAY·muh)—an epidermic scale made up of thin, flat cells.

squamous (SKWAY·mus)—scaly; covered with scales; thin and flat like fish's scales.

square-shaped face (SKWAYR-SHAYPT FAYS)—facial structure characterized by a wide forehead and jaw; usually shorter in length than an oval.

stabilized (STAY·bih·lyzd)—made stable or firm, preventing changes.

stabilizer (STAY·bih·ly·zur)—general name for ingredient that pro-longs lifetime, appearance, and performance of a product. A retarding agent or a substance that preserves a chemical equilibrium. (*See* fixative.)

stable (STAY·bul)—in a balanced condition; not readily destroyed or decomposed; resisting molecular change.

stacking (STAK·ing)—a haircutting technique using a slight grada-tion to achieve volume; an end permanent technique where one roller is stacked and extended above the other.

stack, permanent wave (STAK, PUR·muh·nent WAYV)—a wrap-ping technique to curl ends of long hair; wrapping begins at the hairline and progresses to the crown with sticks used to maintain an even design.

stages (STAY·jez)—the term describing the visible color changes the hair passes through during a lightening process. (*See* degree.)

stagger (STAG·ur)—to arrange rollers on rods in a zigzag order.

stain (STAYN)—an abnormal skin discoloration; hair color technique using a tint alone or mixed conditioner rather than peroxide.

stain remover (STAYN ree·MOOV·ur)—chemical used to remove tint stains from skin.

stand up curl (STAND UP KURL)—cascade curl; a strand of hair held directly up from the scalp and wound with a large cen-ter opening in croquignole fashion and fastened to the scalp in a standing position.

staphylococcus (staf·uh·loh·KOK·us); pl., **staphylococci** (staf·uh·loh·KOK·sye)—cocci that are grouped in clusters like a bunch of grapes; found in pustules and boils.

starch (STARCH)—a white, tasteless, odorless substance found in potatoes, corn, rice, and similar vegetables; used in powders, dentifrices, hair colorings, and many other cosmetic preparations.

starting knot (START·ing NAHT)—the procedure in weaving and securing the first strand of hair.

static electricity (STAT·ik ih·lek·TRIH·sut·ee)—a form of electricity generated by friction.

staying power (STAY·ing POW·ur)—the holding ability or power of a perm or set.

steam (STEEM)—water changed into vapor form when its temperature is raised to boiling.

steamer, facial (STEEM·ur, FAY·shul)—an apparatus, used in place of hot towels, for steaming the scalp or face.

steamer, scalp (STEEM·ur, SKALP)—an apparatus, used in place of hot towels, for steaming the scalp.

stearate (STEE·uh·rayt)—a salt of stearic acid.

stearic acid (stee·AYR·ik AS·ud)—a white, fatty acid, occurring in solid animal fats and in some of the vegetable fats; used in powders, creams, lotions, and soap as a lubricant.

stearrhea (stee·uh·REE·uh)—a form of seborrhea.

steatoma (stee·uh·TOH·muh)—a sebaceous cyst; a fatty tumor.

steatosis (stee·uh·TOH·sis)—fatty degeneration; disease of the sebaceous glands.

stem (STEM)—the strand of hair from the scalp up to but not including the first curvature of a pincurl.

stem direction (STEM dih·REK·shun)—the direction in which the stem moves from the base to the first arc: up, down, forward, and back.

steps (STEPS)—irregular layers in a haircut.

sterile (STAIR·ul)—barren; free from all living organisms.

sterilization (stayr·uh·luh·ZAY·shun)—the process of making sterile; the destruction of all germs, whether beneficial or harmful.

sterilize (STAYR·uh·lyz)—to deprive of production power; to make sterile or free from microorganisms.

sterilizer (STAYR·uh·ly·zur)—an apparatus used to sterilize equipment or other objects by destroying all contaminating microorganisms.

sterilizer cabinet, dry (STAYR·uh·ly·zur KAB·ih·net, DRY)—a closed receptacle containing chemical vapors to keep sterilized objects ready for use.

sterilizer, wet (STAYR·uh·ly·zur, WET)—a receptacle containing a disinfectant for the purpose of sterilizing implements.

sterno (STUR·noh)—a prefix denoting connection with the sternum (breastbone).

sternocleidomastoid artery (STUR·noh·KLEE·ih·doh·MAS·toyd ART·uh·ree)—the artery that supplies blood to the muscles of the neck.

sternocleidomastoideus (STUR·noh·KLEE·ih·doh·mas·TOYD·ee·us) —a muscle of the neck that depresses and rotates the head.

sternomastoid (stur·noh·MAS·toyd)—pertaining to the sternum and the mastoid process.

sternum (STUR·num)—the flat bone or breastbone that forms the ventral support of the ribs.

steroid (STAYR·oyd)—any of a large group of fat soluble organic compounds, including the sterols and sex hormones.

stigma (STIG·muh)—a mark, spot, scar, or other blemish on the skin.

stimulant (STIM·yuh·lent)—an agent that arouses organic activity.

stomach (STUM·uk)—the dilated portion of the alimentary canal, in which one of the processes of digestion takes place.

stopping point (STAHP·ing POYNT)—in massage, a point on a muscle or over a pressure point where pressing movements are made during the facial or scalp massage.

straight (STRAYT)—extending in one direction without a curve or bend; not curly.

straight elevation (STRAYT el·uh·VAY·shun)—in haircutting, a term applied to the method of cutting the hair in a straight sphere or frame.

straightening comb (STRAYT·un·ing KOHM)—also called a pressing comb; a comb constructed of steel or brass with a wood handle, usually heated electrically; used to remove curl from overcurly hair.

straight permanent wave rod (STRAYT PUR·muh·nent WAYV RAHD)—a permanent wave rod that is equal in circumference along the entire curling area.

straight profile (STRAYT PROH·fyl)—a profile that has evenly balanced facial features; being neither concave nor convex, as seen in profile.

straight wave (STRAYT WAYV)—a wave running alongside and parallel to the part.

strand (STRAND)—fibers or hairs that form a unit.

strand test (STRAND TEST)—a test given before tinting, lightening, permanent waving, or hair relaxing to determine the required developing or processing time; a test to determine the degree of porosity and elasticity of the hair, as well as the ability of the hair to withstand the effects of chemicals.

stratum (STRAT·um); pl., **strata** (STRAT·uh)—a layer, as of tissue.

stratum basale (STRAT·um buh·SAY·lee)—basal layer, the cell-producing layer of the epidermis.

stratum corneum (STRAT·um KOR·nee·um)—outer layer of the skin.

stratum germinativum (STRAT·um jur·min·ah·TIV·um)—the deepest layer of the epidermis resting on the corneum.

stratum granulosum (STRAT·um gran·yoo·LOH·sum)—granular layer of the skin.

stratum lucidum (STRAT·um LOO·sih·dum)—the clear, transparent layer of the epidermis under the stratum corneum.

stratum malpighii (STRAT·um mal·PIG·ee)—the germinative or innermost layer of the epidermis including the spinosum or prickle layer.

stratum mucosum (STRAT·um myoo·KOH·sum)—mucous or malpighian layer of the skin.

stratum spinosum (STRAT·um spy·NOH·sum)—the prickle cell layer of the skin often classified with the stratum germinatum to form the basal layer; pricklelike threads join the cells.

streak (STREEK)—to lighten a strand of hair to create a high-lighted effect.

streaking (STREEK·ing)—lightening thin sections of the hair.

streaking cap (STREEK·ing KAP)—also called frosting cap; a plastic or rubber head covering with punctured holes used to lighten or darken strands of hair.

streptococcus (strep·tuh·KOK·us); pl., **streptococci** (strep·tuh·KOK·sye)—pus-forming bacteria that arrange in curved lines resembling a string of beads; found in strep throat and blood poisoning.

stress (STRES)—a situation that causes tension; our body and mind compensate to maintain internal balance and harmony.

stretch wig (STRECH WIG)—a wig that has been constructed with a completely elasticized foundation that will stretch to fit a wide range of head sizes.

striated (STRY·ayt·ud)—marked with parallel lines or bands; striped, as voluntary muscle.

stringy hair (STRING·ee HAYR)—limp hairs matted together forming a ropelike strand.

stripping (STRIP·ing)—the removal of color from the hair shaft; bleaching; lightening; strong shampoos or soap removing some of the color from the hair is also known as stripping. (*See* color remover.)

stroke (STROHK)—the result of a blood clot or ruptured vessel in brain that destroys nerve tissue.

stroking (STROHK·ing)—a gliding movement over a surface; to pass the finger or any instrument gently over a surface; effleurage.

strong hair (STRAWNG HAYR)—hair that is somewhat resistant to treatments, usually coarser than average hair.

strontium sulphide (STRAHN·chum SUL·fyd)—a light gray powder capable of liberating hydrogen sulphide in the presence of water; used as a depilatory.

sty, stye (STY); pl., **sties, styes** (STYZ)—inflammation of one of the sebaceous glands of the eyelid.

style (STYL)—the current, fashionable mode of dress, makeup, or hair design; the specific shape, size, and placement of curls and waves of a finished hairstyle.

style cut (STYL KUT)—a short hair shaping that has the design and style cut into the top, sides, and nape.

style drying (STYL DRY·ing)—the drying and styling of the hair at the same time.

style part (STYL PART)—a planned part in the hair that is visible in the finished hairstyle.

styling chair (STYL·ing CHAYR)—an adjustable chair, usually with a footrest, in which the client sits while the hair is being styled.

styling comb (STYL·ing KOHM)—a comb designed with one half row of thin, close teeth and the other half with wider spaces between the teeth; used to aid in styling hair.

styling gel (STYL·ing JEL)—a jellylike preparation used to aid in styling the hair and add stiffness.

styling iron heater (STYL·ing EYE·urn HEET·ur)—an electric apparatus used to heat thermal curling irons.

styling lotion (STYL·ing LOH·shun)—a liquid preparation used to add body and staying power to the finished hairstyle.

styling station (STYL·ing STAY·shun)—a space or unit in a salon containing the furnishings, implements, and products needed to cut and style hair.

stylist (STYL·ist)—one who develops, designs, advises on, or creates styles.

styptic (STIP·tik)—an agent causing contraction of living tissue; used to stop bleeding; an astringent.

styrofoam (STY·ruh·fohm)—a lightweight plastic foam used for a wig block, used to keep a styled wig in shape.

sub (SUB)—a prefix denoting under; below.

subclavian (sub·KLAY·vee·un)—lying under the clavicle, as the sub-clavian artery.

subcutaneous (sub·kyoo·TAY·nee·us)—under the skin.

subcutis (sub·KYOO·tis)—subdermis; subcutaneous tissue; under or beneath the corium or dermis, the true skin.

subdermis (sub·DUR·mis)—subcutis or subcutaneous tissue of the skin.

subdivide (SUB·dih·vyd)—to divide a section into smaller sections.

submental artery (sub·MEN·tul ART·uh·ree)—artery that supplies blood to the chin and lower lip.

suboccipital nerve (sub·ahk·SIP·ut·ul NURV)—nerve that stimu-lates the deep muscles of the back and the neck.

subsection (SUB·sek·shun)—dividing a section into smaller parts; the part created by this division.

suction machine (SUK·shun muh·SHEEN)—an apparatus used in some facial treatment procedures to dislodge debris from the follicles.

sudamen (soo·DAY·men); pl., **sudamina** (soo·DAM·ih·nuh)—a disorder of the sweat glands with obstruction of their ducts.

sudor (SOO·dor)—sweat; perspiration.

sudoriferous (sood·uh·RIF·uh·rus)—carrying or producing sweat.

sudoriferous ducts (sood·uh·RIF·uh·rus DUKTS)—the excretory ducts of the sweat glands.

sudoriferous glands (sood·uh·RIF·uh·rus GLANDZ)—sweat glands of the skin.

sudorific (sood·uh·RIF·ik)—causing or inducing perspiration.

sulfide (SUL·fyd)—compound of sulfur and an oxide.

sulfite (SUL·fyt)—any salt of sulfurous acid.

sulfonated oil (SUL·fuh·nayt·ud OYL)—an organic substance prepared by reacting oils with sulphuric acid; used as a base in soapless shampoos and in hair sprays as an emulsifier.

sulfur, sulphur (SUL·fur)—a solid, nonmetallic element, usually yellow in color; it is insoluble in water.

sulfur bonds (SUL·fur BAHNDZ)—sulfur cross bonds in the hair, which hold the chains of amino acids together; position determines curl present in the hair.

sulfuric acid (sul·FYOO·rik AS·ud)—oil of vitriol; colorless and nearly odorless, heavy oily corrosive liquid, employed as a caustic.

sulphide (SUL·fyd)—a compound of sulfur with another element or basic radical.

sunburn (SUN·burn)—inflammation of the skin caused by exposure to the sun.

sunburst (SUN·burst)—a special form of hair lightening that creates a sunlike effect, usually in the front of the style.

sunflower seed oil (SUN·flow·ur SEED OYL)—oil obtained from the seeds of sunflowers; a good source of vitamin E; used in soap manufacturing, salad oil, and some food products.

sunlamp (SUN·lamp)—a lamp that radiates ultraviolet rays; used in cosmetic and therapeutic face and body treatments.

sunlighting (SUN·lyt·ing)—the technique of highlighting the top layer of the hair.

suntan (SUN·tan)—a brownish coloring of the skin as a result of sun exposure.

super (SOO·pur)—a prefix denoting over; above; beyond.

superciliary (soo·pur·SIL·ee·ayr·ee)—pertaining to or referring to the region of the eyebrow.

supercilium (soo·pur·SIL·ee·um); pl., supercilia (soo·pur·SIL·ee·uh)—the eyebrow.

superficial (soo·pur·FISH·ul)—pertaining to or being on the surface.

superficial cervical (soo·pur·FISH·ul SUR·vih·kul)—a cranial nerve which supplies the muscle and skin of the neck.

superficial fascia (soo·pur·FISH·ul FAYSH·uh)—a sheet of subcutaneous tissue; tissue that attaches the dermis to underlying structures.

superficial temporal artery (soo·pur·FISH·ul TEM·puh·rul ART·uh·ree)—the artery that supplies blood to the muscles of the scalp and head.

superfluous (soo·PUR·floo·us)—excessive; more than is wanted and needed.

superfluous hair (soo·PUR·floo·us HAYR)—unwanted hair.

superior (soo·PEER·ee·ur)—higher; upper; better or of more value.

superior auricularis (soo·PEER·ur aw·rik·yuh·LAYR·is)—the muscle that draws the ear upward.

superioris (soo·peer·ee·OR·is)—a muscle that elevates.

superior labial artery (soo·PEER·ee·ur LAY·bee·ul ART·ur·ee)—artery that supplies blood to the upper lip and region of the nose.

superior labial nerve (soo·PEER·ee·ur LAY·bee·ul NURV)—nerve that receives stimuli from the skin of the upper lip.

superior maxillary (soo·PEER·ee·ur MAK·suh·layr·ee)—the upper jawbone.

superior palpebral nerve (soo·PEER·ee·ur PAL·puh·brul NURV)—nerve that receives stimuli from the upper eyelid.

superior vena cava (soo·PEER·ee·ur VEE·nuh KAH·vuh)—the large vein that carries blood to the upper right chamber of the heart.

supinate (SOO·puh·nayt)—to turn the forearm and hand so the palmar surface is uppermost.

supinator (SOO·puh·nayt·ur)—a muscle of the forearm, which rotates the radius outward and the palm upward.

supple hair (SUP·ul HAYR)—hair that is easily managed, pliable, and not stiff.

supporting curl (suh·PORT·ing KURL)—a pincurl made in the same direction as the first line of curls.

suppuration (sup·yuh·RAY·shun)—the formation of pus.

supra (SOO·pruh)—a prefix denoting on top of, above, over, beyond, besides; more than.

supraclavicular (soo·pruh·kluh·VIK·yoo·lar)—above the clavicle.

supraclavicular nerve, intermediate (soo·pruh·kluh·VIK·yoo·lar NURV, in·tur·MEE·dee·ut)—nerve that receives stimuli from the lower anterior aspect of the neck and interior chest wall.

supraclavicular nerve, lateral (soo·pruh·kluh·VIK·yuh·lar NURV, LAT·ur·ul)—nerve that receives stimuli from the skin of the lateral aspect of the neck and shoulder.

supraorbital (soo·pruh·OR·bih·tul)—above the orbit or eye.

supraorbital artery (soo·pruh·OR·bih·tul ART·uh·ree)—artery that supplies blood to the upper eyelid and forehead.

supraorbital nerve (soo·pruh·OR·bih·tul NURV)—nerve that receives stimuli from the skin of the upper eyelid and the forehead.

suprascapular artery (soo·pruh·SKAP·yoo·lar ART·uh·ree)—the artery that supplies blood to the shoulder joints and muscles surrounding the area.

supratrochlear (soo·pruh·TRAHK·lee·ur)—above the trochlea or pulley of the superior oblique muscle.

supratrochlear artery (soo·pruh·TRAHK·lee·ur ART·ur·ee)—artery that supplies blood to the anterior scalp.

supratrochlear nerve (soo·pruh·TRAHK·lee·ur NURV)—nerve that receives stimuli from the skin of the medial aspect of forehead, root of the nose, and the upper eyelid.

surface (SUR·fis)—the outer or topmost boundary of an object; the boundary of any three-dimensional figure.

surface tension (SUR·fis TEN·shun)—the tension or resistance to rupture possessed by the surface film of a liquid.

surfactant (sur·FAK·tent)—surface active agent. A molecule that is composed of an oil-loving (oleophilic) part and a water-loving (hydrophilia) part. They act as a bridge to allow oil and water to mix. Wetting agents, emulsifiers, cleansers, solubilizers, dispersing aids, and thickeners are usually surfactants.

surgical glove (SUR·jih·kul GLUV)—a thin, rubber glove with finger and thumb sections, used to protect the hands from stains and irritants.

suspension (sus·PEN·shun)—a state of matter in which the solid particles are dispersed in or distributed throughout a liquid medium; the particles in the medium are large but not large enough to settle to the bottom under the influence of gravity.

swab (SWAHB)—absorbent cotton wrapped around the end of a short, pliable stick; used for the application of solutions and for removing excess makeup.

swathe (SWAHTH)—knotted or woven hair piece usually worn at the nape of the neck.

sweat (SWET)—to exude or excrete moisture from the pores of the skin; perspiration.

sweat gland (SWET GLAND)—small, convoluted tubules that secrete sweat; found in the subcutaneous tissue and ending at the opening of the pores.

Swedish massage (SWEE·dish muh·SAHZH)—a system of passive and active exercise movements and techniques for muscles and joints. Also called Swedish movement cure.

Swedish movements (SWEE·dish MOOV·ments)—a system of muscular movements employed in massage to treat and develop the body.

sweep (SWEEP)—to brush or comb the hair upward, moving or extending in a wide curve or over a wide area; upsweep.

sweet bay oil (SWEET BAY OYL)—an oil produced from the leaves of the laurel; used in soaps, perfumes, and emollients.

swirl (SWURL)—formation of a wave in a diagonal direction from back to side of head.

switch (SWICH)—a long length of wefted hair mounted with a loop on the end; usually constructed with three stem strands to provide flexibility in styling; a separate tress of hair, or of some substitute, worn by women to increase the apparent mass of hair.

swivel clamp (SWIV·ul KLAMP)—a clamp used to secure a wig block or mannikin head to a table top.

sycosis (sy·KOH·sis)—a chronic pustular inflammation of the hair follicles.

sycosis barbae (sy·KOH·sis BAR·bee)—a chronic inflammation of the hair follicles of the beard; barber's itch.

sycosis tinea (sy·KOH·sis TIN·ee·uh)—parasitic ringworm of the beard; barber's itch.

sycosis vulgaris (sy·KOH·sis vul·GAYR·is)—a pustular, follicular lesion caused by staphylococci; nonparasitic sycosis of the beard.

symbol (SIM·bul)—conventional abbreviation; a character, sign, or mark to represent an object, abstract idea, an element, quantity, etc.

symmetrical (sih·MET·rih·kul)—uniform and balanced in proportion and style.

symmetrical hairstyle (sih·MET·rih·kul HAYR·styl)—a hairstyle with a similar design on both sides of the face.

symmetry (SIM·ut·ree)—balanced proportions; harmony of line and form.

sympathetic nervous system (sim·puh·THET·ik NUR·vus SIS·tem)—that part of the autonomic nervous system concerned with mediating involuntary responses of the body such as heart rate, salivary secretion, blood pressure, digestion, etc.

symptomatica alopecia (simp·tum·AT·ih·kuh al·uh·PEE·shun)—loss of hair due to illness.

symptom, objective (SIMP·tum, ahb·JEK·tiv)—a symptom that can be seen, as in pimples or pustules.

symptom, subjective (SIMP·tum, sub·JEK·tiv)—a symptom that can be felt but not seen, such as itching.

syn (SIN)—a prefix denoting along with; together; at the same time.

syndactylism (sin·DAK·tuh·liz·um)—webbed fingers or toes.

synergetic (sin·ur·JET·ik)—working together; the combined action or effect of two or more organs or agents, or to coordination of muscular or organ functions by the nervous system in such a way that specific movements and actions can be performed.

synovia (suh·NOH·vee·uh)—a transparent viscid lubricating fluid secreted by the lining membranes of joints.

synthetic (sin·THET·ik)—produced artificially; not natural.

synthetic hair (sin·THET·ik HAYR)—a manmade, hairlike fiber made from nylon, dynel, rayon, etc., or from any combination of these fibers.

syrian hair (SEER·ee·un HAYR)—a mixture of human hair or animal hair with yak hair.

system (SIS·tum)—a group of bodily organs acting together to perform one or more of the main bodily functions; an arrangement of objects that complete a unit; a procedure or established way of doing something.

systemic (sis·TEM·ik)—pertaining to a system or to the body as a whole; affecting the body generally.

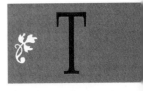

tabes (TAY·beez)—wasting away or atrophy due to disease.

tablespoon (TAY·bul·spoon)—abbr: tbsp; a large spoon used for serving food and in measuring substances; one tablespoonful equals three teaspoons, or 1/2 ounce, or 15 milliliters in metric measure.

tache (TASH)—a small, discolored spot on the skin, such as a freckle; a macule.

tactile (TAK·tul)—pertaining to the sense of touch; capable of being felt.

tactile corpuscle (TAK·tul KOR·pus·ul)—small epidermal structures with nerve endings that are sensitive to touch and pressure.

tag (TAG)—a small appendage, flap, or polyp; skin tag; cutaneous outgrowth of the skin.

tail brush (TAYL BRUSH)—a small, flat brush with stiff bristles and a long, tapering end; used to apply a hair coloring or relaxing product to the hair.

tail comb (TAYL KOHM)—a comb, half of which is shaped into a slender tail-like end. (*See* rat tail comb.)

tailored neckline (TAY·lord NEK·lyn)—a hair shaping in which the hairline is low and angled in the nape area.

talc (TALK)—a soft, white hydrous magnesium silicate used in making powder and soaps.

talcum powder (TAL·kum POW·dur)—finely powdered, purified talc used as a face or body powder.

talipes (TAL·uh·peez)—a deformity of the foot, such as clubfoot.

talipomanus (tal·ih·PAHM·uh·nus)—a deformity of the hand analogous to clubfoot; clubhand.

talus (TAL·us)—bone of the ankle that joins the bones of the leg; the ankle.

tan (TAN)—sunburn; pigmentation of skin from exposure to the sun.

tan color (TAN KUL·ur)—a yellowish-brown color.

tang (TANG)—a projection such as the finger rest on scissors.

tangle (TANG·gul)—a matted mass of hair; snarled hair; to become snarled.

tangled hair (TANG·guld HAYR)—trichonodosis; fraying of the hair resulting in knots, associated with breaking of the hair shaft.

tannic acid (TAN·ik AS·ud)—tannin; an astringent of plant origin.

tanning lotion (TAN·ing LOH·shun)—a sunscreen product, containing oil or other ingredients to assist in the sun-tanning process and to protect the skin while exposed to sun.

tap (TAP)—to touch or strike gently; to pat the face during the application of makeup; in massage, to strike lightly with flexed fingers.

tape (TAYP)—in hairstyling, a narrow strip of material to which adhesive is applied and used to attach false hair to the scalp or face, or to hold flat curls or bangs to the face.

taper (TAY·pur)—a gradual decrease in thickness, narrowing to a point; to become progressively narrower at one end.

tapering (TAY·pur·ing)—in haircutting, to cut the hair at various lengths; to narrow a strand of hair toward the ends.

tapering shears (TAY·pur·ing SHEERZ)—scissors designed for thinning hair and shaping blunt ends.

tapotement (tah·POT·ment)—a massage movement using a short, quick slapping or tapping movement.

tapping (TAP·ing)—a massage movement; striking lightly with the partly flexed fingers.

tar (TAR)—the thick, semisolid brown or black liquid obtained from various species of pine; used to treat certain skin diseases; pine tar.

tarsal artery (TAR·sul ART·uh·ree)—artery that supplies blood to the foot and tarsal joints.

tarsus (TAR·sus)—the root or posterior part of the foot or instep; the seven bones of the instep.

taupe (TOHP)—the color of moleskin, dark gray with a tinge of brown.

taut (TAWT)—tightly drawn; firm; not slack.

teal blue (TEEL BLOO)—a dull greenish-blue color.

tease (TEEZ)—in hairstyling, to comb small sections of hair from the ends toward the scalp to form a cushion or base; also known as ratting, French lacing, or ruffing.

teasing brush (TEEZ·ing BRUSH)—a small brush with short, stiff bristles, and a long, thin handle; used to brush sections of hair from the ends toward the scalp.

teasing comb (TEEZ·ing KOHM)—a comb designed with alternating short and long teeth; used to comb sections of hair from the ends toward the scalp.

teaspoon (TEE·spoon)—1/6 of an ounce. 1/3 of a tablespoon. 5 milliliters in metric measure.

technical (TEK·nih·kul)—relating to a technique; relating to a practical subject organized on scientific principles.

technician (tek·NIH·shun)—an individual trained and expert in a specific skill or subject.

technique (tek·NEEK)—manner of performance; a skill; a process.

tela (TEE·luh)—a weblike structure.

telangiectasis (tel·an·jee·EK·tuh·sus)—loss of hair while hair cells are in the resting stage.

telogen phase (TEL·uh·jen FAYZ)—the final resting phase of the hair cycle in a follicle, lasting until the fully grown hair is shed, at which time anogen begins.

telophase (TEL·uh·fayz)—the final stage of cell mitosis in which the chromosomes reorganize to form an interstage nucleus.

temperature (TEM·pur·uh·chur)—the degree of heat or cold as measured by a thermometer.

temple (TEM·pul)—the flattened space on the side of the forehead.

temporal (TEM·puh·rul)—of or pertaining to the temple.

temporal artery (TEM·puh·rul ART·uh·ree)—deep artery that supplies blood to the temporal muscle, the orbit, and skull.

temporal artery, medial (TEM·puh·rul ART·ur·ee, MEE·dee·ul)—artery that supplies blood to the temporal muscle and eyelids.

temporal artery, superficial (TEM·puh·rul ART·ur·ee, soo·pur·FISH·ul)—artery that supplies blood to the muscles of the head, face, and scalp.

temporal bone (TEM·puh·rul BOHN)—the bone at the side and base of the skull.

temporalis (tem·poh·RAY·lis)—the temporal muscle.

temporal nerve (TEM·puh·rul NURV)—the nerve that receives stimuli from the temporal muscle at the temple.

temporary (TEM·puh·rayr·ee)—not permanent; lasting only for a specific time.

temporary color (TEM·puh·rayr·ee KUL·ur)—a nonpermanent color made from preformed dyes that may be removed by shampooing.

temporary rinse (TEM·puh·rayr·ee RINS)—a nonpermanent color rinse that is used to color the hair and is easily removed by shampoo.

tendon (TEN·dun)—fibrous cord or band connecting muscle with bone.

tendril (TEN·drul)—a small, wispy curl that appears to be falling downward.

tensile (TEN·sul)—capable of being stretched.

tensile strength (TEN·sul STRENGTH)—the resistance of a material to the forces of stress.

tension (TEN·shun)—stress caused by stretching or pulling.

tepid (TEP·ud)—neither hot nor cold; lukewarm.

terminal (TUR·mih·nul)—of or pertaining to an end or extremity; a part that forms the end.

terminal hair (TUR·mih·nul HAYR)—tertiary hair; the long, soft hair found on the scalp; also present on legs, arms, and body of both males and females.

terminology (tur·mih·NAHL·uh·jee)—the special words or terms used in science, art, or business.

terry (TAYR·ee)—a pile fabric in which the loops are uncut; a cotton fabric, very water absorbent; used for towels; terry cloth.

tertiary (TUR·shee·ayr·ee)—third in rank, order, or formation.

tertiary color (TUR·shee·ayr·ee KUL·ur)—an intermediate color achieved by mixing a secondary color and its neighboring primary color on the color wheel in equal amounts; example: blue mixed with green to produce turquoise (blue-green).

Tesla current (TES·luh KUR·unt)—commonly called violet ray; a thermal or heat producing current with a high rate of vibration used by cosmetologists for facial and scalp treatments.

Tesla, Nikola (TES·luh, nih·KOH·luh)—Croatian-American electrical engineer after whom the Tesla high-frequency current is named.

test curls (TEST KURLZ)—a method to predetermine how the client's hair will react to cold waving solution and neutralizer; process of testing the hair to determine curl for motion during the permanent wave.

test strand (TEST STRAND)—a small section of hair on which hair color or chemical relaxer is applied to predetermine how the hair will react.

tetanus (TET·un·us)—an infectious disease that causes spasmodic muscle contractions of voluntary muscles; also called lockjaw.

tetter (TET·ur)—any of various skin eruptions such as herpes, eczema, and psoriasis.

textometer (teks·TAHM·uh·tur)—a device used to measure the elasticity and reaction of the hair to alkaline solutions.

textural combination (TEKS·chur·ul kahm·bih·NAY·shun)—a form incorporating two or more of the basic textures.

texture (TEKS·chur)—the composition or structure of a tissue or organ; the general feel or appearance of a substance.

texture, hair (TEKS·chur, HAYR)—the general quality and feel of the hair such as coarse, medium, fine. The diameter of an individual hair strand.

texture, skin (TEKS·chur, SKIN)—the general feel and appearance of the skin; skin type such as coarse, fine, medium, thin, thick, and degree of elasticity.

texturize (TEKS·chur·yz)—in hairdressing, to cut for effect within the hair length.

thalasso therapy (thal·as·oh THAYR·uh·pee)—water therapy that utilizes sea water and products from the sea.

thallium (THAL·ee·um)—a bluish-white metallic element, the salts of which have been used for epilation; thallium is highly toxic to humans.

thenar (THEE·nar)—the fleshy prominence of the palm corresponding to the base of the thumb.

theory (THEE·uh·ree)—an hypothesis; a reasoned and probable explanation.

therapeutic (thayr·uh·PYOOT·ik)—pertaining to the treatment of disease by remedial agents or methods.

therapeutic lamp (thayr·uh·PYOOT·ik LAMP)—an electrical apparatus producing any of the rays of the spectrum; used for skin and scalp treatments.

therapeutics (thayr·uh·PYOOT·iks)—branch of medical science concerned with the treatment of disease.

therapeutic treatments (thayr·uh·PYOOT·ik TREET·ments)—beneficial treatments for skin, body, or scalp.

therapy (THAYR·uh·pee)—the science and art of healing.

therm (THURM)—a unit of heat to which equivalents have been given, for example, a small calorie, a kilocalorie.

thermal (THUR·mul)—relating to heat.

thermal curling (THUR·mul KURL·ing)—the process of curling straight or pressed hair with a thermal iron.

thermal hairdressing (THUR·mul HAYR·dres·ing)—the art of dressing or setting hair with dry heat.

thermal irons (THUR·mul EYE·urnz)—curling irons.

thermal set (THUR·mul SET)—the technique of setting dry hair with a thermal iron or heated hair rollers.

thermal unit (THUR·mul YOO·nit)—the amount of heat required to raise the temperature of a poind of water one degree Centigrade or Fahrenheit.

thermo cap (THUR·moh KAP)—an insulated cap used in some hair treatments.

thermolysis (thur·MAHL·uh·sus)—the use of high frequency or shortwave current to remove superfluous hair.

thermomassage (THUR·moh·muh·SAHZH)—massage given with the application of heat.

thermometer (thur·MAHM·ut·ur)—any device for measuring temperature.

thermostat (THUR·moh·stat)—an automatic device for regulating temperature.

thiamine (THY·uh·min)—a water-soluble component of vitamin B complex; primary sources are vegetables, egg yolks, organ meats, and whole grains.

thickening agent (THIK·un·ing AY·jent)—a substance that is employed to thicken watery solutions.

thigh (THY)—the part of the lower extremity from the pelvis to the knee.

thighbone (THY·bohn)—the long bone of the thigh; femur.

thinner (THIN·ur)—a product used to thin nail polish.

thinning, hair (THIN·ing, HAYR)—decreasing the thickness of the hair where it is too heavy.

thinning scissors (THIN·ing SIZ·urz)—also called shears; scissors with single or double notched blades; used to thin hair.

thio (THY·oh)—ammonium thioglycolate and thioglycolic acid; used to break down cross linkages of the hair in chemical straightening or cold waving.

thioglycolic acid (thy·oh·GLY·kuh·lik AS·ud)—a colorless liquid or white crystals with a strong unpleasant odor, miscible with water, alcohol or ether; used in permanent wave solutions, hair relaxers, and depilatories.

third-degree burn (THURD-duh·GREE BURN)—a severe burn that destroys the epidermis and underlying tissue, and is more severe than a second-degree burn.

third occipital nerve (THURD ahk·SIP·ut·ul NURV)—nerve that receives stimuli from the skin of the posterior aspect of the neck and scalp.

thoracic (thuh·RAS·ik)—pertaining to the thorax.

thoracic duct (thuh·RAS·ik DUKT)—the common lymph trunk emptying into the left subclavian vein; the principle duct of the lymphatic system.

thorax (THOR·aks)—an elastic bony cage that serves as a protective framework for the heart, lungs, and other internal organs; the chest.

three dimensional (THREE duh·MEN·shun·ul)—having length, width, and depth.

three-dimensional shading (THREE-duh·MEN·shunul SHAYD·ing) —a technique in which hair is bleached and toned with two shades of toner, giving a three-dimensional effect.

throat (THROHT)—the part of the neck leading from the back of the mouth to the stomach and lungs, including the upper larynx, esophagus, and trachea.

thrombocyte (THRAHM·buh·syt)—a blood platelet that aids in clotting.

thumb (THUM)—the short, thick digit next to the forefinger of a human hand.

thumbnail (THUM·nayl)—the nail of the thumb.

thyme (TYM)—a shrub plant of the mint family that produces thyme; used in cosmetics and medicinal preparations.

thymol (THY·mawl)—a compound extracted from the oil of thyme or manufactured synthetically; used in some antiseptics and perfumery.

thymus (THY·mus)—a ductless gland situated in the upper part of the chest; believed to function in the development of the body's immune system.

thyroid cartilage (THY·royd KART·uh·lij)—the largest cartilage of the larynx, composed of two blades that form the Adam's apple.

thyroid gland (THY·royd GLAND)—a large, ductless gland situated in front and on either side of the trachea; it produces the hormone thyroxine, which regulates the growth and metabolism of the body.

thyroxine (thy·RAHK·seen)—a hormone secreted by the thyroid gland; the gland regulating body metabolism and weight control.

tibia (TIB·ee·uh)—the shinbone; the large bone of the leg below the knee.

tibial arteries (TIB·ee·ul ART·uh·reez)—arteries that supply blood to the lower leg and foot.

tibial nerves (TIB·ee·ul NURVZ)—nerves of the leg, sole of the foot, knee, and foot joints.

tight scalp (TYT SKALP)—a scalp that is not easily moved over the underlying structure.

tincture (TING·chur)—an alcoholic solution of a medicinal substance.

tincture of benzoin (TING·chur UV BEN·zuh·wun)—a protective, antiseptic astringent used in healing skin eruptions.

tincture of capsicum (TING·chur UV KAP·sih·kum)—alcoholic solution made from cayenne pepper that is used in a treatment to stimulate hair growth.

tinea (TIN·ee·uh)—a skin disease, especially ringworm.

tinea barbae (TIN·ee·uh BAR·bee)—tinea sycosis.

tinea capitis (TIN·ee·uh KAP·ih·tis)—tinea tonsurans; ringworm of the scalp.

tinea favosa (TIN·ee·uh fah·VOH·suh)—favus; honeycomb ringworm.

tinea pedis (TIN·ee·uh PED·us)—ringworm of the foot.

tinea sycosis (TIN·ee·uh sy·KOH·sus)—parasitic sycosis; ringworm of the beard; barber's itch.

tinea tonsurans (TIN·ee·uh TAHN·syoo·ranz)—tinea capitis; ringworm of the scalp.

tinea unguium (TIN·ee·uh UN·gwee·um)—ringworm of the nail.

tinge (TINJ)—to color or tint slightly.

tint (TINT)—permanent oxidizing hair color product having the ability to lift and deposit color in the same process. (*See* single application color.) To color the hair by means of a permanent hair tint.

tint back (TINT BAK)—to restore the hair to its original color.

tinting (TINT·ing)—the process of adding artificial color to hair.

tip (TIP)—the narrow end of an object; the end of a hair.

tipping (TIP·ing)—similar to frosting, but the darkening or lightening is confined to small strands of hair at the front of the head; lightening the selected ends of the hair.

tipping cap (TIP·ing KAP)—a rubber or plastic head covering designed with small holes all over; hair strands are pulled through the holes and the lightening product applied.

Tirrell burner (tih·REL BURN·ur)—an apparatus used to burn the hair in ash testing.

tis; sis (TIS; SIS)—a word termination added to the name of a part to denote inflammation of that part, such as pityriasis, dermatitis.

tissue (TISH·oo)—a collection of similar cells that perform a particular function.

tissue, connective (TISH·oo, kuh·NEK·tiv)—binding and supporting tissues.

tissue, facial (TISH·oo, FAY·shul)—soft, light absorbent papers, usually of two layers; used as a handkerchief or small towel.

titanium dioxide (ty·TAYN·ee·um dy·AHK·syd)—a white, crystalline powder used in the manufacture of some cosmetics for coverage, especially in foundations, cover sticks, mascara, lipstick, and nail polish.

titian (TISH·un)—a reddish-yellow color.

toenail clipper (TOH·nayl KLIP·ur)—also nipper; an instrument designed for clipping toenails.

tocopherol (toh·KAHF·uh·rawl)—vitamin E; any of a group of four related viscous oils that constitute vitamin E; chief sources are wheat germ and cottonseed oils; used as a dietary supplement, and as an antioxidant in some cosmetic preparations.

toilet (TOY·let)—a cloth cover used in shaving or hairdressing; pertaining to one's grooming regimen.

toilet soap (TOY·let SOHP)—a mild, pure soap containing fats and oils, emollients, preservatives, color, and stabilizers.

toilet water (TOY·let WAW·tur)—a scented liquid containing alcohol; used as an after shave lotion or fragrance; a light, scented water.

toluene diamine (TAHL·yoo·ween DY·uh·min)—a colorless liquid obtained from a coal tar product; used as a solvent in nail polish.

tone or tonality (TOHN or toh·NAL·ut·ee)—in coloring, a term used to describe the warmth or coolness of a color; in muscle tone, healthy functioning of the body or its parts.

tone on tone (TOHN awn TOHN)—a method of coloring hair in which two sections of hair are lightened and toned into two shades of the same color cast.

toner (TOHN·ur)—an aniline derivative tint; a penetrating type used primarily on bleached or pre-lightened hair to achieve pale, delicate colors.

tonic (TAHN·ik)—increasing the strength or tone of the bodily system; an agent or drug that increases body tone.

toning (TOHN·ing)—in hair tinting, adding color to modify the end result. To tone down; to subdue a color to a softer or less emphatic shade; in facials, to tone up; muscle toning; to strengthen and/or invigorate the muscles of the face.

top coat (TAHP KOHT)—liquid, colorless nail enamel applied over polish to prevent chipping and to impart a high gloss.

topette (tahp·ET)—a hair piece such as a wig; wiglet; cascade or fall.

topical (TAHP·ih·kul)—pertaining to the surface; limited to a spot or part of the body.

top of the head (TAHP UV THE HED)—the uppermost front section of the head.

topper (TAHP·ur)—a hair piece, generally made on a round or oval base and designed for use on the top of the head.

topping (TAHP·ing)—the process of cutting the hair on top of the head.

torsade (tor·SAHD)—a woven or foundational hair piece, dressed into a variation of coils or curls.

tortoise-shelling (TOR·tus-SHEL·ing)—the shell of the tortoise (turtle), used for combs and ornaments; in tinting, the use of varying shades of golden blond and platinum on dark and medium dark hair for contrast.

Touch for Health (TUCH FOR HELTH)—a simplified form of kinesiology to relieve stress on muscles and internal organs.

touch up (TUCH up)—to brighten or refresh a recent set; the process of coloring the new growth of tinted or lightened hair. (*See* retouch.)

toupee (too·PAY)—a small wig used to cover the top or crown of a man's head.

toupee adhesive (too·PAY ad·HEE·siv)—a substance used to adhere the hair piece to the scalp.

toupet (too·PET)—a lady's frontal hair piece, larger than a fringe but not as large as semitransformation.

towel blot (TOW·ul BLAHT)—the technique of gently pressing a towel over the hair to remove excess moisture or lotion.

towel dry (TOW·el DRY)—to remove excess moisture from the hair with a towel.

toxemia (tahk·SEE·mee·uh)—form of blood poisoning.

toxic (TAHK·sik)—due to, or of the nature of poison; poisonous.

toxicoderma (tahk·sih·koh·DUR·muh)—disease of the skin due to poison.

toxin (TAHK·sin)—any of various poisonous substances produced by some microorganisms; many are proteins capable of stimulating the production of antibodies or antitoxins.

"T" pin (TEE PIN)—a pin resembling the letter *T*; used to secure a hair piece to the block.

trachea (TRAY·kee·uh)—windpipe; air passage from the larynx to the bronchi and the lungs.

trachoma (truh·KOH·muh)—a contagious disease of the inner eyelids and cornea characterized by scar formation and granulation.

tragacanth (TRAJ·uh·kanth)—a gummy exudation from the stems of Astragalus gummifier; used as a thickener and as an emulsifier.

Trager method (TRAY·gur METH·ud)—movement exercises and gentle shaking of the body to eliminate and prevent tension.

tranquil (TRANG·kwil)—quiet, calm; free from agitation, as a calm atmosphere.

tranquilizer (TRANG·kwuh·ly·zur)—any of a class of drugs having the properties of reducing nervous tension and anxiety.

trans (TRANS)—a prefix used to signify over, across, beyond, through.

transfer rod permanent wave (TRANZ·fur RAHD PUR·muh·nent WAYV)—a permanent wave technique in which the hair is rolled on a small rod, transferred to a large rod, and then neutralized.

transformation (tranz·for·MAY·shun)—a change in the external appearance of an object; an artificial band of hair worn over a person's own hair; a foundational hair piece completely encircling the hairline.

transformer (tranz·FOR·mer)—a device used for increasing or decreasing the voltage of the current used; it can only be used on an alternating current.

translucent (tranz·LOO·sent)—somewhat transparent. The property of letting diffused light pass through.

translucent powder (tranz·LOO·sent POW·dur)—a powder containing the same ingredients as other face powders but to which more titanium dioxide has been added to give the powder an opaque, colorless quality.

transmission (tranz·MISH·un)—passing on of anything; often said of disease.

transmit (tranz·MIT)—to cause to go across; to send over; dispatch.

transmitter (tranz·MIT·ur)—one who or that which transmits.

transparent (tranz·PAYR·ent)—allowing light to pass through; clear.

transplant (TRANZ·plant)—removal of hair from a part of the body or head by surgical means and affix it to a bald area of the scalp; to transfer tissue or organ from one part of the body to another; graft.

transverse (tranz·VURS)—lying or being across or crosswise.

transverse facial artery (tranz·VURS FAY·shul ART·ur·ee)—artery supplying the skin, the parotid gland, and the masseter muscle.

transverse nerve (tranz·VURS NURV)—nerve that receives stimuli from the skin of the neck.

trapezius (truh·PEE·zee·us)—muscle that draws the head backward and sideways; covers the upper and middle back and back of neck.

trapezoid (TRAP·uh·zoyd)—a small bone in the second row of the corpus.

trauma (TRAW·muh)—a wound or injury.

treatment (TREET·ment)—a substance, technique, or regimen used in therapeutic practices.

tremble (TREM·bul)—to shake or quiver involuntarily.

tremor (TREM·ur)—an involuntary trembling or quivering.

trend (TREND)—the general direction, course, or tendency of fashion or style.

treponema pallida (trip·uh·NEE·muh PAL·ih·duh)—bacteria causing syphilis.

tress (TRES)—a lock or ringlet of hair.

tressed (TREST)—hair arranged in braids; long hair.

triangular (try·ANG·gyuh·lur)—having three sides joined at three angles or corners.

triangularis (try·ang·gyuh·LAY·rus)—depressor anguli oris; a muscle that pulls down corners of the mouth.

triangular-shaped face (try·ANG·gyuh·lur-SHAYPT FAYS)—a face with a narrow forehead, having the greater width at the jawline.

triceps (TRY·seps)—a large three-headed muscle at the back of the arm that extends the forearm.

trichiasis (trik·EYE·uh·sus)—a condition in which hairs, especially the eyelashes, turn inward causing irritation of the eyeball.

trichology (trih·KAHL·uh·jee)—the science dealing with the hair, its disease and care.

trichomadesis (trik·uh·muh·DEE·sus)—abnormal hair loss.

trichonosis (trik·uh·NOH·sis)—any disease of the hair.

trichopathy (trih·KAHP·uh·thee)—pertaining to diseases of the hair.

trichophytina (trik·oh·fih·TEE·nuh)—a fungus that thrives in the hair follicles, causing tinea.

trichophyton (try·KAWF·ih·tahn)—a fungus that attacks the hair, skin, and nails, causing dermatophytosis.

trichophytosis (trih·KAWF·ih·TOH·sus)—ringworm of the skin and scalp due to invasion by fungus.

trichoptilosis (trih·kahp·tih·LOH·sus)—a splitting of the hair ends, giving them a feathery appearance.

trichorrhea (trik·uh·REE·uh)—a rapid loss of hair.

trichorrhexis (trik·uh·REK·sis)—brittleness of the hair.

trichorrhexis nodosa (trik·uh·REK·sis nuh·DOH·suh)—a hair disease characterized by brittleness and the formation of nodular swellings on the hair shafts.

trichosiderin (trih·kuh·SID·ur·un)—a pigment containing iron found in human red hair.

trichosis (trih·KOH·sus)—any diseased condition of the hair.

trichromat (TRY·kroh·mat)—a person with normal color vision; the ability to distinguish the primary colors: red, yellow, and blue.

trichromatic (try·kroh·MAT·ik)—three-colored; having three standard colors.

tricuspid (try·KUS·pid)—having three points, as the right auriculoventricular valve of the heart.

trifacial nerve (try·FAY·shul NURV)—the fifth cranial nerve; trigeminus nerve; receives stimuli from the face and scalp.

trigeminal (try·JEM·un·ul)—relating to the fifth cranial or trigeminus nerve, which divides into three division: mandibular, maxillary, and ophthalmic.

triglyceride (try·GLIS·ur·yd)—a fat found in adipose cells; a compound consisting of three molecules of fatty acid linked to glycerol.

trim (TRIM)—a haircut in which the hair is cut without altering the shape of the existing lines; to remove a small amount of hair from the ends.

triolein (try·OH·lee·un)—glyceryl trioleate; an olive oil used in nondrying creams, lotions, and other cosmetic preparations.

triphase (TRY·fayz)—a method of color application; first to the midshaft then to ends of hair and finally to the hair nearest the scalp.

trochlea (TRAHK·lee·uh)—a pulleylike process; a smooth articular surface of bone upon which another glides.

trochlea muscularis (TRAHK·lee·uh mus·kyuh·LAYR·us)—an attachment that changes the direction of the pull of a muscle.

trochlear nerve (TRAHK·lee·ur NURV)—the fourth cranial nerve.

trophedema (troh·fuh·DEE·muh)—chronic edema of the feet or legs due to damage to nerves or blood-supplying vessels in the area.

trophic (TROH·fik)—pertaining to nutrition and its processes.

trophodynamics (trohf·uh·dy·NAM·iks)—the branch of medical science dealing with the forces governing nutrition.

trophology (troh·FAHL·uh·jee)—the science of nutrition.

trophopathy (troh·FAHP·uh·thee)—a disorder caused by improper or inadequate nutrition, such as a vitamin or mineral deficiency.

trough (TRAWF)—the semicircular area of a wave between two ridges.

true fixative (TROO FIKS·uh·tiv)—substance that makes something permanent; or holds back evaporation of other materials.

true skin (TROO SKIN)—the corium; dermis.

trunk (TRUNK)—the human body exclusive of the extremities (arms, legs, neck, head).

trypsin (TRIP·sun)—an enzyme in the digestive juice secreted by the pancreas; trypsin changes proteins into peptones.

tryptophan (TRIP·tuh·fan)—an amino acid existing in proteins; essential in human nutrition.

Tshanpau (TSHAN·pow)—the Hindu method of massage at the bath.

tubercle (TOO·bur·kul)—an abnormal rounded, solid lump on the skin, bone, or an organ.

tuberculosis (tuh·bur·kyoo·LOH·sus)—an infectious disease due to a specific bacillus; characterized by the formulation of tubercles, usually in the lungs.

tuberculosis cutis (tuh·bur·kyoo·LOH·sis KYOO·tis)—tuberculosis of the skin.

tuberose oil (TOOB·uh·roz OYL)—oil obtained from the Mexican plant of the agave family; used in perfumes.

tubular (TOOB·yuh·lur)—tube shaped; resembling a long, hollow, cylindrical body.

tuck (TUK)—reducing the size of a wig cap by folding the netting into a tuck formation and sewing the fold together.

Tui-na (QE)—the Chinese method of massage using pressure points of the body.

tumefacient (too·muh·FAY·shunt)—swollen; tending to cause swelling.

tumid (TOO·mud)—swollen; enlarged; puffy.

tumor (TOO·mur)—a swelling; an abnormal cell mass resulting from excessive multiplication of cells, varying in size, shape, and color.

turbinal; turbinate (TUR·buh·nul; TUR·buh·nayt)—a bone in the nose; turbinated body.

turbinated (TUR·buh·nayt·ud)—shaped like a top; scroll-shaped.

turning (TURN·ing)—in wiggery, the procedure by which root ends are arranged to prevent hair from tangling and to ensure correct positioning in weaving; to align the roots all on one end.

turpentine gum (TUR·pen·tyn GUM)—the brownish-yellow, sticky oleoresin from the terebinth pine and other coniferous trees; used as a solvent in hair preparations and some kinds of soap.

tweezers (TWEEZ·urz)—a pair of small forceps to remove hair.

tweezing (TWEEZ·ing)—removing hair with the use of a tweezer.

twice-in-weft (TWYS-in-WEFT)—a more widely spaced method of weaving than once-in weaving.

twine (TWYN)—to form a coil of hair; to interlace.

twist (TWIST)—in hairdressing, to form the hair into a roll or spiral shape; an overlapping of a section of hair as a French twist or roll.

two dimensional (TOO·duh·MEN·shun·ul)—having length and width.

two-dimensional shading (TOO-duh·MEN·shun·ul SHAYD·ing)—a hair coloring effect using two or more colors to add dimension or accentuate a style.

typhoid (TY·foyd)—acute, infectious fever with intestinal lesions and an eruption of rose-colored spots on the chest and abdomen.

Tyrosinase (TY·ruh·sin·ays)—the enzyme that reacts together with the amino acid tyrosine to form the hair's natural melanin pigment.

tyrosine (TY·ruh·seen)—an amino acid widely distributed in proteins, particularly in casein. Reacts together with the enzyme tyrosinase to form hair's natural melanin pigment.

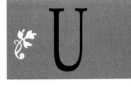

ulcer (UL·sur)—an open sore on an internal or external part of the body.

ulceroglandular (ul·sur·uh·GLAN·dyuh·lur)—pertaining to ulcers involving lymph nodes.

ulna (UL·nuh)—the inner and larger bone of the forearm, attached to the wrist and located on the little finger side.

ulnar (UL·nur)—pertaining to the ulna or to the ulnar, or medial aspect of the arm as compared to the radial (lateral) aspect.

ulnar artery (UL·nur ART·ur·ee)—artery that supplies blood to the muscle of the little finger, side of the arm, and the hand.

ulnar nerve (UL·nur NURV)—the nerve that affects the muscles of the little finger, side of the arm and the hand.

ulodermatitis (yoo·loh·dur·muh·TY·tis)—inflammation of the skin with formation of cicatrices.

ultra (UL·truh)—a prefix denoting beyond; on the other side; excessively.

ultramarine blue (ul·truh·muh·REEN BLOO)—a blue pigment obtained by grinding lapis lazula or produced synthetically; used in eyeshadows, powders, and mascara.

ultraviolet (ul·truh·VY·uh·let)—invisible rays of the spectrum that are beyond the violet rays; used for germicidal purposes.

un (UN)—a prefix denoting not; contrary.

unadulterated (un·uh·DUL·tur·ayt·ud)—pure, unmixed.

unciform (UN·sih·form)—hook-shaped, the bone on the inner side of the second row of the carpus.

unctuous (UNG·chuh·wus)—greasy; oily.

undercut (UN·dur·kut)—to cut hair from the underside or the nape area.

underdirected (un·dur·dih·REK·tud)—having less than the usual or normal amount of direction.

underelevation (un·dur·el·uh·VAY·shun)—hair-shaping technique in which hair is cut on top of the head, longer at the crown, then progressively shorter to create overlapping.

underknotting (un·dur·NAHT·ing)—fine knotting used under the hairline of foundational hair pieces.

underprocessing (un·dur·PRAH·ses·ing)—insufficient exposure of the hair to the chemical action of the waving solution, resulting in little or no change in hair structure and condition of the hair.

undertint (UN·dur·tint)—a subdued tint; not bright.

undertone (UN·dur·tohn)—a subdued shade of a color; a color upon which another color has been imposed and which can be seen through the other color. The underlying color that emerges during the lifting process of melanin, that contributes to the end result. When lightening hair, a residual warm tone occurs. Also called contributing pigment.

undulation (un·juh·LAY·shun)—a wavelike movement or shape.

unguent (UN·gwunt)—an ointment or salve.

unguentum (un·GWEN·tum); pl., **unguenta** (un·GWEN·uh)—a salve or ointment.

unguis (UN·gwis)—the nail of a finger or toe.

unguis incarnatus (UN·gwis in·kar·NAY·tus)—ingrown fingernails or toenails.

unguium, tinea (UN·gwee·um, TIN·ee·uh)—ringworm of the nails.

uni (YOO·nih)—a prefix denoting one; once.

unidirectional (yoo·nih·dih·REK·shun·ul)—moving in one direction.

unidirectional current (yoo·nih·dih·REK·shun·ul KUR·rent)—an electric current of uniform direction; a direct current.

uniform layering (YOO·nih·form LAY·ur·ing)—the effect produced by sculpting the hair at the same length consistently; using a 90° (normal) projection angle.

unipolar (yoo·nih·POH·lur)—having or acting by a single magnetic pole; the application of one electrode of a direct current to the body during a treatment.

unisex (YOO·nih·seks)—cosmetology services suitable for both men and women.

unit (YOO·nit)—a single thing or value.

United States Pharmacopeia (USP) (yoo·NYT·ud STAYTS far·muh·kuh·PEE·uh)—an official book of drug and medicinal standards.

unprofessional (un·pruh·FESH·un·ul)—in violation of ethical codes and standards of conduct of a profession.

unstable (un·STAY·bul)—not firm; not constant; readily decomposing or changing in chemical composition or biological activity.

unwind (un·WYND)—to unwrap hair from a permanent wave or hair-setting rod.

upangle cutting (up·ANG·gul KUT·ing)—cutting subsections of hair into layers, longer by degrees from the innermost to the outermost layers of hair.

upblending (up·BLEND·ing)—blending the hair upward from the nape.

upelevation (up·el·uh·VAY·shun)—a technique in which hair is cut in graduated lengths, shorter to longer; upangle cutting.

upstroke (UP·strohk)—stroking upward, as in shaving.

upsweep (UP·sweep)—a hairstyle combed up from the nape of the neck toward the crown.

urea (yoo·REE·uh)—a colorless crystalline compound; the chief solid component of urine and an end product of protein metabolism; used in some cosmetic and medicinal products.

urea peroxide (yoo·REE·uh puh·RAHK·syd)—a combination of urea and peroxide in the form of a cream developer or activator; occasionally employed in hair coloring. When added to an alkaline mixture, it releases oxygen.

uric acid (YOO·rik AS·ud)—a crystalline acid contained in urine; a product of protein metabolism.

uridrosis, urhidrosis (yoo·ry·DROH·sis, yur·hy·DROH·sis)—the presence of urea in the sweat in excess of normal.

urticaria (urt·uh·KAYR·ee·uh)—a skin condition characterized by smooth and slightly elevated patches sometimes whiter or redder than the surrounding skin, with severe itching; hives; nettle rash.

urticaria medicamentosa (ur·tih·KAYR·ee·uh med·ih·kuh·ment·TOH·suh)—skin eruptions due to the ingestion of a drug to which the individual is allergic.

urticaria papulosa (ur·tih·KAYR·ee·uh pap·yoo·LOH·suh)—a pruritic skin eruption usually in children, related to insect bites and characterized by papules.

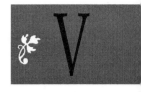

vaccination (vak·sih·NAY·shun)—inoculation; administration of any vaccine.

vaccine (vak·SEEN)—any substance used for preventive inoculation.

vacuum (VAK·yoom)—a space entirely devoid of matter; a space from which the air has been exhausted.

vacuum procedure (VAK·yoom pruh·SEE·jur)—the use of a suction-type apparatus to cleanse the pores during a facial treatment.

vagus (VAY·gus)—pneumogastric nerve; tenth cranial nerve.

valence (VAY·lens)—the capacity of an atom to combine with other atoms in definite proportions.

valine (VAL·een)—amino acid essential in human nutrition.

value (VAL·yoo)—*see* level; depth.

valve (VALV)—a structure that temporarily closes a passage or orifice or permits flow in one direction only.

vanishing cream (VAN·ish·ing KREEM)—a skin cream formulated to leave no oily residue on the surface of the skin.

vapor (VAY·pur)—a gas; the gaseous form of a substance that at ordinary temperature is liquid or a solid.

vaporization (vay·pur·ih·ZAY·shun)—act or process of converting a solid or liquid into a vapor.

vaporizer (VAY·pur·eye·zur)—an apparatus designed to turn water or other substance into vapor; used in hair and skin treatments; a vaporizing machine.

variable (VAYR·ee·uh·bul)—changeable; subject to variations or changes.

variation (vayr·ee·AY·shun)—changes of differences, as in procedures or styles.

varicolored (VAYR·ee·kul·urd)—having various or several colors.

varicophlebitis (vayr·ih·koh·fluh·BY·tis)—inflammation of a varicose vein or veins.

varicose veins (VAYR·ih·kohs VAYNZ)—swollen or knotted veins.

varicosis (vayr·ih·KOH·sis)—a dilated or varicose state of a vein or veins.

variegating (VAYR·ee·uh·gayt·ing)—lightening small sections or strands of hair throughout the head; also known as frosting.

varnish (VAR·nish)—a product used to give the nails a smooth, glossy appearance; nail polish.

vasa lymphatica profunda (VAY·suh lim·FAT·ih·kuh proh·FUN·duh)—the deep lymphatic vessels.

vasa lymphatica superficialia (VAY·suh lim·FAT·ih·kuh soo·pur·FISH·ee·AY·lee·uh)—the superficial lymphatic vessels.

vascular (VAS·kyoo·lur)—supplied with small blood vessels; pertaining to a vessel for the conveyance of a fluid, such as blood or lymph.

vascular bed (VAS·kyoo·lur BED)—the total blood supply system of an organ or region of the body: arteries, capillaries, veins.

vascularity (vas·kyuh·LAYR·ih·tee)—the condition of being vascular.

vascularization (vas·kyuh·lar·ih·ZAY·shun)—the formation of capillaries; the process of becoming vascular.

vascular system (VAS·kyuh·lur SIS·tem)—the organs of the body involved in the circulation of the blood: heart, arteries, veins, and capillaries.

vasoconstrictor (vay·zoh·kun·STRIK·tur)—a nerve or agent that causes narrowing of blood vessels.

vasodilator (vas·oh·dih·LAY·tur)—a nerve or agent that causes expansion of the blood vessels.

vegetable dye (VEJ·tuh·bul DYE)—a natural organic coloring obtained from the leaves or bark of plants; examples are henna and camomile, which are used to tint hair.

vegetable facial mask (VEJ·tuh·bul FAY·shul MASK)—a mask made of fresh vegetables such as cucumber or avocado; used on the face for their beneficial enzyme action.

vegetable oil (VEJ·tuh·bul OYL)—any of various liquid fats obtained from seeds of certain plants; examples are peanut, olive, and sesame seed oil; used in hypoallergenic and a wide variety of other cosmetics including baby preparations, creams, lotions, powders, and hair-grooming products.

vegetable peel (VEJ·tuh·bul PEEL)—a mild skin peeling process using creams or lotions containing vegetable enzymes.

vegetable sponge (VEJ·tuh·bul SPUNJ)—a genus of the gourd family producing a fibrous fruit used as a sponge; a loofah.

vegetable tints (VEJ·tuh·bul TINTS)—tints comprised of Egyptian henna, indigo, or camomile; used as hair tints or hair rinses.

vein; vena (VAYN; VEE·nuh)—a blood vessel carrying blood toward the heart.

vellus (VEL·us)—the fine, downy hair that appears on the body, with the exception of the palms of the hands and soles of the feet.

vena cava (VEE·nuh KAH·vuh)—one of the two large veins that carry the blood to the right auricle of the heart.

vena cutanea (VEE·nuh kyoo·TAY·nee·uh)—a cutaneous vein.

venenata, dermatitis (VEN·uh·nah·tuh dur·muh·TY·tus)—inflammation produced by local action of irritating substances.

venous (VEE·nus)—pertaining to or marked with veins.

ventilate (VEN·tuh·layt)—to renew the air in a place; to oxygenate the blood in the capillaries of the lungs.

ventilated (VEN·tuh·layt·ud)—describes a method of knotting single strand groups of hair individually to the net foundation of a wig.

ventilating needle (VEN·tuh·layt·ing NEE·dul)—a miniature crocheting needle, made of spring steel; used in attaching hair to a foundation.

ventricle (VEN·truh·kul)—a small cavity, particularly in the brain or heart; one of the two lower chambers of the heart.

venule (VEEN·yool)—a small vein or smallest branch of a vein.

vermillion (vur·MIL·yun)—a bright orange-red color; also called Chinese red and cinnabar.

verruca (vuh·ROO·kuh)—a wart; a circumscribed hypertrophy of the papillae and epidermis.

verrucose; verrucous (VUR·oo·kohs, vur·OO·kohs, vur·OO·kus)—warty; presenting wartlike elevations.

versicolor (VUR·sih·kul·ur)—having a variety of colors; iridescent; changing color under different light.

vertebra (VUR·tuh·brah); pl., **vertebrae** (VUR·tuh·bree)—a boney segment of the spinal column.

vertebral artery (VUR·tuh·brul ART·ur·ee)—artery that supplies blood to the muscles of the neck.

vertex (VUR·teks)—the crown or top of the head; top; highest point.

vertical (VUR·tih·kul)—in an upright position; usually described in terms of up and down as opposed to left and right.

vertical base (VUR·tih·kul BAYS)—a vertical section of a hair form used in practical exercises.

vesicant (VES·ih·kent)—an agent that produces blisters on the skin.

vesicle (VES·ih·kul)—a small blister or sac with clear fluid in it.

vesicle bulla (VES·ih·kul BOOL·uh)—a large vesicle; blister.

vesicular (vuh·SIK·yuh·lur)—relating to or containing vesicles.

vesiculopapular (veh·sik·yuh·loh·PAP·yuh·lur)—consisting of both vesicles and papules.

vesiculopustular (vuh·sik·yuh·loh·PUS·tyoo·lur)—consisting of both vesicles and pustules.

vessel (VES·ul)—tube or canal in which blood, lymph, or other fluid is contained or conveyed or circulated.

vibex (VIH·beks); pl., **vibices** (VY·bih·seez)—a narrow linear mark on the skin; stretchmark; a condition generally caused by pregnancy or rapid weight gain.

vibrate (VY·brayt)—to swing; to mark or to measure by oscillation.

vibration (vy·BRAY·shun)—shaking; a to-and-fro movement.

vibration, massage movement (vy·BRAY·shun, muh·SAHZH MOOV·ment)—also called shaking movement; consists of pressing fingertips to the point of application and shaking the arms to produce a stimulating effect on tissues.

vibration treatment (vy·BRAY·shun TREET·ment)—massage by rapid shaking of the body part; given by hand, machine or oscillator.

vibrator (VY·bray·tur)—an electrically driven apparatus used in some massage procedures.

vibrator scalp treatment (VY·bray·tur SKALP TREET·ment)—massage for the scalp given with the aid of a hand vibrator.

vibratory (VY·bruh·toh·ree)—vibrations or light, rapid percussion used in massage, and given by hand or an electrical apparatus.

vibrissa (vy·BRIS·uh); pl., **vibrissae** (vy·BRIS·ee)—stiff hairs in the nostrils.

vibroid (VY·broyd)—a vibratory movement in massage.

villus (VIL·us); pl., **villi** (VIL·eye)—minute, fingerlike processes covering the surface of the mucous membrane of the small intestine.

vinegar (VIN·uh·gur)—a sour liquid used as a condiment or as a preservative, formed by fermentation of dilute alcoholic liquids as wine, cider, etc.; it contains acetic acid.

violet (VY·uh·let)—a bluish-red color; bluish-purple hue.

violet-ray (VY·uh·let-ray)—high frequency; an electric current of medium voltage and medium amperage; also called Tesla current.

virgin bleaching (VUR·jin BLEECH·ing)—first bleaching (lightening) of the hair.

virgin hair (VUR·jin HAYR)—natural hair that has had not previous bleaching or tinting treatments, chemical or physical abuse.

virgin tint (VUR·jin TINT)—first time the hair has been tinted.

virulent (VEER·yuh·lent)—extremely poisonous; marked by a rapid, severe course, as an infection; able to overcome bodily defense mechanisms.

virus (VY·rus)—the causative agent of an infectious disease; any of a large group of submicroscopic structures capable of infesting almost all plants and animals, including bacteria.

viscera (VIS·uh·ruh)—plural of viscus; the organs enclosed within the cranium, thorax, abdomen, or pelvis, especially the organs within the abdominal cavity.

visceral (VIS·ur·ul)—pertaining to viscera.

visceral cranium (VIS·ur·ul KRAY·nee·um)—the part of the skull that forms the face and jaws.

viscid (VIS·ud)—sticky or adhesive; glutinous.

viscosity (vis·KAHS·ut·ee)—the degree of density, thickness, stickiness, and adhesiveness of a substance.

viscous (VIS·kus)—sticky or gummy.

viscus (VIS·kus); pl., **viscera** (VIS·ur·uh)—an internal organ located in the cavity of the trunk or in the thorax, cranium, or pelvis.

visible rays (VIZ·uh·bul RAYZ)—light rays that can be seen.

vital (VY·tul)—relating to life; concerned with or necessary to the maintenance of life.

vitality (vy·TAL·ut·ee)—vigor; to grow, develop, and perform the functions of a living body.

vitamin (VY·tuh·min)—one of a group of organic substances present in a very small quantity in natural food stuffs, which are essential to normal metabolism and the lack of which causes deficiency diseases.

vitamin chart (VY·tuh·min CHART)—a chart showing the essential vitamins and minerals, their sources, and benefits.

vitiligines (vit·ih·LIH·jih·neez)—depigmented areas of the skin.

vitiligo (vih·til·EYE·goh)—milky-white spots of the skin.

volatile (VAHL·uh·tul)—easily evaporating; diffusing freely; explosive.

volt (VOLT)—the unit of electromotive force; the electromotive force that, steadily applied to a conductor with a resistance of one ohm, will produce a current of one ampere.

voltage (VOL·tij)—electrical potential difference expressed in volts.

voltage drop (VOL·tij DRAHP)—the decrease in the potential energy in an electric circuit due to the resistance of the conductor.

voltaic cell (vohl·TAY·ik SEL)—a receptacle for producing direct electric current by chemical action.

voltaic current (vohl·TAY·ik KUR·ent)—galvanic current.

voltaic electricity (vohl·TAY·ik ih·lek·TRIS·ut·ee)—galvanic electricity.

voltmeter (VOHLT·mee·tur)—an instrument used for measuring (in volts) the differences of potential between different points of an electrical circuit.

volume (VAHL·yoom)—amount (bulk or mass); quantity; space occupied, as measured in cubic units; the lift, elevation, and height created by the formation of curls or waves in the hair; measure of potential oxidation of varying strengths of hydrogen peroxide. Expressed as volumes of oxygen liberated per volume of solution; 20 vol. peroxide would thus liberate 20 pints (99.4 liters) of oxygen gas for each pint (liter) of solution.

volume curl (VAHL·yoom KURL)—a pincurl with the stem moving upward from the scalp to create fullness.

volume of peroxide (VAHL·yoom UV pur·AHK·syd)—the concentration of hydrogen peroxide in water solution; as 20 volume peroxide.

voluntary (VAHL·un·tayr·ee)—under the control of the will; being done by choice.

voluntary muscle (VAHL·un·tayr·ee MUS·ul)—striated muscle under the control of the will.

vomer (VOH·mur)—the thin plate of bone between the nostrils.

vortices pilorum (VORT·uh·seez py·LOH·rum)—hair whorls; commonly called a cowlick.

vulgaris, acne (vul·GAYR·is AK·nee)—common pimple condition.

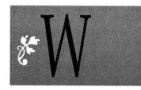

wall plate (WAWL PLAYT)—an apparatus equipped with indicators and controlling devices to produce various currents, used for facial treatments.

wall socket (WAWL SAHK·ut)—a wall receptacle into which may be fitted the plug of an electrical appliance.

walnut (WAWL·nut)—a warm, reddish-brown color.

walnut stain (WAWL·nut STAYN)—one of the wood extracts historically used as a hair coloring.

warm (WORM)—having the color or tone of something that imparts heat, as in the range of colors from yellow or gold through orange and red.

wart (WORT)—verruca; a circumscribed hypertrophy of the papillae of the corium, usually of the hand, covered by thickened epidermis.

water blister (WAW·tur BLIS·tur)—a blister with watery contents.

water, hard (WAW·tur, HARD)—water containing certain minerals; does not lather with soap.

water, soft (WAW·tur, SAWFT)—water that lathers easily with soap and is relatively free of minerals.

water softener (WAW·tur SAWF·un·ur)—certain chemicals, such as the carbonate or phosphate of sodium, used to soften hard water to permit the lathering of soap.

water soluble (WAW·tur SAHL·yoo·bul)—able to dissolve in water.

water vapor (WAW·tur VAY·pur)—water diffused in a vaporous form; used in some facial treatments.

water-wrapped perm (WAW·tur-RAPT PURM)—a permanent wave wrapped with water and the waving lotion applied after the entire head is wrapped; this is done to control timing during the process.

watt (WAHT)—the electrical unit of energy; the power required to cause a current of one ampere to flow between points differing in potential by one volt; a measurement of how much electric energy is being used in one second.

wattage (WAHT·ij)—amount of electric power expressed in watts.

watt hour (WAHT OW·ur)—one watt of power expended for one hour.

wave (WAYV)—two connecting c-shapings placed in alternating directions.

wave clip (WAYV KLIP)—a clamplike device with rows of small teeth used to hold a wave in place while the hair dries.

wave, cold (WAYV, KOHLD)—a method of permanent waving using chemicals instead of heat.

wave, croquignole marcel (WAYV, KROH·ken·yoh mar·SEL)—a wave produced with the marcel iron, using the croquignole winding.

wave, marcel (WAYV, mar·SEL)—a wave that resembles a perfect natural wave; produced by means of heated irons.

waves (WAYVZ)—hair formation resulting in a side-by-side series of S-like movements or half-circles going in opposite directions.

wave, shadow (WAYV SHAD·oh)—a wave with low ridges and shallow waves.

wax (WAKS)—a substance insoluble in water but soluble in most organic solvents; derived from animal sources such as beeswax, stearic acid, and Chinese wax; vegetable sources such as carnauba, bayberry, etc.; mostly composed of fatty acid esters and alcohol; waxes are used in cosmetics, packaging, candles, and many other products; in cosmetology, waxes are used for facial masks and as aid to the removal of superfluous hair.

wax depilatory (WAKS dih·PIL·uh·tor·ee)—a soft wax applied to remove superfluous hair.

wax heater (WAKS HEET·ur)—a thermostatically controlled heating pot used to warm wax to be used for a facial or depilatory treatment.

wax mask (WAKS MASK)—a special mixture of oils and waxes used to form a facial mask for facial treatments; these waxes may be combinations of beeswax, mineral oil, and similar oils and waxes.

weave (WEEV)—a technique in hair styling accomplished by interlacing strands of hair to form intricate patterns.

weaving, hair (WEEV·ing, HAYR)—a special technique of sewing or weaving, wefts of matched hair into a net-shaped base, of nylon thread, which had previously been tied into the remaining hair on the head.

weaving silk (WEEV·ing SILK)—a strong, fine silk used on weaving sticks when weaving hair into a weft.

wedged parting (WEJD PART·ing)—a triangular sectioning pattern used as a base for a standup curl.

weft (WEFT)—an artificial section of woven hair used for practice work or as a substitute for natural hair.

weft wig (WEFT WIG)—a wig made of wefts of hair sewn into a wig base; a machine-made wig.

weight (WAYT)—mass in form and space; the length concentration in a hair design.

weight (WAYT LYN)—the line of maximum length within the weight area.

welt (WELT)—a ridge of lump usually on the scalp.

wet pack (WET PAK)—packing the body or a part in towels that have been saturated in water or other fluids for therapeutic purposes.

wet sanitizer (WET SAN·ih·ty·zur)—a container filled with a germicidal solution into which implements are placed for sanitizing, and can be completely immersed.

wetting agent (WET·ing AY·jent)—a substance that causes a liquid to spread more readily on a solid surface, chiefly through a reduction of surface tension.

wheal (WHEEL)—a raised ridge on the skin, usually caused by a blow, a bite of an insect, urticaria, or a sting of a nettle.

wheat germ oil (WHEET JURM OYL)—the oil of the wheat embryo used in oils, fats, food, and cosmetic products as a stabilizer.

white (WHYT)—the color produced by reflection of all the light rays in the spectrum; the absence of pigment; having light-colored skin; having the color of milk or new snow.

white corpuscle (WHYT KOR·pus·ul)—leukocyte; cell in the blood whose function is to destroy disease germs.

whitehead (WHYT·hed)—milium.

whiten (WHYT·un)—to make white or lighter as in the use of a white lead to whiten tips of the fingernails.

whorl (WHORL)—hair that forms in a swirl effect, as on the crown.

widow's peak (WIH·dohz PEEK)—a "V" shaped growth of hair at the center of the forehead. (*See* peak.)

wig (WIG)—an artificial covering for the head consisting of a network of interwoven hair.

wig bar (WIG BAR)—a showcase or counter for the sale of ready-to-wear wigs and hair pieces.

wig block (WIG BLAHK)—a head-shaped block (which may be constructed of wood, cork-filled cloth, plastic, or other materials) on which hair pieces and wigs are formed or dressed.

wig brush (WIG BRUSH)—a brush with semistiff bristles used to comb and disentangle a wig after cleaning.

wig cap (WIG KAP)—the foundation to which the hair or fiber of a wig is attached.

wig cleaner (WIG KLEEN·ur)—any type of dry-cleaning fluid that may be used to clean wigs and hair pieces.

wig conditioner (WIG kuh·DIH·shun·ur)—a product, in cream, lotion, or spray form, which is used to restore life and add luster to wigs or hair pieces.

wiglet (WIG·lut)—a hair piece with a flat base that is used in special areas of the head.

wig net (WIG NET)—a soft, narrow-meshed net of silk, cotton, linen, or nylon, used in the base of a wig or hair piece.

wig pin (WIG PIN)—a steel pin about two inches in length with a "T" shaped head, used to secure a wig to a canvas head-block while combing and styling.

wig spray (WIG SPRAY)—a hair spray used to hold coiffures set in wigs.

wig spring (WIG SPRING)—a small spring inserted into a wig or hair piece to hold it to the head.

wig stand (WIG STAND)—a head-shaped stand designed for keeping wigs in the proper shape when not being worn.

winding, croquignole (WYND·ing, KROH·ken·yohl)—winding the hair from the hair ends towards the scalp.

windpipe (WIND·pyp)—the trachea.

wine color (WYN KUL·ur)—the color of red wine; dark purplish-red, similar to burgandy wine.

wintergreen oil (WIN·tur·green OYL)—an oil made from the leaves of the wintergreen shrub or bark of sweet birch; used in flavorings, mouthwashes, toothpastes, and some medicinal products.

wire mesh roller (WYR MESH ROHL·ur)—a hair roller made of wire open-work mesh to allow for faster drying of the hair.

wiry hair (WYR·ee HAYR)—a hair fiber that is strong and resilient, difficult to form into a curl formation, and having a smooth, hard, glossy surface.

wisp (WISP)—a small, lightweight, thin strand of hair; light, fluffy curls.

witch hazel (WICH HAY·zul)—an extract with alcohol and water of the bark of the hamamelis shrub; soothing and mildly astringent; used as a lotion and mild medication.

wood's lamp (WOODZ LAMP)—a light used to study and analyze skin conditions.

wool crepe (WOOL KRAYP)—a material used to keep hair ends smooth when winding in permanent waving.

wooly hair (WOOL·ee HAYR)—short, overcurly hair.

wrap (RAP)—to wind the hair on permanent wave rods.

wrapping (RAP·ing)—winding hair on rollers or rods in order to form curls.

wring (RING)—to squeeze or compress by twisting.

wrinkle (RINK·ul)—a small ridge or furrow on the skin.

wrinkle remover (RINK·ul ree·MOOV·ur)—a cream or lotion claimed to be formulated to puff up and fill out lines in the face; there is no scientific evidence to support claims that such products actually remove wrinkles from the skin.

wrist (RIST)—the joint between the hand and arm.

wrist electrode (RIST ih·LEK·trohd)—an electrode for high-frequency current attached to the wrist to produce mild current during a phase of a facial treatment.

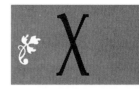

xanthochroid (ZAN·thuh·kroyd)—characterized by a light yellow or fair complexion.

xanthochromia (zan·thoh·KROH·mee·uh)—a yellowish discoloration of the skin or cerebrospinal fluid.

xanthoma (zan·THOH·muh)—a skin disease characterized by the presence of yellow nodules or slightly raised plates in the subcutaneous tissue, often around tendons.

xanthoma palpebrarum (zan·THOH·muh pal·puh·BRAY·rum)—yellowish, raised patches occurring around the eyelids resulting from lipid-filled cells in the dermis.

xanthosis (zan·THOH·sis)—a discoloration of the skin caused by eating an overabundance of carotene-producing foods, such as squash, carrots, etc.; the condition is reversible.

xanthous (ZAN·thus)—having yellowish skin tone.

xerasia (zuh·RAY·zee·uh; zuh·RAH·zhuh)—a disease of the hair marked by cessation of growth, dryness, and general lifeless appearance.

xeroderma (zee·roh·DUR·muh)—a condition of excessively dry skin; a mild form of ichthyosis marked by a dry, discolored, rough condition of the skin.

xerosis (zee·ROH·sis)—a condition of abnormal dryness of tissue such as the eyes, skin, or mucous membranes.

x rays (EKS RAYZ)—Roentgen rays; electromagnetic radiations of very short wave length; rays used in some medical therapy procedures.

xyrospasm (ZY·roh·spazm)—a spasm of the wrist and forearm muscles; an occupational condition that may affect cosmetologists, estheticians, and barbers.

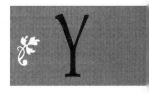

yak (YAK)—the long-haired ox of Tibet and central Asia; hair used for making wigs.

yak hair (YAK HAYR)—hair from the yak; this long, coarse, curly hair is used in the manufacture of inexpensive wigs and hair pieces; it is often mixed with the soft hair from the Angora sheep to add body and strength to Angora hair.

yang and yin (YANG and YIN)—a Chinese philosophy often applied to personality and fashion theories; yang is active, positive, masculine, and a source of heat and light, contrasted with an complimentary to yin; yin is the passive, negative, feminine force, and source of heat and light, contrasted with and complimentary to yang.

yard (YARD)—a standard English-American measure of length equal to 3 feet or 36 inches.

yeast (YEEST)—a substance consisting of minute cells of fungi; used to promote fermentation; a high source of vitamin B.

yellow (YEL·oh)—one of the three primary colors; having the color of ripe lemons.

yin (YIN)—pertaining to the Chinese philosophy and art of yin and yang.

ylang ylang (EE·lahng EE·lahng)—an Asiatic tree producing greenish-yellow flowers from which a perfume oil is produced.

yoga (YOH·guh)—a Hindu system of philosophy that involves physical and mental disciplines; a system of exercise.

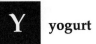

yogurt (YOH·gurt)—A thick, curdled milk regarded as a nutritious
and beneficial food; sometimes used as a facial mask.

zeis's glands (ZYS·uz GLANDZ)—the sebaceous glands associated with the cilia.

zeolite (ZEE·uh·lyt)—a chemical mixture of natural or synthesized silicates used to soften hard water.

zero projection (ZEE·roh pruh·JEK·shun)—in haircutting, no elevation or projection; hair held as close to the scalp as possible.

zigzag (ZIG·zag)—pertaining to short, sharp, angled partings used during some roller settings to prevent separation of strands during comb-out.

zinc (ZINGK)—a white crystalline metallic element; used in some cosmetics such as powders and ointments; salts of zinc are used in some antiseptics and astringents.

zinc ointment (ZINGK OYNT·ment)—a medicated ointment containing zinc oxide and petrolatum, used for skin disorders.

zinc oxide (ZINGK AHK·syd)—a fine, white compound used as a mild antiseptic and astringent.

zinc sulphate (ZINGK SUL·fayt)—a salt often employed as an astringent, both in lotions and creams.

zinc sulphocarbonate (ZINGK sul·fuh·KAR·bun·ayt)—a fine, white powder having the odor of carbolic acid; used as an antiseptic and astringent in deodorant preparations.

zoodermic (zoh·oh·DUR·mik)—pertaining to skin graft done with the grafts from the tissue or skin of an animal.

zoster herpes (ZAHS·tur HUR·peez)—an acute viral infectious disease affecting the skin and mucous membranes.

zygoma (zy·GOH·muh)—a bone of the skull that extends along the front or side of the face, below the eye; the molar or cheekbone.

zygomatic (zy·guh·MAT·ik)—pertaining to the zygoma (the molar or cheekbone).

zygomatic artery (zy·guh·MAT·ik ART·uh·ree)—superficial temporal artery supplying blood to the orbit and orbicularis.

zygomatic bone (zy·goh·MAT·ik BOHN)—the cheekbone.

zygomatic nerve (zy·goh·MAT·ik NURV)—temporal nerve that supplies stimuli to the skin of the temple area.

zygomatic process (zy·goh·MAT·ik PRAH·ses)—the process of the temporal bone that helps to form the zygoma.

zygomaticus (zy·goh·MAT·ih·kus)—a muscle that draws the upper lip upward and outward.

zymosis (zy·MOH·sis)—fermentation; any infectious or contagious disease; the development or spread of an infectious disease.